Studying for the Boards: Pediatric Radiology Cases

AF882246

Studying for the Boards: Pediatric Radiology Cases

STUDYING FOR THE BOARDS:

PEDIATRIC RADIOLOGY

Heike E. Daldrup-Link, M.D.

First published in the United States of America
by Monasteria Press LLC, San Francisco
© Monasteria Press 2022

This book is protected under the copyright laws of the United States and other countries throughout the world. No part of this publication may be reproduced or transmitted, in any form or by any means, electronic, mechanical, photocopying, recording or otherwise, without the prior written permission of Monasteria Press.

Thank you for reading an authorized copy of this book. You are supporting our authors and allowing Monasteria Press to continue to publish new books for future readers.

Every effort has been made in preparing this book to provide accurate and up-to-date information about the nomenclatures and appearances of normal findings, abnormal findings and medical conditions on pediatric imaging studies, which is in accord with accepted standards and medical practices at the time of publication. Nevertheless, the author and publisher can make no warranty that the information contained herein is totally free from error, not least because accepted standards and practices are constantly changing through research and regulation. The author and publisher therefore disclaim any and all liability for direct or consequential damages resulting from the use of material contained in this book. Readers are strongly advised to pay careful attention to the most current policies and regulations of their institution and relevant medical boards/societies as well as information provided by the manufacturer of any diagnostic devices, medical treatments, or medical equipment they plan to use.

ISBN 978-1-958277-01-0

Monasteria Press LLC

DEDICATION

Being a student is not a matter of age or status or experience, but rather a philosophy of curiosity and continuous intellectual growth. I hope that this case collection will help you preparing for the board exams, and - more importantly – providing the correct diagnosis for your next patient who entrusts themselves into your care.

INTRODUCTION

This collection of more than 200 case studies reviews typical pediatric imaging diagnoses based on ultrasound, radiography, fluoroscopy, computed tomography (CT), magnetic resonance imaging (MRI), molecular imaging, and interventional radiology technologies. The cases are organized according to the American Board of Radiology (ABR) study guide and presented in multiple choice format in order to facilitate preparations for the ABR core exam, the ABR certifying exam and the continued added qualification (CAQ) exam in Pediatric Radiology. We included a few duplicate cases to prevent an exclusion bias when answering multiple choice questions. This should enable the reader to equally consider all answer options, including previously presented diagnoses. While a case collection cannot be encompassing, our multidisciplinary author team took great care to assemble typical cases seen by pediatric radiologists in order to prepare aspiring trainees for the ABR exam. In addition, the cases presented here may be also of interest to pediatric radiologists, general radiologists and pediatricians who want to refresh and expand their knowledge in the area of pediatric imaging diagnoses.

CONTENTS

STUDYING
FOR THE BORDS:

PEDIATRIC
RADIOLOGY

Heike E. Daldrup-Link, M.D.

Chest, Cardiac, Facial Bones, ENT, Airway

1) Facial bones, sinuses, mastoids

Patient 1: Adolescent male, nasal stuffiness, and headaches
Author: Heike E. Daldrup-Link, M.D.

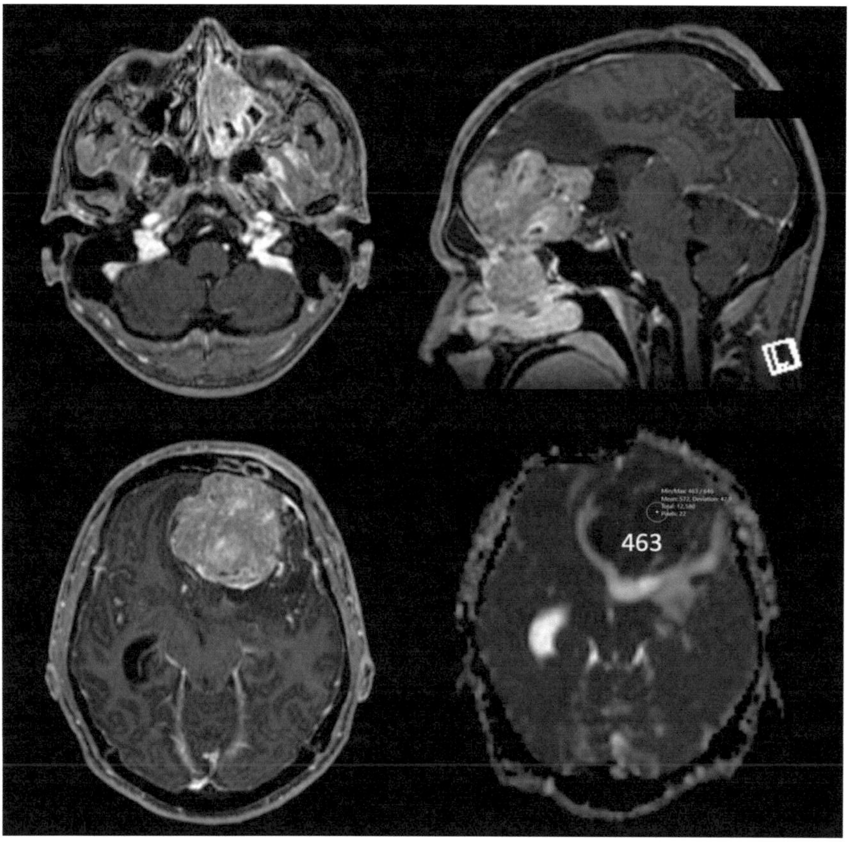

What is the most likely diagnosis:

a) Rhinocerebral Mucormycosis
b) Juvenile Angiofibroma
c) Rhabdomyosarcoma
d) Chordoma

Case 1: Paranasal Rhabdomyosarcoma

a) Rhinocerebral mucormycosis typically occurs in patients with an underlying immune deficiency, such as leukemia, diabetes, or autoimmune diseases. The lesions typically demonstrate moderate or absent enhancement on contrast-enhanced MRI, along with vessel wall enhancement due to an accompanying vasculitis. Brain involvement is devastating, and a lesion of the size seen here would be lethal.

b) A juvenile angiofibroma would be more posteriorly located and demonstrate less restricted diffusion with ADC values above 1000 mm^2/s. T2-weighted MRI images can show characteristic flow voids within these vascular lesions.

c) Rhabdomyosarcoma: Correct! The contrast-enhanced T1-weighted MRI demonstrates a soft tissue mass in the left nasal cavity and ethmoid cells, which extends into the adjacent left maxillary sinus and superiorly into the cranial fossa with a large extra-axial left frontal soft tissue component. The lesion shows markedly restricted diffusion with an ADC value of less than 1000 mm^2/s, which is indicative of a high-grade malignant tumor. There is also contrast enhancement of the meninges, indicating meningeal involvement. In an adolescent patient, the most common diagnosis would be a rhabdomyosarcoma. Another differential diagnosis would be an esthesioneuroblastoma, which would typically demonstrate intermediate ADC values around 1000 mm^2/s.

d) A chordoma would be more posteriorly located and involve the sphenooccipital bone. They typically demonstrate inhomogeneous enhancement on contrast-enhanced T1-weighted MRI scans, with a honeycomb appearance. Conventional chordomas demonstrate relatively high ADC values above 1000 mm^2/s. However, dedifferentiated chordomas can demonstrate restricted diffusion with ADC values of less than 1000 mm^2/s.

Patient 2: Adolescent male with facial swelling
Author: Heike E. Daldrup-Link, M.D.

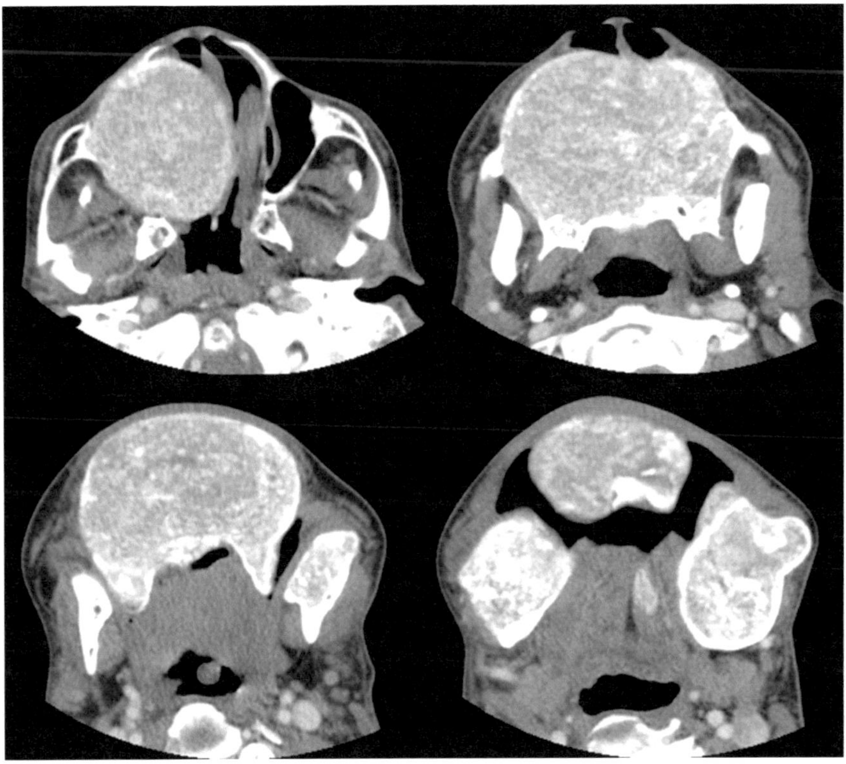

What is the most likely diagnosis:

a) Ewing Sarcoma
b) Juvenile Angiofibroma
c) Rhabdomyosarcoma
d) Fibrous Dysplasia

Case 2: Craniofacial Fibrous Dysplasia

a) Ewing sarcoma would present with aggressive bone destruction, disruption of the cortex of the bone, malignant periosteal reactions, and a para-osseous soft tissue component. The ground glass matrix shown here suggests a different diagnosis.

b) A juvenile angiofibroma would be centered in the nasal cavity, not the bone.

c) A rhabdomyosarcoma would be centered in the soft tissues. While rhabdomyosarcomas can infiltrate adjacent bones primarily or secondarily, through bone marrow metastases, they would not demonstrate the expansile, ground-glass pattern shown here.

d) Fibrous Dysplasia: Correct! Fibrous dysplasia is a benign proliferation of fibrous tissue which grows within the intramedullary cavity and expands the affected bone(s). Up to 25% of cases affect the craniofacial bones. The CT scan demonstrates an expansile lesion in the mandibula and maxilla, which significantly expands the affected bone. The lesion has a bubbly ground glass matrix. There is no periosteal reaction. Craniofacial fibrous dysplasia can present as an isolated, monostotic form or as part of the McCune Albright Syndrome (Polyostotic fibrous dysplasia, precocious puberty, and café-au-lait skin pigmentations).

Patient 3: Ten-month-old male with asymmetric forehead

Authors: Shakthi Kumaran Ramasamy, M.D., Wipawee Morakote, M.D.

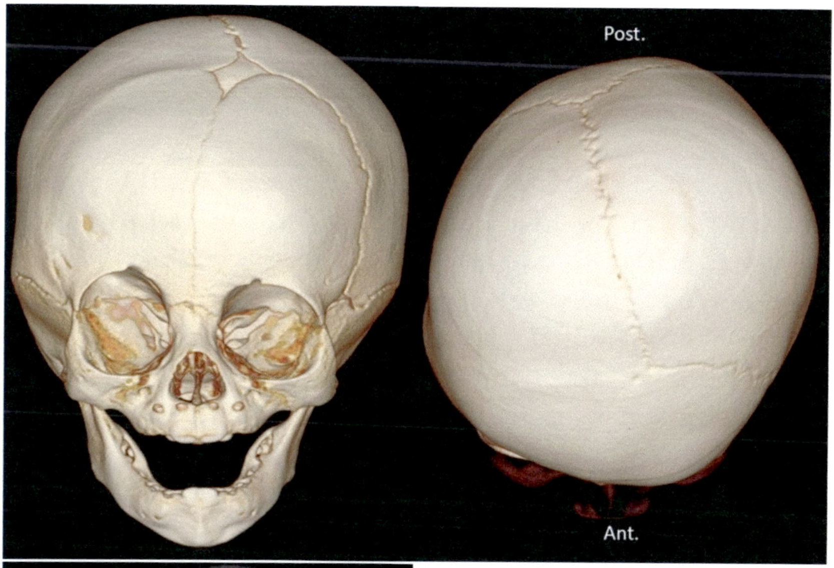

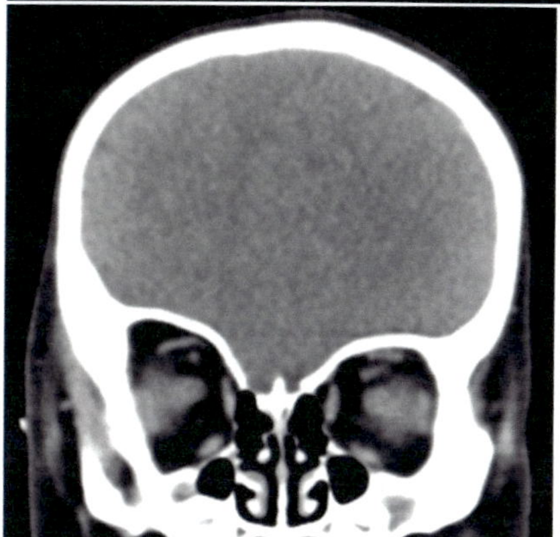

What is the most likely diagnosis:

a) Brachycephaly
b) Frontal Plagiocephaly
c) Cloverleaf Skull
d) Occipital Plagiocephaly

Case 3: Craniosynostosis - Frontal plagiocephaly

a) Brachycephaly describes a shortened anteroposterior and widened mediolateral diameter if the infant skull. A premature closure (craniosynostosis) of the coronal and lambdoid sutures leads to brachycephaly.

b) Correct! Plagiocephaly describes a flattened skull. It may be either unilateral or bilateral. The underlying cause can be positional or due to craniosynostosis of the lambdoid suture (posterior/occipital plagiocephaly) or craniosynostosis of the coronal suture (frontal plagiocephaly). The CT images here demonstrate an unilateral right coronal suture synostosis, causing unilateral right frontal flattening (plagiocephaly), elevation of the superolateral corner of the right orbit (harlequin eye deformity), and rightward displacement of the unfused sagittal suture.

c) A cloverleaf skull is a severe form of craniosynostosis which occurs because of intrauterine premature closure of the sagittal, coronal, and lambdoid sutures. It is associated with Aperts syndrome, Crouzon syndrome and several other genetic syndromes.

d) Occipital plagiocephaly is seen in patients with craniosynostosis of the lambdoid suture.

Patient 4: Infant with spontaneous periorbital ecchymosis

Authors: Wipawee Morakote, M.D., Pannee Visrutaratna, M.D.

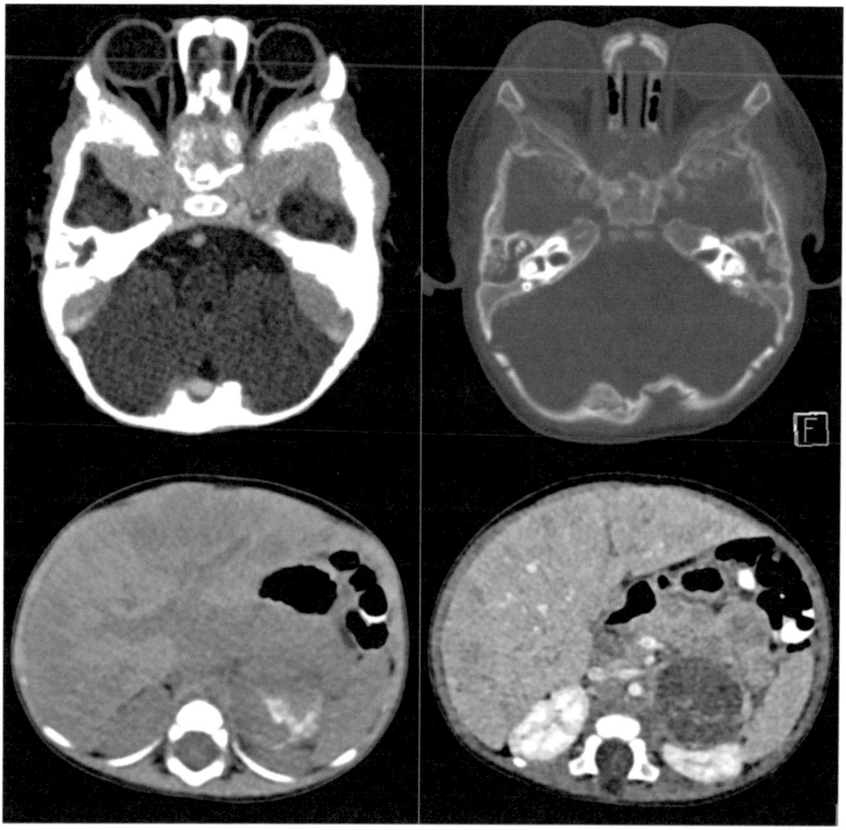

What is the most likely diagnosis:

a) Lymphoma
b) Neuroblastoma
c) Langerhans cell histiocytosis (LCH)
d) Ewing sarcoma

Case 4: Neuroblastoma

a) Lymphoma usually presents with lymphadenopathy, although extra nodal disease of lymphoma can be seen. Calcification is uncommon in lymphomas unless there is post-treatment change.

b) Neuroblastoma: Correct! The contrast enhanced axial CT scan of the brain shows permeative osteolytic lesions with sun-burst periosteal reaction involving all bones of the skull base, including the bilateral sphenoid and temporal bones. There is associated extraconal soft tissue and epidural soft tissue. The axial unenhanced and contrast enhanced CT of the abdomen demonstrate a left suprarenal mass with internal calcifications. Multiple ill-defined hypodense nodules in the liver are compatible with hepatic metastasis. Also note the infiltrative periaortic soft tissue that pushes the aorta away from the spine. Over 90% of neuroblastomas of the adrenal glands contain calcifications. Metastatic neuroblastoma in the orbital region can induce periorbital ecchymosis, so called "raccoon eyes".

c) Langerhans cell histiocytosis (LCH) is a multisystemic disease. Skull involvement typically presents as well-defined osteolytic lesions. The calvarium is more frequently affected than the skull base. The characteristic appearance of calvarial LCH is single or multiple punched-out lesions with beveled-edges. The mastoid part of the temporal bone is the most common site of skull base involvement which can be seen as destructive bone lesion with soft tissue.

d) Ewing sarcoma is a primary malignant bone tumor. The most common site of Ewing sarcoma is lower extremities, followed by pelvis, upper extremities, spine and rib, and skull. Common metastatic sites are lungs, other bones, and bone marrow. It rarely spreads to the liver, brain, and lymph nodes.

Patient 5: 4-year-old male, cannot open right eye

Author: Heike E. Daldrup-Link, M.D.

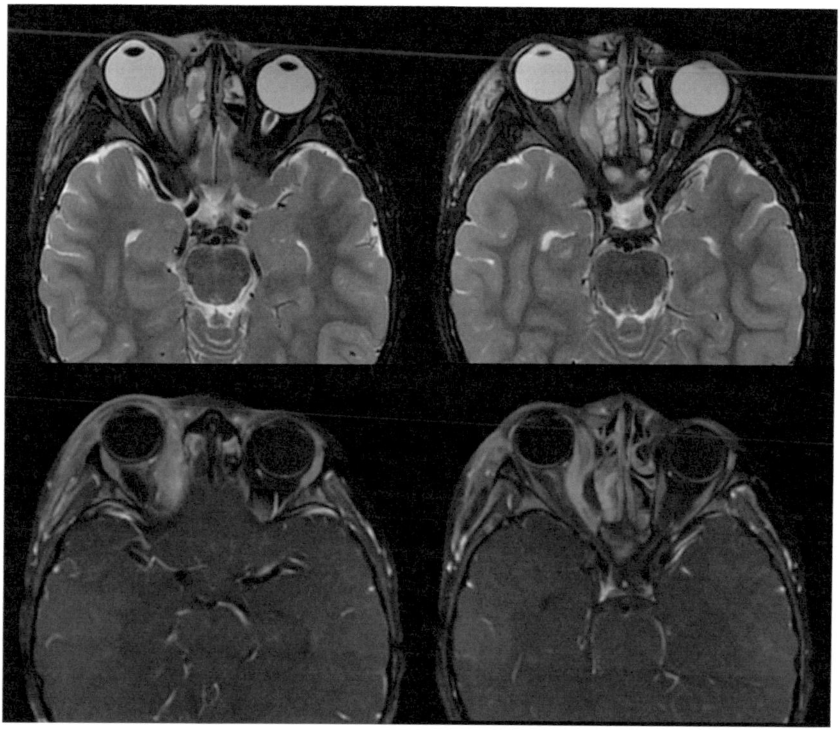

What is the most likely diagnosis:

a) Thyroid Associated Orbitopathy
b) Nonspecific Orbital Inflammation
c) Optic Neuritis
d) Orbital Cellulitis

Case 5: Orbital Cellulitis

a) A thyroid-associated orbitopathy presents in patients with Graves disease with symmetric bilateral enlargement of the extraocular muscles. Importantly, the tendons of these muscles are not involved. There is often also an increased amount of intraorbital fat and proptosis of the ocular globe.

b) Non-specific orbital inflammation or orbital pseudotumor is a benign, non-infectious inflammatory enlargement of the extraocular muscles and tendons. The inflammation can extend to surrounding tissues and cause a proptosis. An abscess formation would not be typical for this condition.

c) Optic Neuritis is an inflammation of the optic nerve which presents with T2-hyperintense signal and marked contrast-enhancement of the optic nerve. There is no optic nerve signal abnormality noted here.

d) Orbital Cellulitis: Correct! The axial T2-weighted and contrast-enhanced T1-weighted MRI demonstrates edema and enhancement of the periorbital soft tissues consistent with right periorbital cellulitis (i.e., an inflammation of the preseptal soft tissues). In addition, there is edema and enhancement of the right superior oblique and right medial rectus muscle with formation of a subperiosteal abscess, mass effect on the right optic sheath and proptosis of the right globe, consistent with a right orbital cellulitis (i.e., an inflammation/infection of the postseptal soft tissues). The process is likely due to extension of sinusitis through the lamina papyraceae. and no intracranial extension.

Patient 6: Two-year-old male, white reflection in the left pupil

Author: Heike E. Daldrup-Link, M.D.

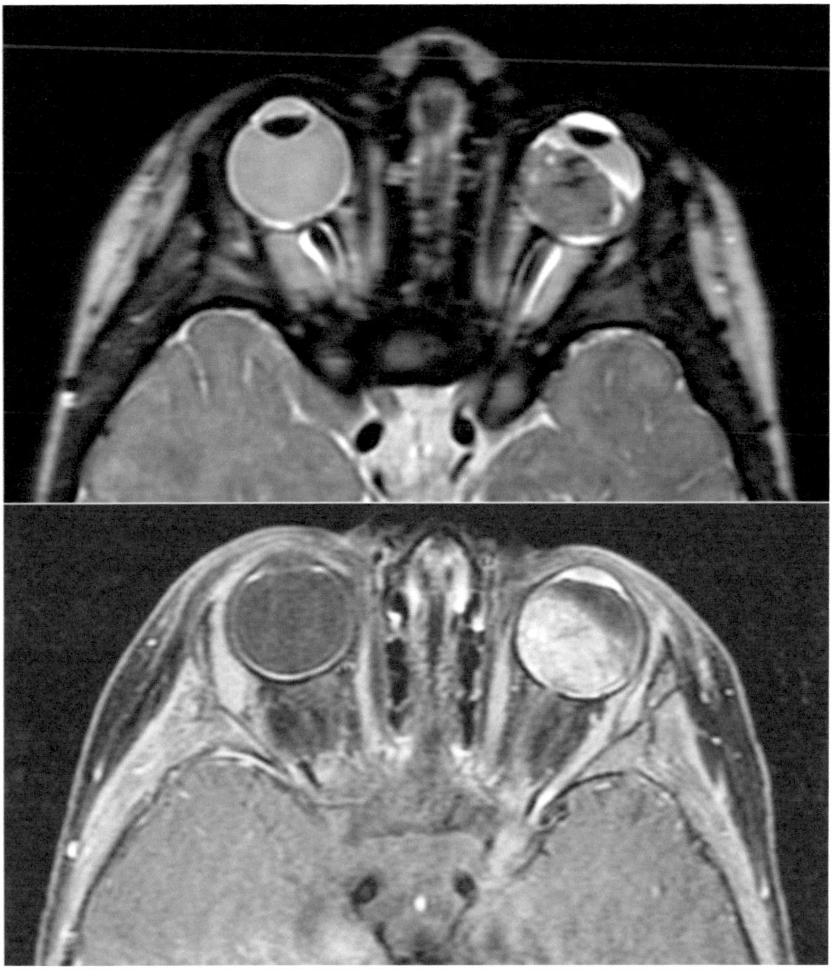

What is the most likely diagnosis:

a) Coats Disease
b) Persistent Fetal Vasculature
c) Retinoblastoma
d) Coloboma of the Choroid

Case 6: Retinoblastoma

a) Coats disease is a congenital vascular malformation of the retina which leads to retinal detachment and a subretinal fluid collection. The subretinal fluid collection often contains hemorrhagic elements and then presents with hyperintense signal on T1-weighted MR images and mildly hypointense signal on T2-weighted images. The lesion does not enhance with contrast and does not contain calcifications.

b) Persistent fetal vasculature is due to persistence and proliferation of the primary vitreous and leads to development of fibrovascular tissue along the hyaloid canal, a T2-hypointense triangular midline structure between the optic disc and the lens. On MRI scans, the affected globe is abnormally small. The lesion contains the hyaloid artery, which can lead to enhancement of the vitreal abnormalities on contrast-enhanced MRI. There can be an associated retinal detachment and subretinal hemorrhage. But there is no localized mass.

c) Retinoblastoma: Correct! The MRI of the orbit demonstrates a large unilateral soft tissue mass in the posterior chamber left globe, which demonstrates decreased signal compared to the vitreus on the axial T2-weighted scan and inhomogenous enhancement on the contrast-enhanced fat-saturated T1-weighted MRI. Note that there is T2-hyperintense signal and contrast enhancement of the iris, which indicates angiogenesis in the anterior chamber and is considered an indirect sign of large tumors with poor prognosis.

d) A coloboma represents a gap in the choroidal layer of the globe and presents as an outpouch or bulge of the sclera on MRI scans. A coloboma can lead to leukocoria, but it is not associated with a soft tissue mass in the globe.

Patient 7: 11-year-old male, swelling of the right eye

Author: Heike E. Daldrup-Link, M.D.

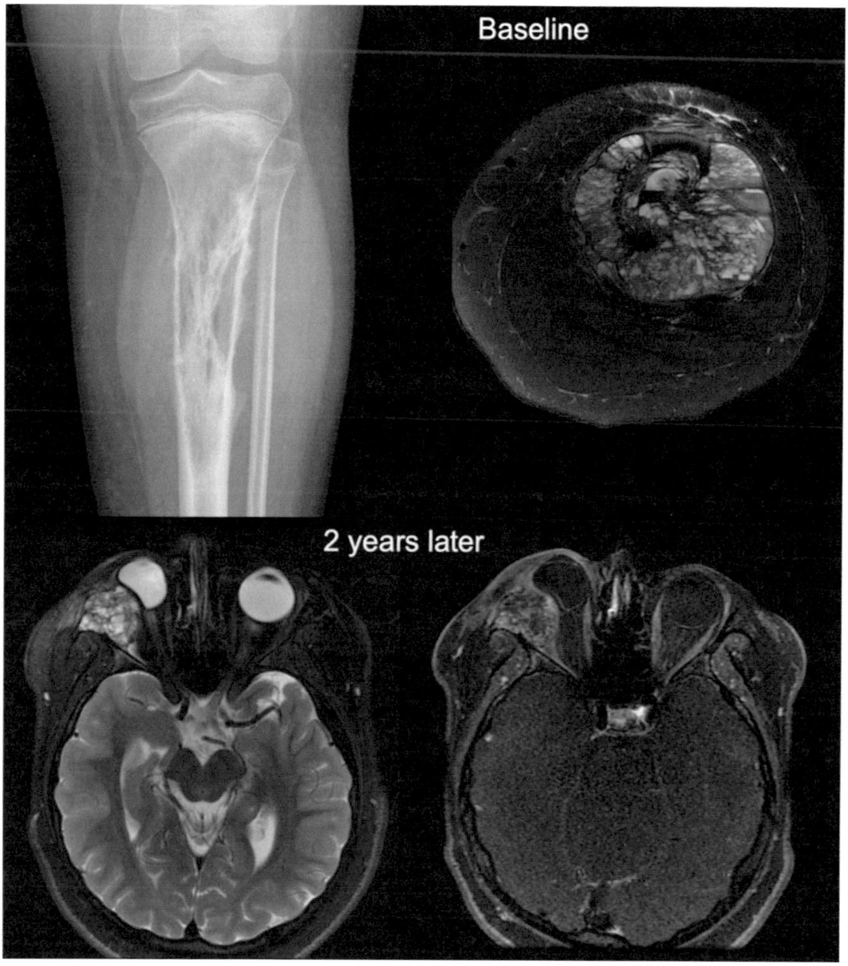

What is the most likely diagnosis:

a) Thyroid Associated Orbitopathy
b) Osteosarcoma Metastasis
c) Retinoblastoma
d) Periorbital Cellulitis

Case 7: Osteosarcoma Metastasis

a) A thyroid-associated orbitopathy presents in patients with Graves disease with symmetric bilateral enlargement of the extraocular muscles. There is often also an increased amount of intraorbital fat and proptosis of the ocular globe.

b) Osteosarcoma Metastasis: Correct! The x-ray demonstrates an aggressive osteolysis in the proximal tibia metaphysis and diaphysis with wide zone of transition, cortical destruction, and sunburst periosteal reaction. The axial T2-weighted MRI of the lower leg shows an intra- and extraosseous lesion with multiple fluid-fluid levels, consistent with a large telangiectatic osteosarcoma. The patient did not have lung metastases or any other bone metastases at the time of the diagnosis. However, pulmonary metastases and multiple bone metastases developed two years later. The axial T2-weighted MRI and contrast-enhanced T1-weighted MRI of the orbits demonstrate a mass in the lateral wall of the orbit, which extends into the orbit and causes significant mass effect and proptosis of the right globe. The orbital metastases also demonstrate fluid-fluid levels on the T2-weighted MRI scan. The findings are consistent with a right orbital metastasis of the osteosarcoma. By contrast, muti-focal osteosarcomas represent multiple synchronous or metachronous osteosarcomas without visceral involvement.

c) Patients with hereditary retinoblastoma related to RB1 germline mutations have an increased risk of developing osteosarcomas later in life. There is no retinoblastoma noted here.

d) Periorbital cellulitis present with edema and enhancement of the preseptal periorbital soft tissues. Orbital cellulitis present with edema and enhancement of the postseptal soft tissues.

Chest, Cardiac, Facial Bones, ENT, Airway

2) Airway, tongue, nasopharynx

Patient 8: Newborn baby with severe dyspnea at birth.
Authors: Desiree R. Eshraghi, Soni C. Chawla, M.D.

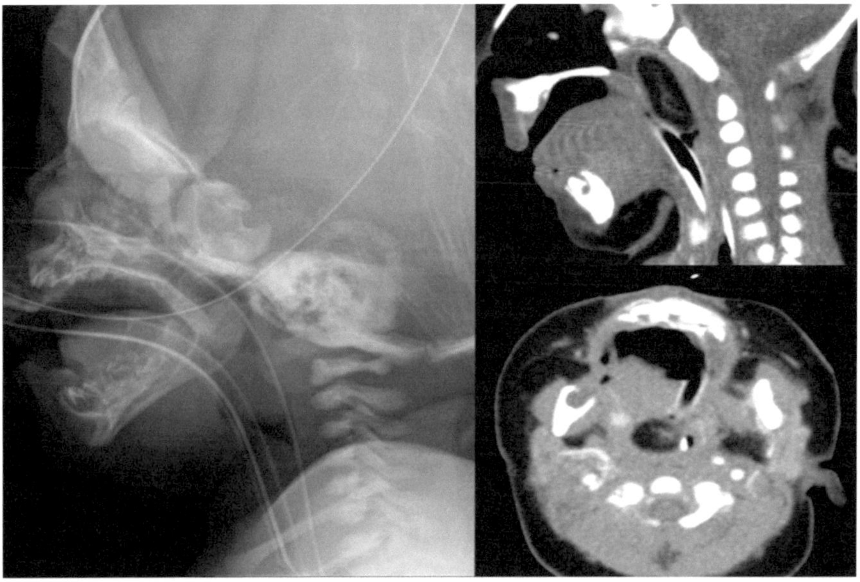

What is the most likely diagnosis:

a) Retropharyngeal abscess
b) Nasopharyngeal teratoma/epignathus
c) Tonsillar and adenoidal hypertrophy
d) Hemangioma

Case 8: Nasopharyngeal Teratoma/Epignathus

a) A retropharyngeal abscess manifests as thickened precervical prevertebral soft tissues with mass effect on the airway. Intra-lesional fat would be unusual.

b) Nasopharyngeal teratoma/epignathus: Correct! A nasopharyngeal epignathus is a very rare teratoid tumor. The scout lateral view of the CT exam demonstrates a focal mass-like soft tissue density in the oropharynx. The nasogastric tube is traversing through the nasal cavity into the esophagus and the endotracheal tube is noted in the airway in appropriate position. The tubes are not significantly displaced or deviated. Axial and sagittal postcontrast CT scans of the neck demonstrate a well defined oval solid mass in the region of the nasopharynx and oropharynx, which obliterates the nasopharyngeal airway. The lesion is composed of small areas of enhancing soft tissue and large areas of internal fat, which is most consistent with a nasopharyngeal teratoma/epignathus.

c) A tonsillar and adenoidal hypertrophy manifests as diffuse prominence of the adenoidal soft tissues at the skull base and diffuse prominence of the palatine tonsillar soft tissues in the oropharynx. Enlarged tonsils and adenoids demonstrate soft tissue density on a CT scan, while the lesion here demonstrates fat density.

d) A hemangioma presents as a highly vascular, avidly enhancing lobulated lesion in the airways. The term hemangioma has often been misapplied to other non-neoplastic vascular malformations in the airways. The lesion shown here demonstrates limited contrast enhancement and large components of fat.

Patient 9: An infant with swollen neck and fever

Authors: Wipawee Morakote, M.D.

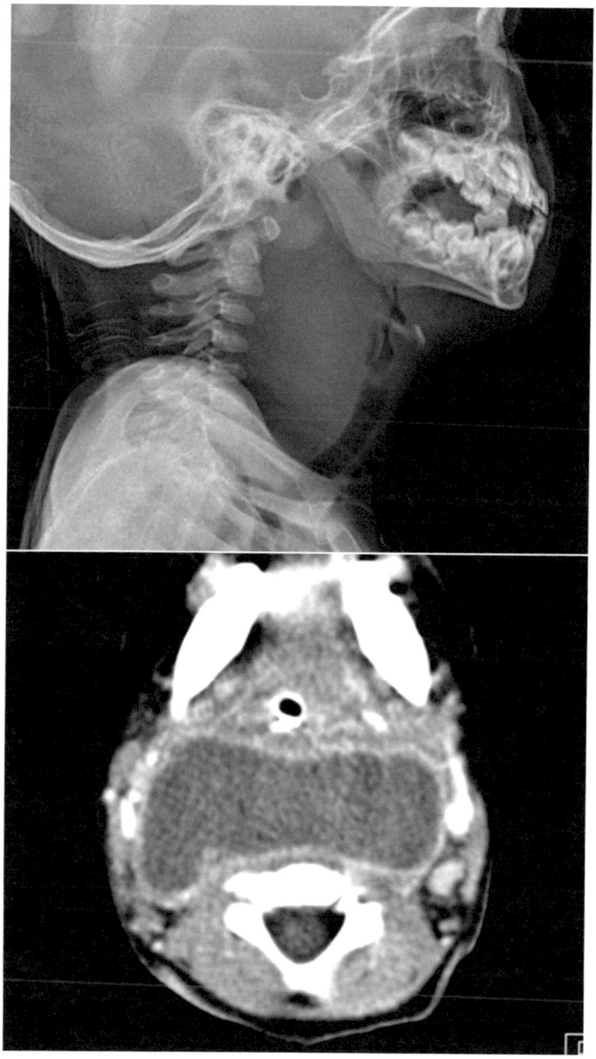

What is the most likely diagnosis:

a) Lymphoma
b) Neuroblastoma
c) Retropharyngeal Abscess
d) Branchial Cleft Cyst

Case 9: Retropharyngeal Abscess

a) The lesion is not composed of soft tissue. There is no lymphadenopathy.

b) Most neuroblastomas are soft tissue masses. Rarely, cystic neuroblastomas or neuroblastomas with large necroses can occur. These tumors typically encase vessels and airways rather than displacing them.

c) Retropharyngeal Abscess. Correct! The lateral radiograph of the neck shows marked thickening of the prevertebral soft tissue. The axial CT image demonstrates a rim-enhancing fluid-containing lesion in the retropharyngeal space which causes anterior displacement of the trachea. These findings are consistent with a retropharyngeal abscess.

d) A branchial cleft cyst is typically found in a lateral or paramedian location in the head or neck, not the midline.

Patient 10: Young child with cough

Author: Heike E. Daldrup-Link, M.D., Jayne Seekins, D.O.

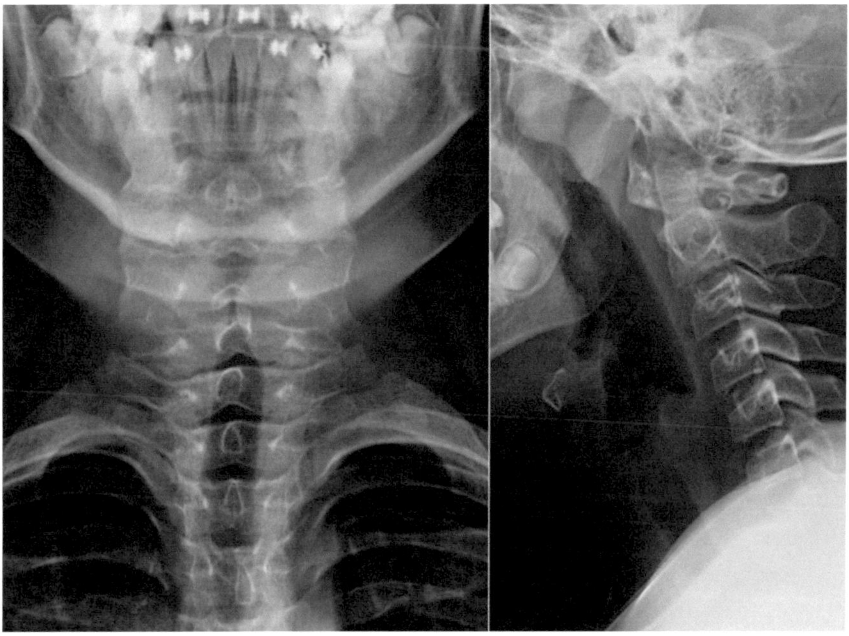

What is the most likely diagnosis (ultrasound of the neck):

a) Epiglottitis
b) Retropharyngeal Abscess
c) Croup
d) Foreign body

Case 10: Croup

a) An epiglottitis presents with a thickened epiglottis on the lateral radiograph of the neck, causing the "thumb sign". In this case, the lateral radiograph of the upper airway shows a normal epiglottis.

b) A retropharyngeal abscess presents with prevertebral soft tissue swelling on a lateral neck radiograph and a rim-enhancing fluid-collection in the retropharyngeal space on CT or MRI scans.

c) Croup (Laryngotracheobronchitis): Correct! The frontal radiograph shows a steeple sign, i.e., a uniform narrowing of the subglottic airway. The normal convex shape of the subglottic airway is lost and narrowing of the subglottic trachea demonstrates an inverted V configuration which is reminiscent of a church steeple. On the lateral radiograph, there is air-distension of the hypopharynx. The epiglottis is normal. The most common cause of croup is a viral infection of the upper airway, such as parainfluenza virus or respiratory syncytial virus (RSV) infection.

d) There is no foreign body noted on the radiographs shown.

Patient 11: 14-year-old teenager with neck swelling

Author: Heike E. Daldrup-Link, M.D.

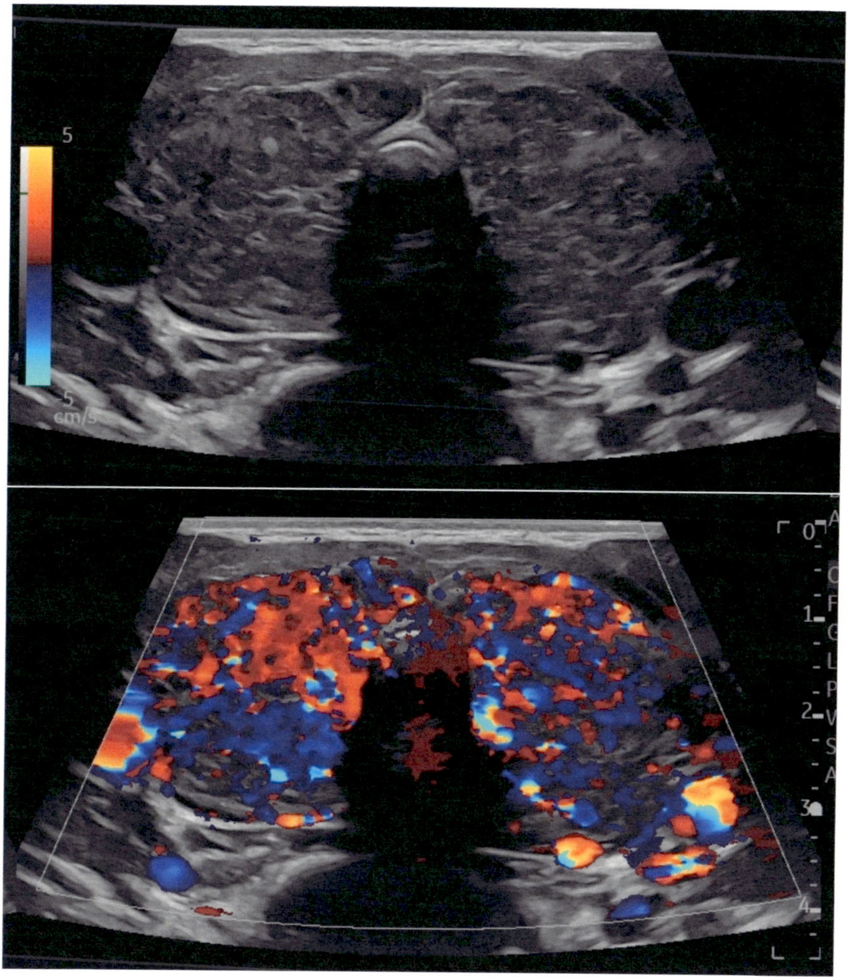

What is the most likely diagnosis (ultrasound of the neck):

a) Papillary cancer
b) Neuroblastoma
c) Hashimoto Thyroiditis
d) Vascular Malformation

Case 11: Hashimoto Thyroiditis

a) A papillary thyroid cancer would present as a focal lesion within the thyroid gland. The lesion may contain small calcifications. Enlarged lymph node may be also seen, indicating metastases.

b) A neuroblastoma would present as a soft tissue mass with irregular borders, inhomogeneous echotexture, and moderate vascularity on Doppler ultrasound. A neuroblastoma of the neck would infiltrate or displace the thyroid gland. Enlarged lymph node may be also seen, indicating metastases.

c) Hashimoto Thyroiditis. Correct! The grayscale ultrasound demonstrates a diffusely enlarged thyroid gland with inhomogeneous parenchyma, multiple hypoechoic micronodules and surrounding echogenic septations, causing a so-called giraffe echotexture. Color Doppler ultrasound most frequently demonstrates decreased flow but can occasionally also demonstrate increased flow. This case here shows a "thyroid inferno", multiple small vessels and arteriovenous shunting throughout the gland. Differential consideration includes Graves disease.

d) A vascular malformation would demonstrate fluid filled vascular spaces on grayscale ultrasound. The structure shown here is located in front of the trachea and has the shape of the thyroid gland, because it is an enlarged thyroid gland.

Patient 12: Newborn premature infant, respiratory distress

Author: Heike E. Daldrup-Link, M.D.

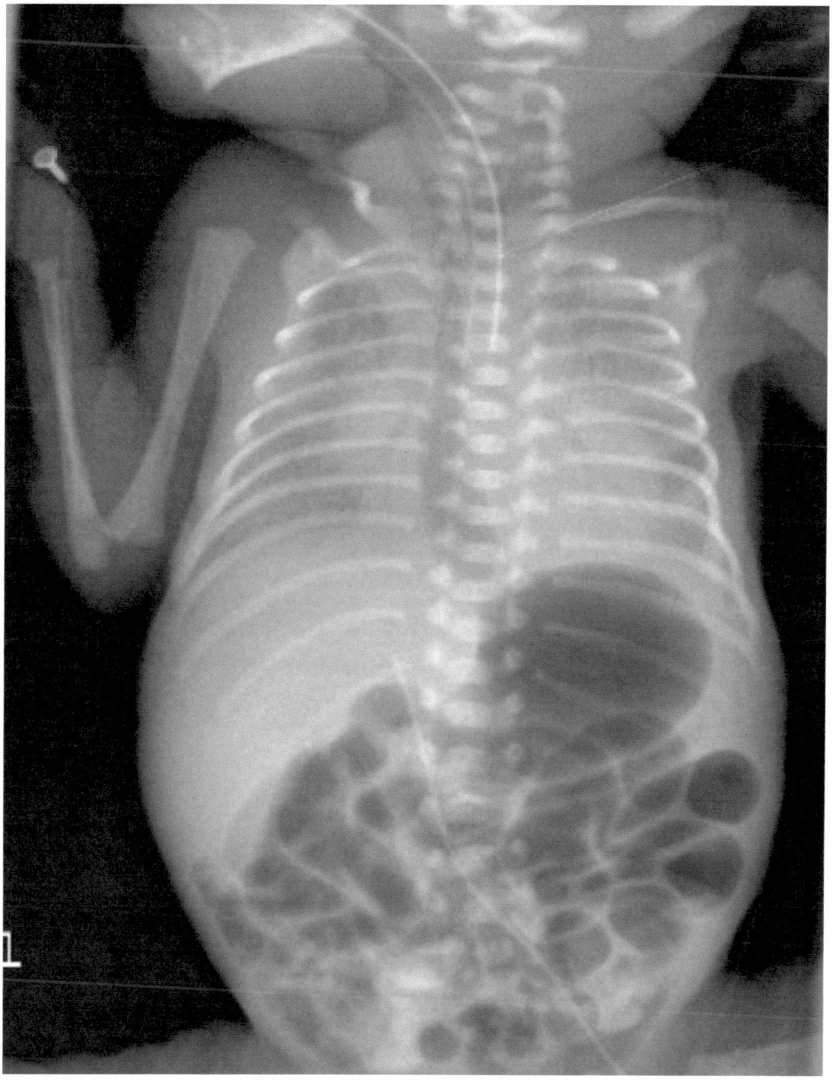

What is the most likely diagnosis:

a) Hiatal hernia
b) Pneumomediastinum
c) Tracheoesophageal fistula
d) Esophageal Intubation

Case 12: Esophageal Intubation

a) The radiograph of the chest demonstrates air in the esophagus. This is because air is insufflated into the esophagus via a misplaced endotracheal tube. The gas-distended stomach is located below the left diaphragm.

b) Pneumomediastinum: There is no free air in the mediastinum. The air noted in the midline of the chest colocalizes to the location of the esophagus.

c) Tracheoesophageal fistula: There is no evidence for a fistula between the trachea and the esophagus. The most common type (type C) would present with a blind ending, gas distended upper esophagus and decompressed lower esophagus, which is attached to the trachea. The diagnosis of a tracheoesophageal fistula can be confirmed with an upper GI fluoroscopy exam.

d) Esophageal Intubation: Correct! The radiograph demonstrates the gas-filled trachea in front of the endotracheal tube, which projects on the esophagus. The esophagus, stomach and bowel loops are gas-distended because they are ventilated through the misplaced tube. The lungs demonstrate diffuse airspace opacities and positive aerobronchograms, consistent with diffuse bilateral microatelectases.

Chest, Cardiac, Facial Bones, ENT, Airway

3) Cardiovascular (in chest)

Patient 13: Four-year-old female

Authors: Heike E. Daldrup-Link, M.D.

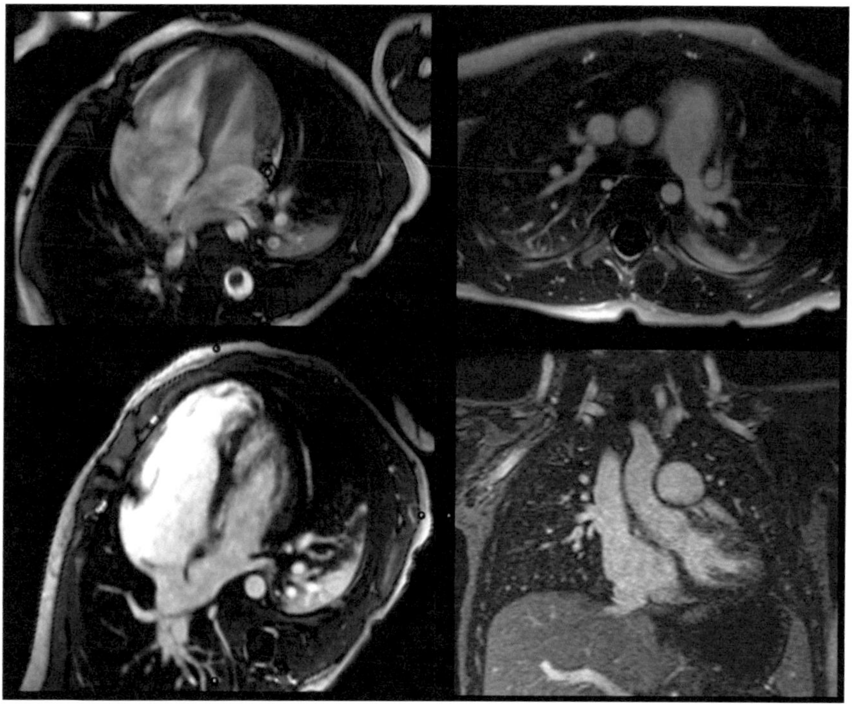

What is the most likely diagnosis:

a) Ventricular septal defect and partial anomalous pulmonary venous return
b) Atrial septal defect and partial anomalous pulmonary venous return
c) Scimitar Syndrome
d) Pulmonary Sequestration

Case 13: Atrial Septal Defect and Partial Anomalous Pulmonary Venous Return

a) The images here show an atrial septal defect rather than a ventricular septal defect. Note that partial anomalous venous return is associated with atrial septal defects.

b) Atrial septal defect and partial anomalous pulmonary venous return: Correct! The MRI demonstrates a sinus venosus atrial septal defect (ASD) and drainage of the right upper and right middle pulmonary vein into SVC. The right ventricle is enlarged.

c) Scimitar Syndrome is defined as hypoplastic lung and partial anomalous pulmonary venous return, most commonly involving an abnormal vein in the right lower lobe which drains into the inferior vena cava or the right atrium.

d) A pulmonary sequestration involves an abnormal segment of lung, which is supplied by an abnormal artery that arises directly from the aorta. The abnormal lung segment is not connected to the tracheobronchial tree. It is most common in the left lower lobe. Venous drainage can occur through the pulmonary veins (intralobar sequestration) or systemic veins (extralobar sequestration).

Patient 14: Two-month-old male infant
Author: Heike E. Daldrup-Link, M.D.

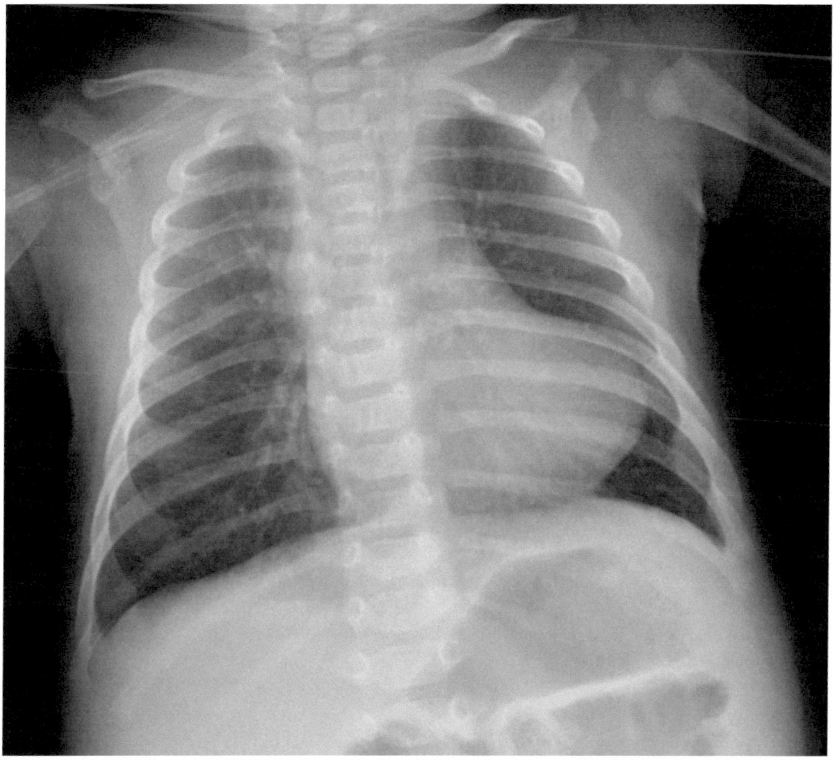

Tetralogy of Fallot is defined as:

a) Ventricular Septal Defect, Right Ventricular Outflow Tract Obstruction, Overriding Aorta, Right Ventricular Hypertrophy
b) Ventricular Septal Defect, Right Ventricular Outflow Tract Obstruction, Overriding Aorta, Left Ventricular Hypertrophy
c) Ventricular Septal Defect, Right Ventricular Outflow Tract Obstruction, Overriding Aorta, Open ductus arteriosus
d) Atrial Septal Defect, Right Ventricular Outflow Tract Obstruction, Overriding Aorta, Right Ventricular Hypertrophy

Case 14: Tetralogy of Fallot

a) Correct! Tetralogy of Fallot is the most common cyanotic heart disease in infants and is defined by four (tetralogy) findings: (1) Ventricular Septal Defect, (2) Right Ventricular Outflow Tract Obstruction, (3) Overriding Aorta, (4) Right Ventricular Hypertrophy. The chest x-ray shows a typical boot-shaped heart with upturned cardiac apex due to the underlying right ventricular hypertrophy and a concave pulmonary arterial segment due to pulmonary hypoplasia. The lungs show asymmetric pulmonary vascular markings with increased blood flow to the right lung and decreased blood flow to the left lung.

d) A left ventricular hypertrophy is not part of the tetralogy of Fallot.

c) The four findings above plus an atrial septal defect or persistent ductus arteriosus define a Pentalogy of Fallot.

d) The four findings above plus an atrial septal defect or persistent ductus arteriosus define a Pentalogy of Fallot.

Patient 15: Five-year-old male with chest pain

Authors: Heike E. Daldrup-Link, M.D.

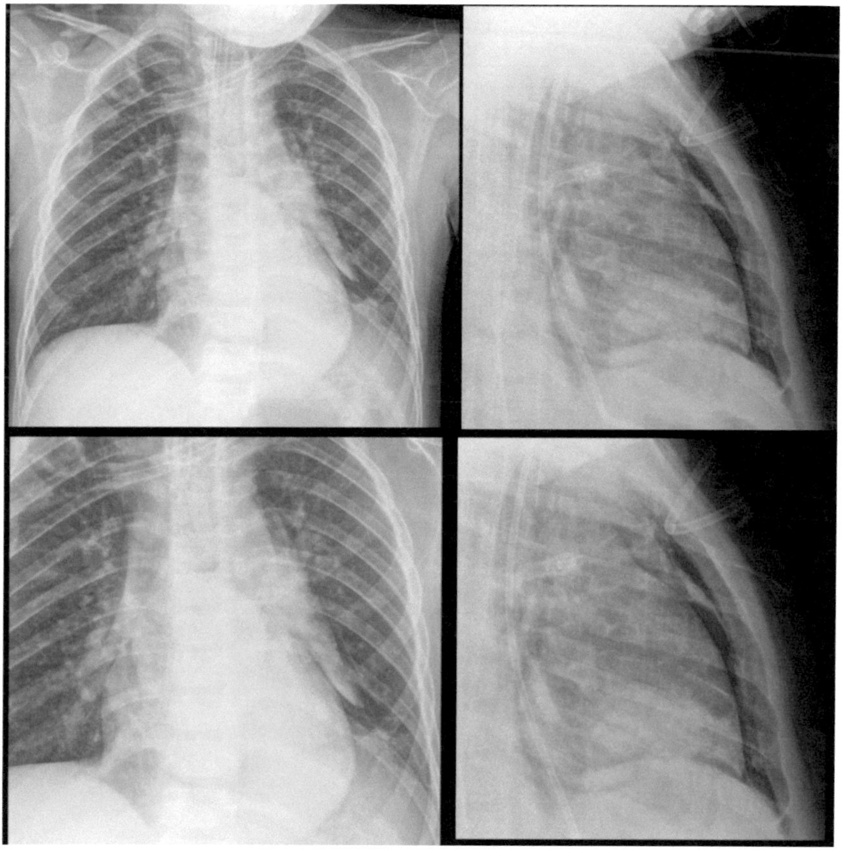

What is the most likely diagnosis:

a) Pneumothorax
b) Pneumomediastinum
c) Atelectasis
d) Pneumopericardium

Case 15: Pneumomediastinum

a) A pneumothorax can be located medially but would extend along the pleural space. In this case, free air is noted on both sides of the mediastinum.

b) Pneumomediastinum: Correct! The x-rays demonstrate extraluminal air surrounding the heart and thymus. On the frontal view, the thymus is lifted upwards, leading to a characteristic "angel wing" or "spinnaker" appearance. There is also a "continuous diaphragm sign" due to gas extending along the surface of the diaphragm, below the heart.

c) Atelectases are not noted on this radiograph. The dense structure above the heart is the thymus.

d) A pneumopericardium would surround the heart and not extend superiorly beyond the pericardial reflections. In this case here, free air surrounds the thymus.

Patient 16: Seven-year-old female with dysphagia

Authors: Heike E. Daldrup-Link, M.D.

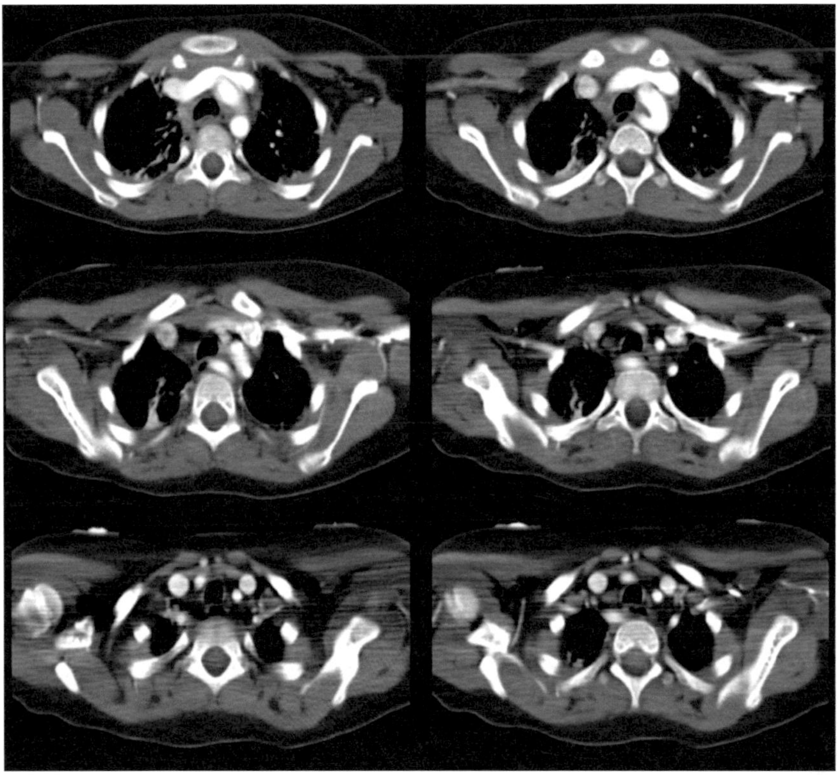

What is the most likely diagnosis:

a) Aberrant left subclavian artery
b) Aberrant right subclavian artery
c) Bovine aortic arch
d) Ductus diverticulum

Case 16: Aberrant Right Subclavian Artery

a) An aberrant left subclavian artery arises from a right aortic arch.

b) Aberrant right subclavian artery: Correct! The CT scan demonstrates an aberrant branch arising from the distal left aortic arch and coursing behind the esophagus to the right.

c) A bovine aortic arch is the most common variant of the aortic arch. It describes a common origin of the innominate and left common carotid arteries. Rather than arising directly from the aortic arch as a separate branch, the left common carotid artery origin merged with the origin of the innominate artery.

d) A ductus diverticulum represents a bling ending smooth outpouch of the anteromedial thoracic aorta, at the insertion site of the ligamentum arteriosum.

Patient 17: Two-year old female with dyspnea

Author: Heike E. Daldrup-Link, M.D.

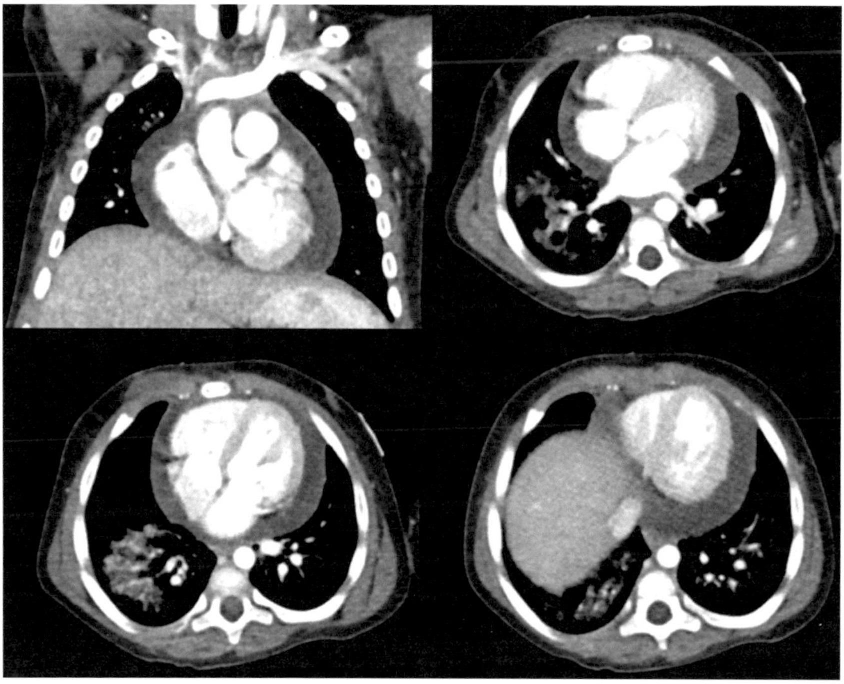

What is the most likely diagnosis:

a) Pericardial cyst
b) Large thymus
c) Pericardial hematoma
d) Pericardial effusion

Case 17: Pericardial Effusion

a) Pericardial cyst are benign fluid-containing lesions, most commonly located at the cardiophrenic angles. They typically demonstrate a hypodense center and a thin wall, which may or may not enhance with contrast. The effusion here is not localized but surrounds the entire heart.

b) A large thymus would involve the anterior-superior mediastinum. It can wrap around the heart silhouette anteriorly and laterally, but usually not circumferentially. In addition, a thymus would demonstrate soft tissue attenuation on the CT scan.

c) A pericardial hematoma would present with increased attenuation on the CT scan, with a density of > 35 Hounsfield units (HU).

d) Pericardial effusion: Correct! The CT scan demonstrates fluid surrounding the heart. The normal pericardium measures 2 mm or less. The effusion here measures 10 mm. Underlying etiologies can be infection, fluid overload/renal disease, pulmonary hypertension, trauma, or neoplasms, among others. A pericardiocentesis is indicated for clinical tamponade, suspicion of purulent or neoplastic pericarditis, and treatment of patients who have symptoms despite treatment for more than one week.

Patient 18: Six-month old infant with shortness of breath

Author: Heike E. Daldrup-Link, M.D.

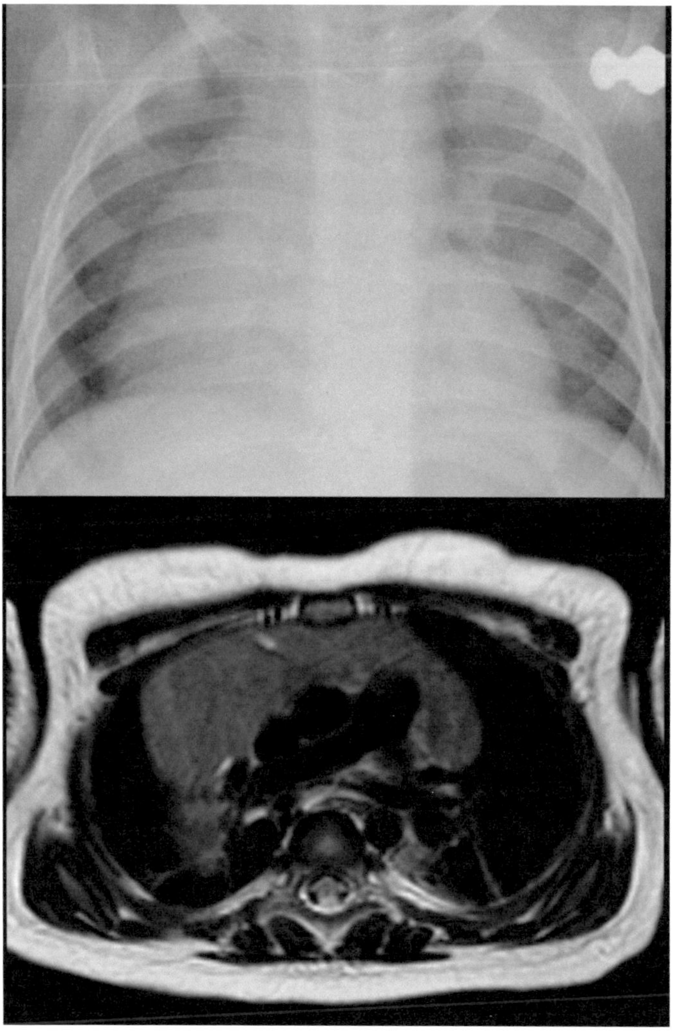

What is the most likely diagnosis:

a) Malignant Lymphoma
b) Thymoma
c) Normal Thymus
d) Neuroblastoma

Case 18: Normal Thymus

a) Malignant lymphoma. Malignant lymphoma is very rare in children less than one year of age and typically presents in older children. It would present as a soft tissue mass in the anterior and middle mediastinum, which encases and compresses adjacent vessels. Often, additional enlarged lymph nodes are noted.

b) A thymoma is rare in children and would present as a slow growing, more nodular and inhomogeneous soft tissue mass in the anterior mediastinum. It typically presents in young adults. Only about 50 cases in children have been reported in the literature. Patients typically present with clinical signs of myasthenia gravis.

c) Normal thymus: Correct! The radiograph demonstrates a widened mediastinum with lobulated right-lateral border, indicative of the soft texture of the thymus. The lungs are normally ventilated, suggesting that there is no compression or impairment of the airways. The axial MRI demonstrates homogeneous soft tissue in the anterior mediastinum, which does not compress, encase, or displace the mediastinal vessels. This is typical of a normal thymus.

d) A neuroblastoma presents as a posterior mediastinal mass. The thymus shown here is centered in the anterior mediastinum.

Patient 19: Adolescent female with dyspnea

Author: Heike E. Daldrup-Link, M.D.

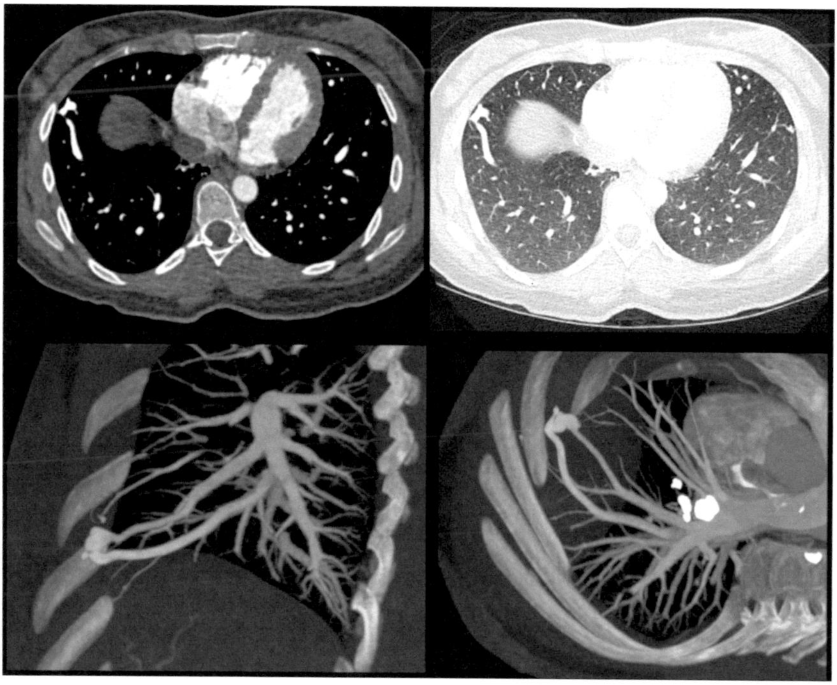

What is the most likely diagnosis:

a) Pulmonary Sequestration
b) Scimitar Syndrome
c) Bronchial Atresia
d) Pulmonary Arteriovenous Malformation

Case 19: Pulmonary Arteriovenous Malformation

a) A pulmonary sequestration is characterized by an abnormal segment of lung, which is supplied by an abnormal artery that arises directly from the aorta. The abnormal lung segment is not connected to the tracheobronchial tree. It is most common in the left lower lobe. Venous drainage can occur through the pulmonary veins (intralobar sequestration) or systemic veins (extralobar sequestration).

b) A Scimitar Syndrome is defined as hypoplastic lung and partial anomalous pulmonary venous return, most commonly involving an abnormal vein in the right lower lobe which drains into the inferior vena cava or the right atrium.

c) Bronchial atresia presents with a mucus-filled blind ending bronchus and surrounding oligemia and hyperinflation of the adjacent lung. The serpiginous structure seen here enhances on contrast-enhanced images, consistent with a vascular lesion.

d) Pulmonary Arteriovenous Malformation: Correct! The axial CT scan demonstrates a well-circumscribed, non-calcified pulmonary nodule in the right lower lobe, which is connected with a serpiginous blood vessel. The 3D reconstruction shows that the lesion is composed of a feeding artery, the aneurysmal portion, and a draining vein.

Patient 20: 7-day old male with cyanosis

Author: Heike E. Daldrup-Link, M.D.

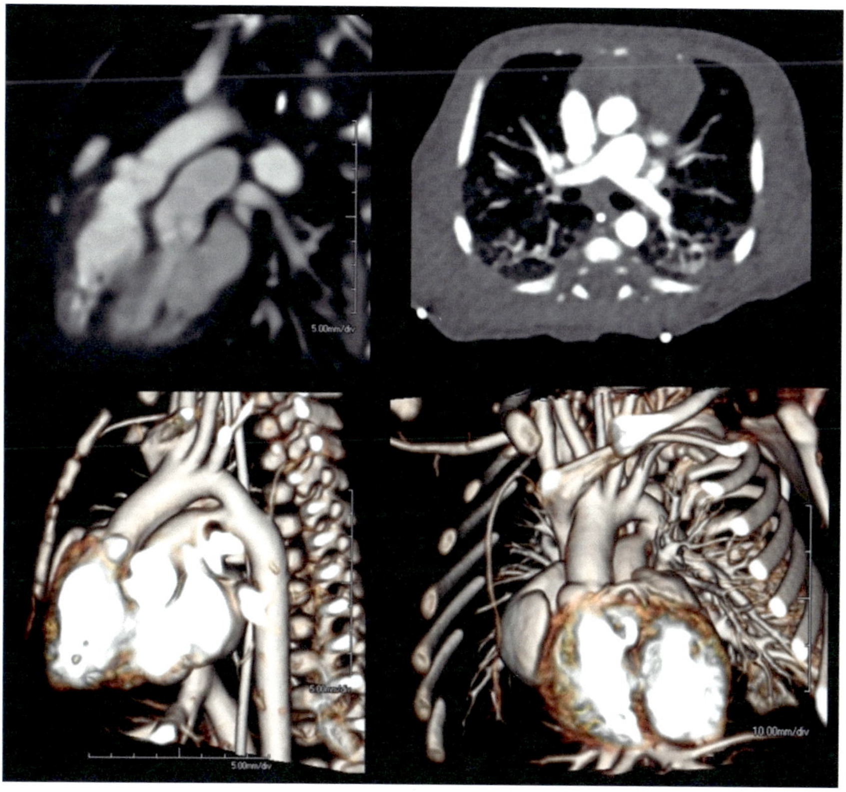

What is the most likely diagnosis:

a) L-Transposition of the Great Arteries
b) D-Transposition of the Great Arteries
c) Tetralogy of Fallot
d) Coarctation of the Aorta

Case 20: D-Transposition of the Great Arteries

a) L-Transposition of the Great Arteries is characterized by reverse position of the ventricles: Deoxygenated systemic blood enters a correctly located right atrium to a discordant left ventricle through the mitral valve into a discordant pulmonary artery into the pulmonary circulation. Oxygenated blood from the pulmonary veins flow from a correctly located left atrium to a discordant right ventricle through a tricuspid valve into a discordant aorta into the systemic circulation.

b) D-Transposition of the Great Arteries: Correct! The CT scan demonstrates a discordant ventricular arterial connection: The aorta arises from the right ventricle and is located anterior to the main pulmonary artery, which arises from the left ventricle. The main pulmonary artery courses anterior and to the left of the ascending aorta, consistent with D-position of the great arteries. The ascending aorta and pulmonary artery are in parallel position. The left-sided aortic arch demonstrates a normal branching pattern. The patient also had a ventricular septal defect and an open ductus arteriosus. D-TGA is the most common congenital cyanotic heart disease. Treatment options include an initial Rashkind atrial septostomy and a Jatene arterial switch procedure.

c) Tetralogy of Fallot is defined by a ventricular septal defect, right ventricular outflow tract obstruction, an overriding aorta and right ventricular hypertrophy.

d) Coarctation of the aorta in a neonate is characterized by a discrete narrowing of the thoracic aorta, causing obstruction of blood flow to the systemic circulation. The most common location for an aortic coarctation is just distal to the left subclavian artery at the insertion site of the ductus arteriosus. Clinically, neonates may be asymptomatic or show weak/absent femoral pulses with delayed capillary refill.

Patient 21: 11-year-old male with dyspnea

Author: Heike E. Daldrup-Link, M.D.

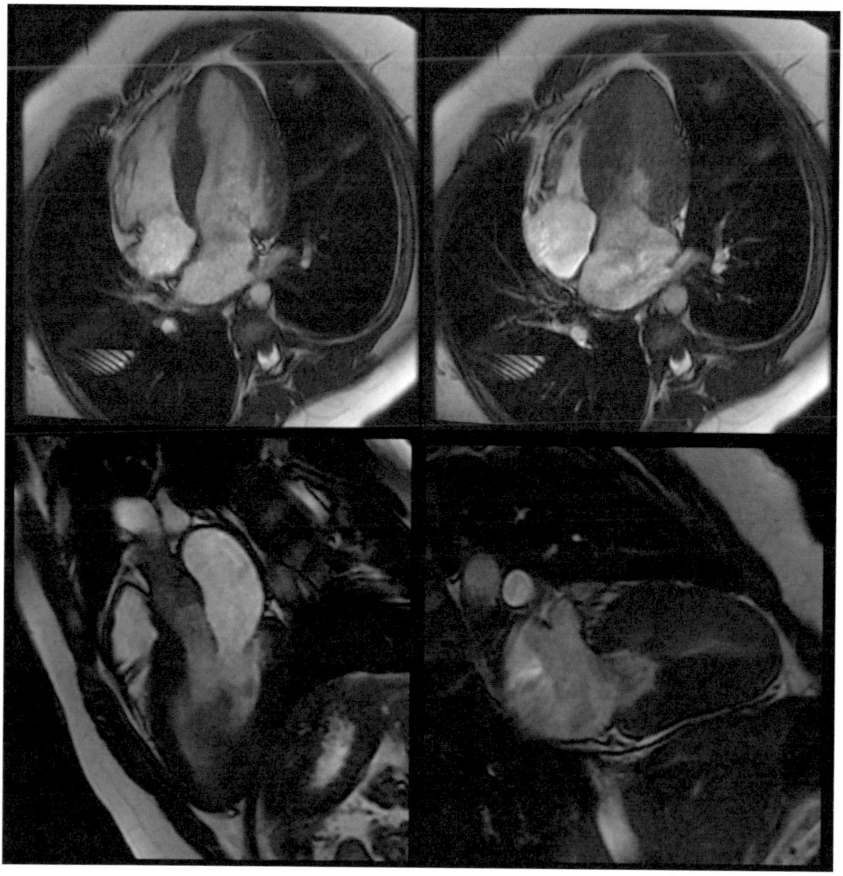

What is the most likely diagnosis:

a) Hypertrophic Cardiomyopathy
b) Athletes Heart
c) Kawasaki Disease
d) Tetralogy of Fallot

Case 21: Hypertrophic Cardiomyopathy

a) Hypertrophic Cardiomyopathy (HCM): Correct! The MRI scan demonstrates a marked, asymmetric hypertrophy of the myocardium with greatest involvement of the mid inferoseptum and basal anteroseptum. The maximum septal wall thickness was measured up to 23 mm (normal < 12 mm). The thickened myocardium caused a narrowing of the left ventricular outflow tract that reduced the blood flow from the left ventricle to the aorta.

b) An athletes' heart leads to mild myocardial thickening, 2-3 mm above normal values.

c) Kawasaki disease represents an autoimmune vasculitis, which can affect the coronary arteries, leading to coronary aneurysms and calcifications. Myocardial hypertrophy is not usually associated with Kawasaki disease.

d) Tetralogy of Fallot is defined by a ventricular septal defect, right (not left) ventricular outflow tract obstruction, an overriding aorta and right (not left) ventricular hypertrophy.

Patient 22: 2-year-old male with recent viral infection

Author: Heike E. Daldrup-Link, M.D.

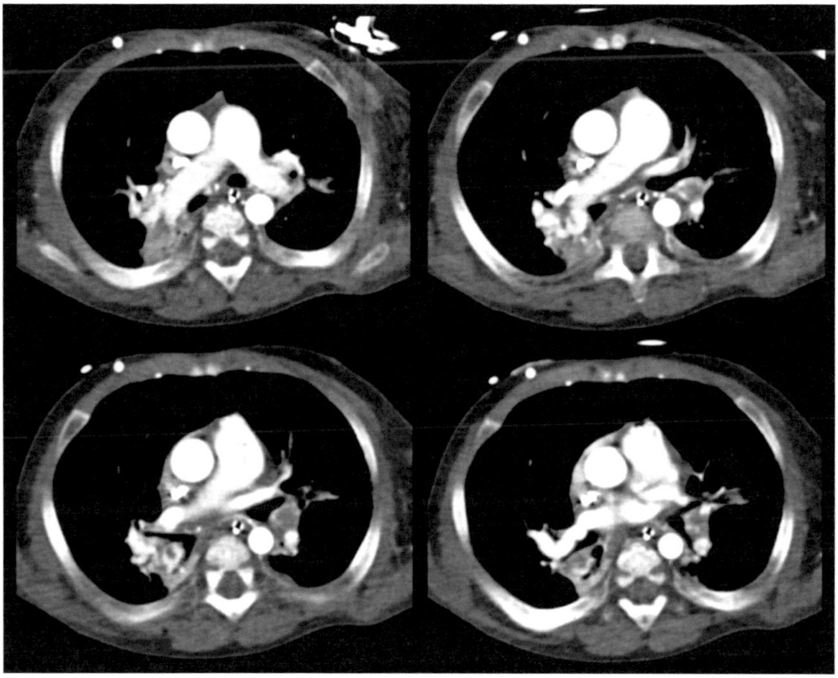

What is the most likely diagnosis:

a) Tuberculosis
b) Coarctation
c) Pulmonary Embolism
d) Transposition of the Great Arteries

Case 22: Pulmonary Embolism

a) Tuberculosis can be associated with necrotic mediastinal lymph nodes. However, the CT scan here shows thrombi in branches of the pulmonary artery.

b) Coarctation of the aorta is characterized by narrowing of the thoracic aorta, causing obstruction of blood flow to the systemic circulation. The most common location for an aortic coarctation is just distal to the left subclavian artery, at the insertion site of the ductus arteriosus.

c) Pulmonary Embolism: Correct! The contrast-enhanced CT scan demonstrates a central filling defect in the left lower lobe pulmonary artery and an additional central filling defect in the right lower lobe pulmonary artery. A small rim of contrast material surrounds the filling defects, consistent with a thrombus in branches of the pulmonary artery. Risk factors for the development of pulmonary emboli include genetic factors (e.g., antithrombin III, protein S and/or C deficiency), COVID-19 infection, recent surgery, prolonged immobility, oral contraceptives in adolescents.

d) A transposition of the great arteries involves discordant ventricular arterial connections. The relative position of the aorta and pulmonary artery shown here is normal.

Chest, Cardiac, Facial Bones, ENT, Airway

4) Lungs and chest wall

Patient 23: Newborn premature infant, shortness of breath
Author: Heike E. Daldrup-Link, M.D.

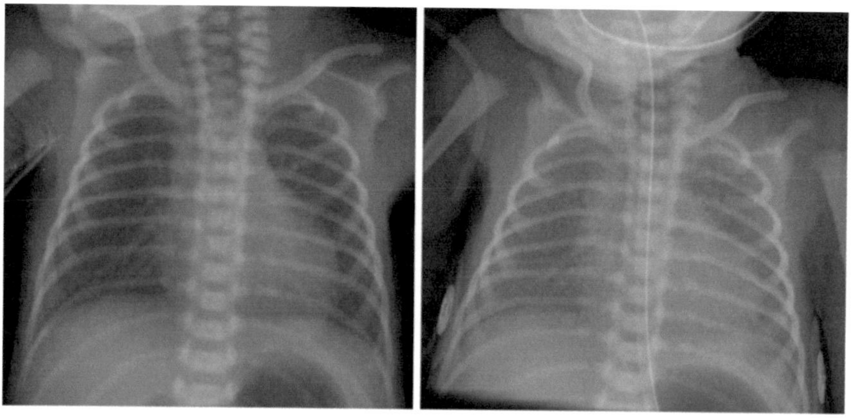

1 hour after birth **24 hours after birth**

What is the most likely diagnosis:

a) Respiratory Distress Syndrome
b) Transient Tachypnea of the Newborn
c) Pulmonary Edema due to Patent Ductus Arteriosus
d) Normal radiographs

Case 23: Respiratory Distress Syndrome

a) Respiratory Distress Syndrome (Synonyms: Hyaline Membrane Disease, Lung Disease of Prematurity): Correct! The radiograph demonstrates a typical ground glass opacity of the lungs bilaterally which classically worsens over 48-72 hours, plateaus for one or more days, then improves. Positive bronchograms are also noted. The ground glass opacity can have a granular texture. The opacity is due to insufficient production of surfactant by type II pneumocytes.

b) Transient tachypnea of the newborn is typically seen in term babies due to retained fetal fluid in the lungs. It often also presents with bilateral ground glass opacities of the lungs shortly after birth. Small pleural effusions can also be present. However, these opacities typically improve on subsequent radiographs.

c) A pulmonary edema due to patent ductus arteriosus typically develops after several days of live. In term infants, the ductus closes within 48 hours after birth. In preterm infants it can stay open. During the first days of life, there is typically limited shunt vascularity due to the high pressure in the lungs. Over subsequent days, the shunt vascularity across the open ductus increases, which leads to an increased heart size and pulmonary edema with a peek around day 7 to 10 after birth.

d) These radiographs are not normal, as detailed above.

Patient 24: Four-month-old male with respiratory distress

Author: Heike E. Daldrup-Link, M.D.

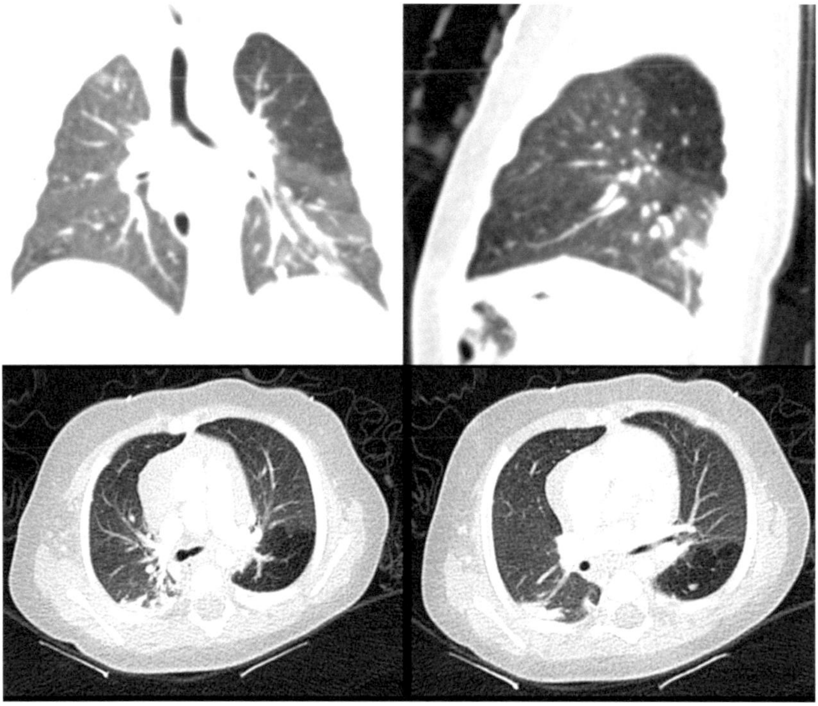

What is the most likely diagnosis:

a) Swyer James syndrome
b) Poland syndrome
c) Congenital lobar overinflation (CLO)
d) Congenital Pulmonary Airway Malformation (CPAM)

Case 24: Congenital lobar hyperinflation (CLO)

a) A Swyer James syndrome is an acquired form of segmental or lobar overinflation after a bronchopulmonary infection, which led to a bronchiolitis obliterans. Imaging studies would typically show sequelae of prior pneumonia, bronchial wall thickening and/or bronchiectasis.

b) Poland syndrome is characterized by an apparent unilaterally hyperlucent lung on chest x-rays due to hypo- or agenesis of anterior chest wall muscles. The chest wall muscles here are symmetric and normal.

c) Congenital lobar overinflation (CLO): Correct! The CT images show an hyperexpanded left upper lobe which contains diminished vessels (oligemia) compared to the normal contralateral lung. A location in the left upper lobe us most common. A frequent association is a bronchial atresia with a bling ending, mucus-filled bronchus, which causes air-trapping.

d) Congenital pulmonary airway malformation (CPAM) is characterized by multiple thin-walled cysts of variable sizes. There is no focal cystic mass noted here.

Patient 25: 14-year-old female, long-standing dyspnea

Author: Heike E. Daldrup-Link, M.D.

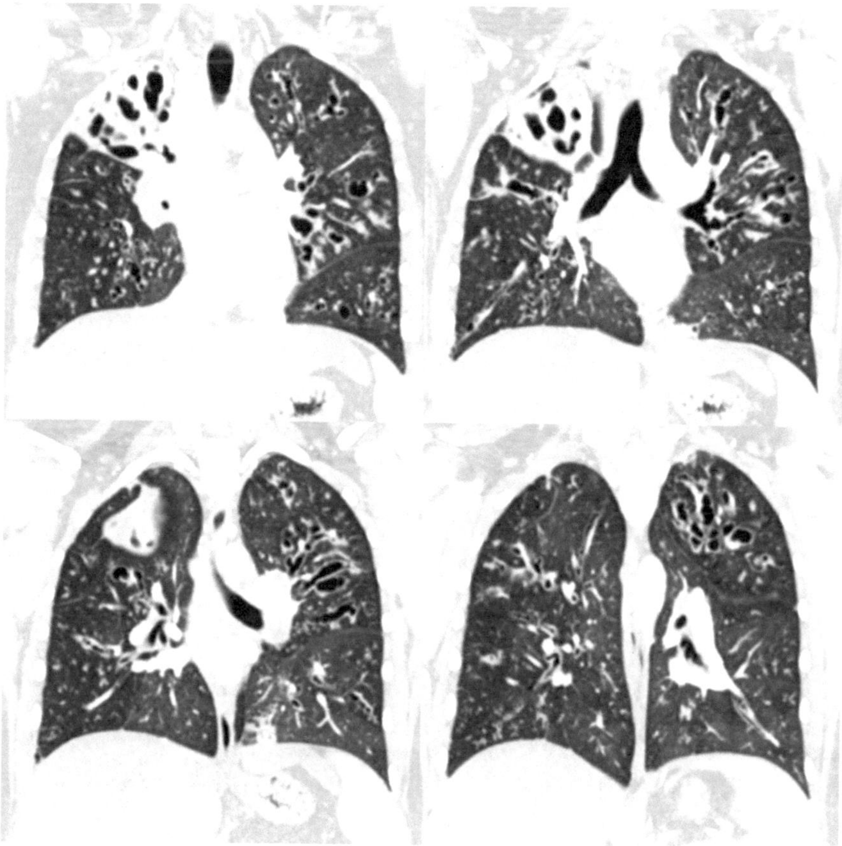

What is the most likely diagnosis:

a) Tuberculosis
b) Cystic Fibrosis
c) Kartagener syndrome
d) Lymphangioleiomyomatosis

Case 25: Cystic Fibrosis

a) Pulmonary tuberculosis can have many different appearances. However, the bilateral extensive bronchiectasis and air trapping seen here suggest a different diagnosis.

b) Cystic Fibrosis. Correct! Cystic fibrosis is an autosomal recessive disorder that leads to abnormal electrolyte transport and production of thick mucus by glands in the respiratory, digestive, and reproductive system. The CT scan demonstrates typical findings of bronchial wall thickening and bronchiectasis of the lungs bilaterally, most predominant in the upper lobes and perihilar areas. In addition, the lungs are hyperinflated and the pulmonary artery appears enlarged due to pulmonary hypertension. Note that the shape of bronchiectasis can evolve over time from cylindrical to varicose and cystic. Several bronchiectasis in the right upper and left mid lung contain dense material, consistent with mucus plugging. There is dense consolidation and atelectasis of the right upper lobe, with elevation of the minor fissure.

c) Kartagener syndrome is an autosomal recessive disorder that leads to immotile cilia. The condition can be also associated with bronchial wall thickening, bronchiectasis and mucus plugging. However, in addition, Kartagener syndrome is associated with a situs inversus which is not seen here. Patients with Kartagener syndrome also typically have a history of chronic sinusitis since glands in the sinus are affected as well.

d) Lymphangioleiomyomatosis in children is typically associated with tuberous sclerosis and can present with cystic lung disease. A CT scan would show pulmonary hyperinflation with scattered thin-walled, air-filled cysts throughout the lungs. An accompanying pneumothorax or chylus effusion may be also to seen.

Patient 26: Teenage female with cystic fibrosis

Author: Heike E. Daldrup-Link, M.D.

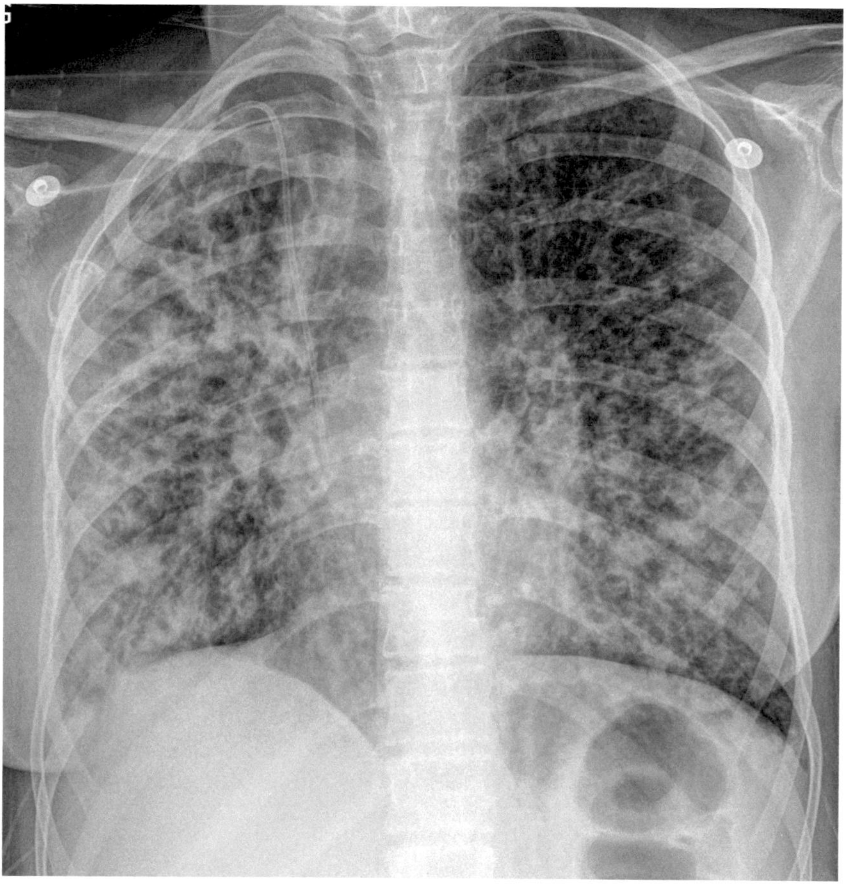

The Brasfield system scores which findings:

a) Overinflation, bronchial line shadows, ring shadows, mottled shadows, large soft shadows.
b) Air trapping, linear markings, cystic lesions, nodular lesions, general severity
c) Air trapping, linear markings, nodular cystic lesions, large lesions, general severity
d) Overinflation, linear markings, bronchiectasis, mucous plugging, general severity

Case 26: Cystic Fibrosis, Brasfield Scoring System

a) The criteria listed here represent the Crispin-Norman score, a different scoring system that is also used to assess the severity of pulmonary findings in patients with cystic fibrosis.

b) The criteria listed here represent some but not all criteria that are scored with the Brasfield Scoring system.

c) Brasfield scoring system. Correct! The criteria listed here represent the Brasfield scoring system. The score is based on radiographic findings on chest x-rays. The maximum score is 25 and points are subtracted based on the severity of findings under each of the listed five categories.

d) The criteria listed here represent some but not all criteria that are scored with the Brasfield Scoring system. Bronchiectasis and mucus plugging are covered by "nodular cystic lesions" in the actual scoring system. Bronchiectases are scored with and without lucent centers.

Patient 27: Newborn, serial x-rays over the first days of life

Author: Heike E. Daldrup-Link, M.D.

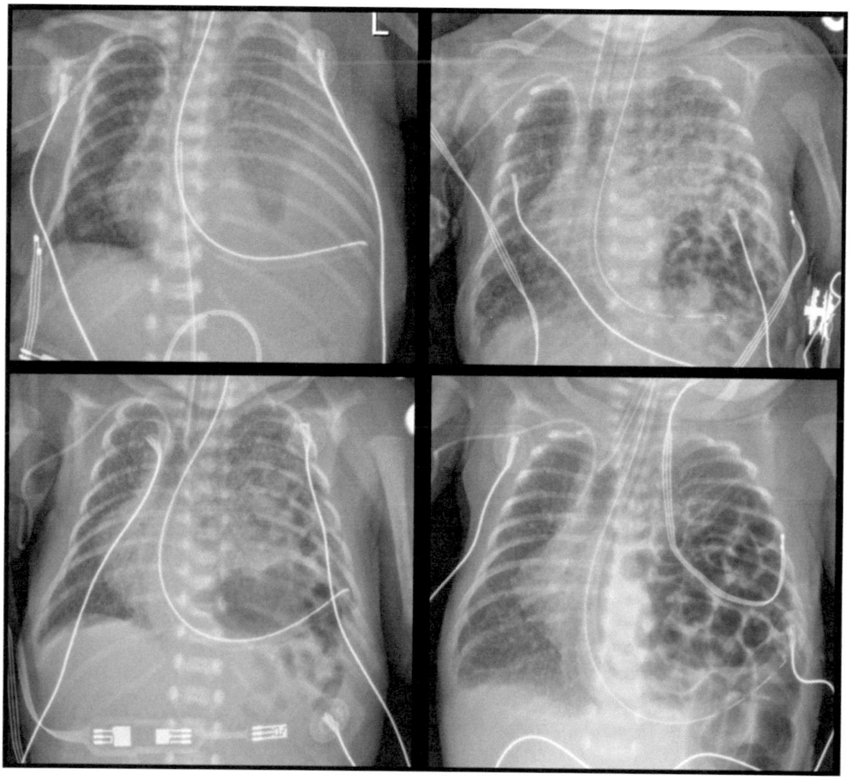

What is the most likely diagnosis:

a) Congenital diaphragmatic hernia
b) Pneumonia with pneumatoceles
c) Congenital lobar overinflation
d) Congenital Pulmonary Airway Malformation

Case 27: Congenital Diaphragmatic Hernia

a) Congenital diaphragmatic hernia: Correct! The radiograph directly after birth shows an opacification in the left lower hemithorax and an unusual high location of the distal feeding tube in the left lower hemithorax. The mediastinum is shifted to the right. Serial subsequent images demonstrate an air-filled stomach in the left hemithorax and multiple air-filled tubular structures in the left hemithorax, which are most consistent with bowel loops. The left lung is hypoplastic. More than 80% of diaphragmatic hernias involve a defect of the left side of the diaphragm. The most common location of the defect is posterolateral (Bochdalek hernia).

b) A pneumonia can present with a consolidation of an entire lung. Pneumatoceles can develop after pneumonia. However, in this case here, the feeding tube and stomach are clearly located in the left lower hemithorax, suggesting a different diagnosis.

c) Congenital lobar overinflation is characterized by segmental or lobar hyperinflation of the lung. The hyperinflated lung can cause mass effect with lateral shift of the mediastinum, flattening of the ipsilateral diaphragm and caudal (rather than cranial) displacement of the stomach.

d) Congenital pulmonary airway malformation would present with multiple thin-walled cysts of variable sizes. However, in this case here, the feeding tube and stomach are clearly located in the left lower hemithorax, suggesting a different diagnosis.

Patient 28: A newborn with respiratory distress

Author: Wipawee Morakote, M.D.

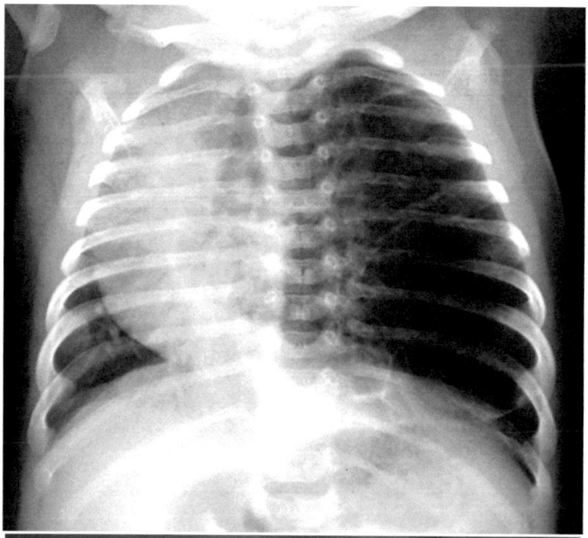

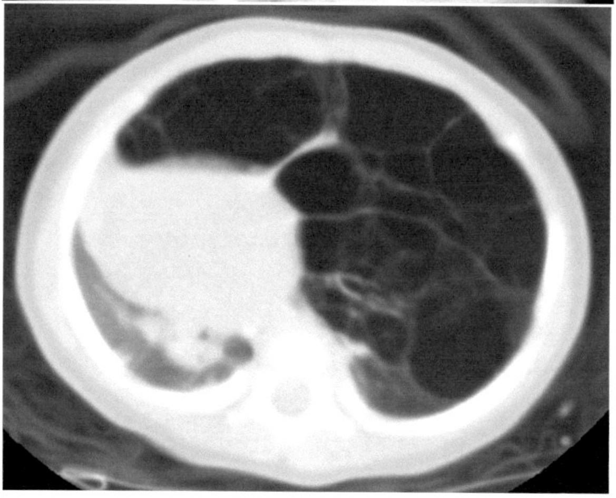

What is the most likely diagnosis:

a) Simple lung cyst
b) Pneumatoceles
c) Congenital lobar overinflation (CLO)
d) Congenital Pulmonary Airway Malformation (CPAM)

Case 28: Congenital pulmonary airway malformation

a) A simple lung cyst presents typically as a single unilocular thin walled (< 2mm) round intrapulmonary lesion containing air.

b) Pneumatoceles can develop after pneumonia or lung injury. Imaging demonstrates a single or multiple discrete thin-walled round air-containing intrapulmonary lesions. Adjacent consolidations or ground glass opacities may be noted. Most pneumatoceles resolve spontaneously or after an underlying infection has been treated.

c) Congenital lobar overinflation (CLO) is characterized by hyperinflation of a lung segment or lobe with visualized normal bronchovascular marking within the affected lung. CLO may occur because of airway cartilage abnormalities, extrinsic airway compression, or bronchial atresia. These pathologies lead to air-trapping and resultant overinflation of the alveoli; however, the alveolar walls are intact. A cyst formation is not noted in CLO.

d) Congenital pulmonary airway malformation (CPAM): Correct! The radiograph and axial CT image show an hyperexpanded left upper lobe which contains multiple thin-walled cysts of variable sizes. The hyperexpanded lung demonstrates mass effect on the mediastinum and right lung. These findings are consistent with CPAM type 1 since the largest cyst is greater than 2 cm in size. CPAM is the most common congenital lung abnormality. On imaging studies, CPAM has been classified into three types based on size of the cysts. Type 1 consists of cysts larger than 2 cm. Type 2 consists of cysts smaller than 2 cm. Type 3 consists of microscopic cysts and appears solid on medical imaging studies.

Patient 29: 21-month-old child with cough and fever

Author: Heike E. Daldrup-Link, M.D.

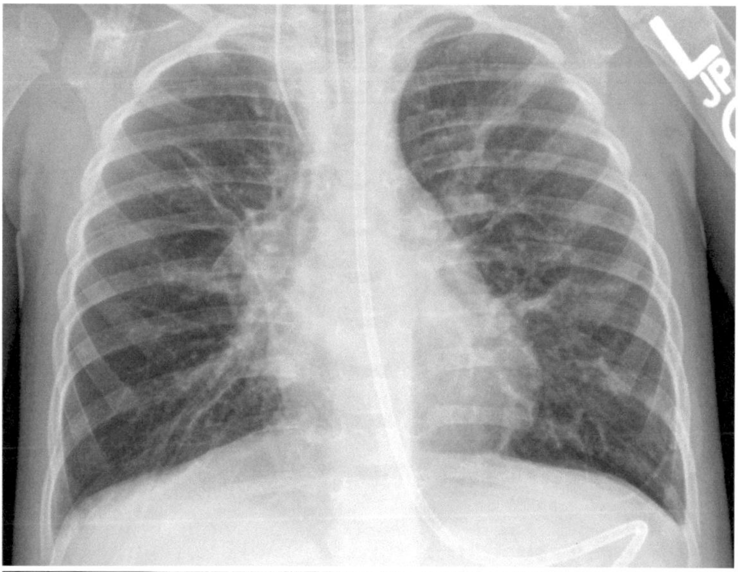

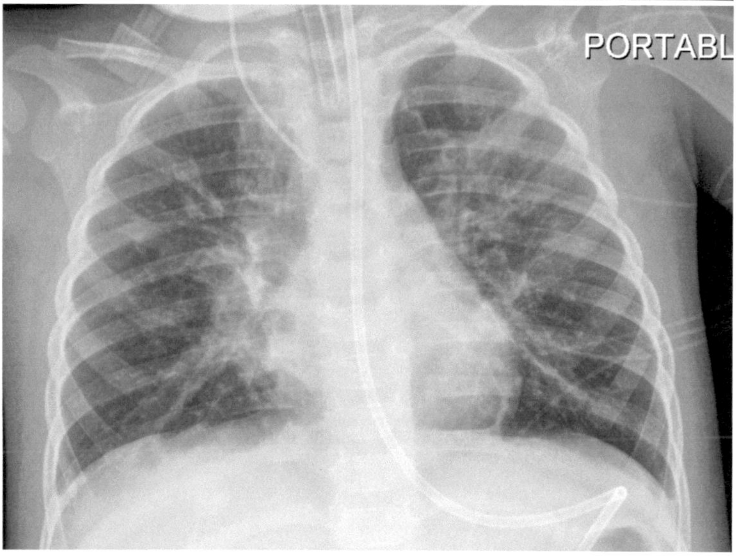

What is the most likely diagnosis:

a) Bacterial Pneumonia
b) Tetralogy of Fallot
c) Cystic fibrosis
d) Viral Pneumonia

Case 29: Viral Pneumonia

a) A bacteria pneumonia typically presents with a segmental or multisegmental airspace opacity and positive air bronchograms. A pleural effusion may also be present.

b) Tetralogy of Fallot classically present with a boot-shaped heart with an elevated cardiac apex due to right ventricular hypertrophy. The pulmonary vessels are small due to the underlying pulmonary stenosis.

c) Cystic fibrosis is characterized by bronchial wall thickening and bronchiectasis, which is usually most pronounced in the upper lobes. Areas of air trapping, mucus plugging, and nodular cystic lesions can also be seen. The findings here are centered around the hili.

d) Viral pneumonia: Correct! The chest radiographs show peribronchial thickening of central bronchi, areas of distal air tracking and streaky perihilar opacities, which are due to atelectasis distal to obstructed bronchi. Bronchial wall swelling leads to a ventil mechanism and air trapping. When the bronchial wall swells more, then air cannot enter the lung any more and flat atelectasis develop distal to the affected bronchus. These atelectases can shift from one radiograph to another. With further progression, perihilar interstitial infiltrates and consolidations can be seen. Hilar lymphadenopathy or pleural effusions are not usually seen in viral pneumonias.

Patient 30: 17-year-old, two-week history of fever, headache, and malaise

Author: Lisa Adams, M.D., Shakthi Kumaran Ramasamy, M.D.

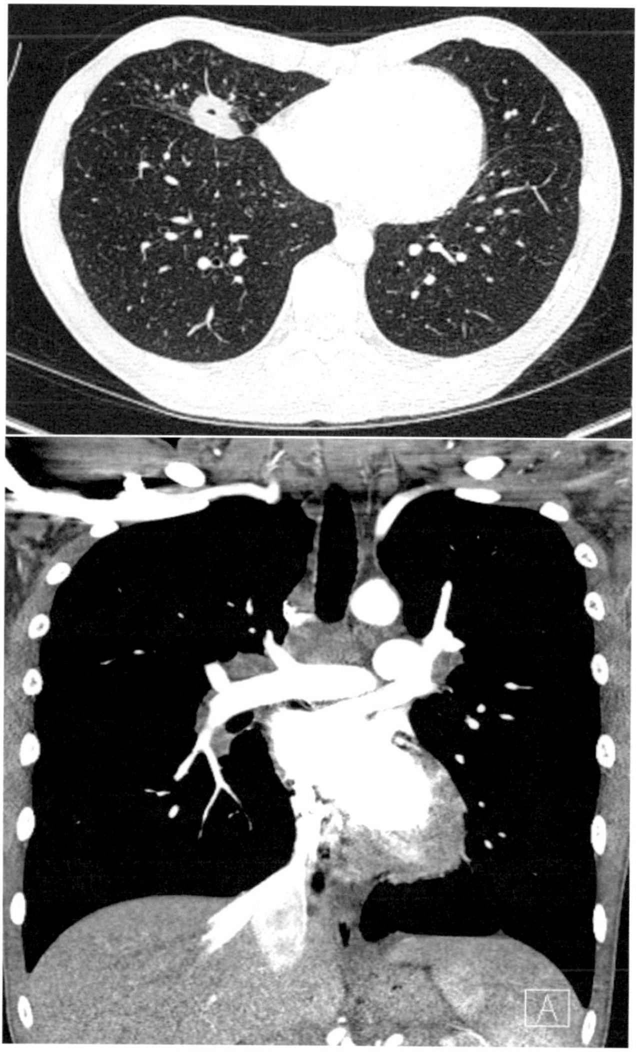

What is the most likely diagnosis:

a) Coccidiomycosis
b) Bacterial pneumonia
c) Cystic fibrosis
d) Mediastinal lymphoma

Case 30: Coccidiomycosis

a) Coccidioidomycosis - Correct! The CT scan demonstrates multiple enlarged mediastinal lymph nodes and an ill-defined pulmonary nodule in the right middle lobe with central cavitation and surrounding micronodules. Tuberculosis could be considered in the differential diagnosis.

b) A bacterial pneumonia would typically present as a segmental or lobar pulmonary consolidation with air bronchograms. The degree of lymphadenopathy shown here would be unusual.

c) Cystic fibrosis is characterized by bronchial wall thickening and bronchiectasis, which is usually most pronounced in the upper lobes. Areas of air trapping, mucus plugging, and nodular cystic lesions can also be seen. In the absence of an acute infection, the degree of lymphadenopathy shown here would be unusual.

d) Mediastinal lymphoma characteristically presents with a large soft tissue mass in the mid mediastinum. There can be associated pulmonary involvement. However, the combination of multiple enlarged lymph nodes, cavitating pulmonary nodule and fever suggest a different primary diagnosis.

Patient 31: Teenage female with shortness of breath
Author: Heike E. Daldrup-Link, M.D.

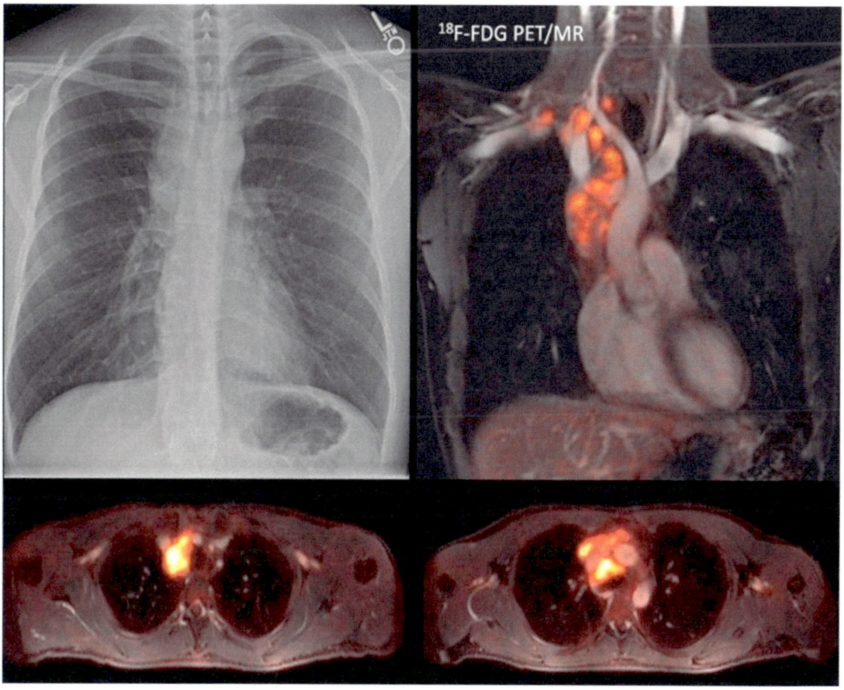

What is the most likely diagnosis:

a) Thymoma
b) Neuroblastoma
c) Teratoma
d) Hodgkin Lymphoma

Case 31: Hodgkin Lymphoma

a) A thymoma is rare in children. It represents a slow growing tumor in the anterior mediastinum which demonstrates limited or no 18F-FDG uptake. Associated lymph nodes would be uncommon

b) A neuroblastoma presents as a posterior mediastinal mass. The lesion shown here is centered in the mid and anterior mediastinum.

c) A mediastinal teratoma typically presents as an inhomogeneous mass in the anterior mediastinum, which contains cystic components, macroscopic fat and/or calcifications. 18F-FDG uptake is variable. The majority of mediastinal teratomas are benign and associated lymph nodes would be uncommon.

d) Hodgkin Lymphoma. Correct! The CT scan demonstrates multiple enlarged lymph nodes in the anterior and mid mediastinum, which demonstrate increased metabolic activity on the 18F-FDG PET scan. This finding is most consistent with a Hodgkin Lymphoma.

Patient 32: 17-year-old female with shortness of breath

Author: Heike E. Daldrup-Link, M.D.

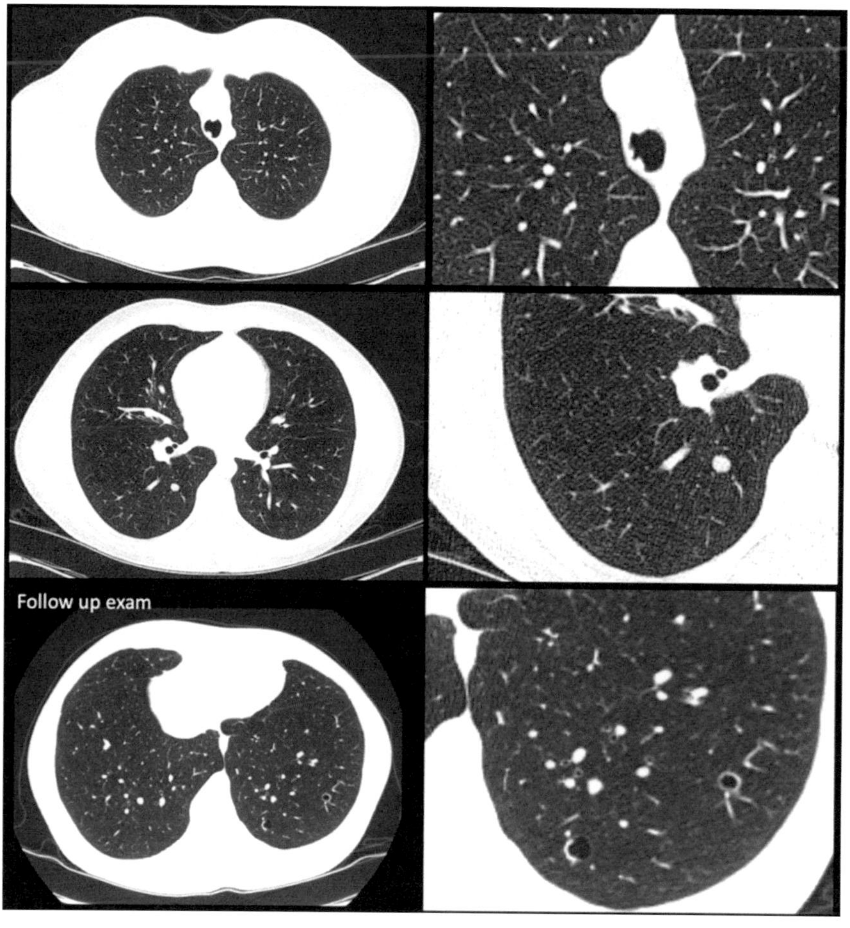

What is the most likely diagnosis:

a) Bronchial Carcinoid
b) Recurrent Respiratory Papillomatosis
c) Aspirated Foreign Bodies
d) Coccidiomycosis

Case 32: Recurrent Respiratory Papillomatosis

a) A bronchial carcinoid would present as a single focal mass in the trachea or one of the main stem bronchi.

b) Recurrent Respiratory Papillomatosis: Correct! The CT scan demonstrates multiple nodules in the trachea, consistent with papillomas, i.e., benign squamous cell tumors. The lower cuts through the lung tissue demonstrate multiple small round pulmonary nodules, which start to cavitate. A follow up scan several months later demonstrates thin-walled cysts. The disease is due to infection by human papillomavirus (HPV), usually types 6 and 11. The juvenile onset form presents before age 12, is more aggressive than the adult-onset form, and symptoms are more severe. Inoculation of children typically occurs through the placenta or through the birth canal.

c) There are multiple nodules noted in the trachea. There is no evidence for a foreign body.

d) Coccidiomycosis can present with micronodules and centrally cavitating nodules. However, intra-tracheal lesions would not be a typical feature. Coccidiomycosis is often associated with enlarged mediastinal lymph nodes which are not noted here.

Patient 33: Five-day old premature infant, respiratory distress

Author: Heike E. Daldrup-Link, M.D.

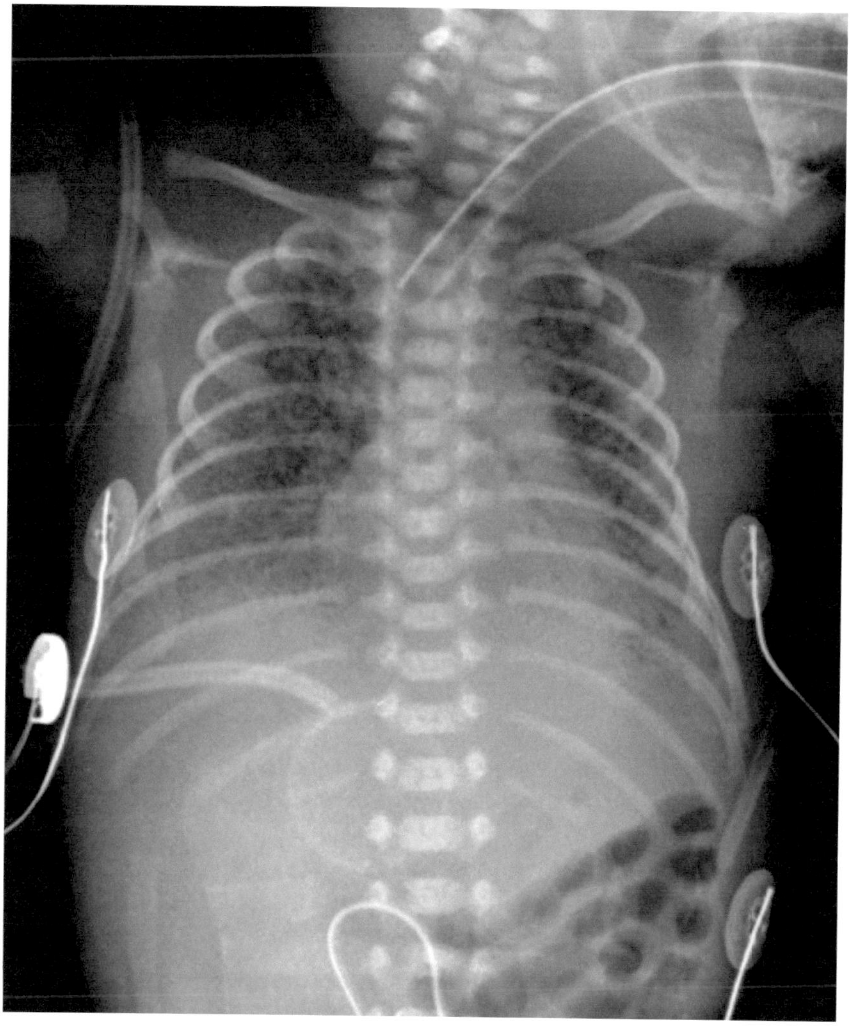

What is the most likely diagnosis:

a) Patent ductus arteriosus
b) Diaphragmatic hernia
c) Spinal dysraphism
d) Pulmonary interstitial emphysema (PIE)

Case 33: Pulmonary Interstitial Emphysema (PIE)

a) A patent ductus arteriosus would present with an increasing pulmonary edema over the course of the first one to two weeks of life. This is not shown here.

b) The radiograph does not show bowel loops or other abdominal organs in the chest.

c) Spinal dysraphism: The radiograph shows normal ossification centers of the vertebral bodies.

d) Pulmonary interstitial emphysema (PIE): Correct! The chest radiograph demonstrates multiple focal and linear lucencies of the lungs bilaterally on a background of fine granular microatelectasis. The lucencies are darker than the air in the main stem bronchi. The patient has an endotracheal tube and has been ventilated since birth. Positive pressure ventilation of premature lungs can lead to dissection of air from the bronchi into the interstitium of the lungs where it gets trapped as PIE.

Patient 34: 2-year-old female, shortness of breath

Author: Heike E. Daldrup-Link, M.D.

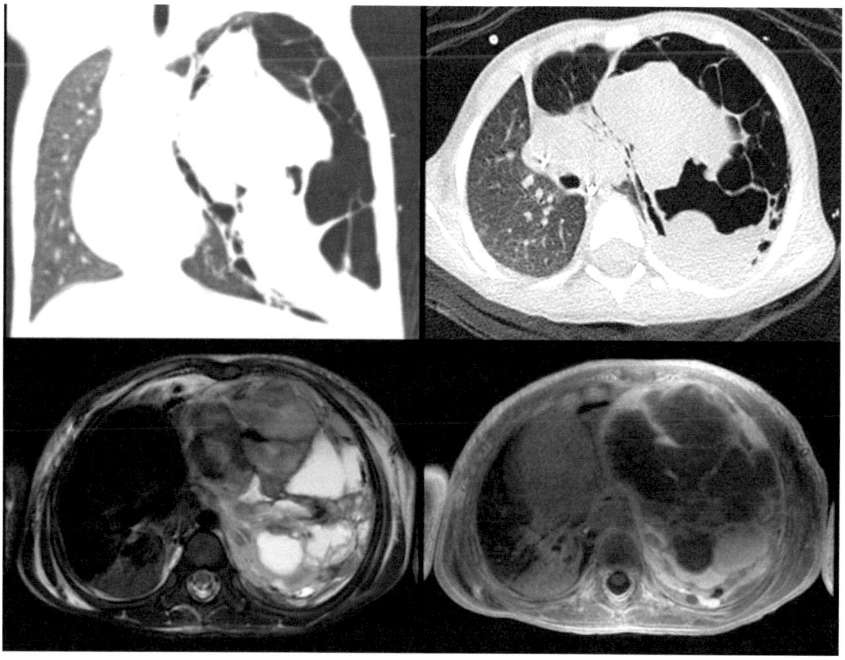

What is the most likely diagnosis:

a) Pneumonia
b) Pleuropulmonary blastoma
c) Congenital pulmonary airway malformation
d) Congenital diaphragmatic hernia

Case 34: Pleuropulmonary Blastoma

a) Necrotizing pneumonia can present with consolidations (which do not enhance with contrast), pneumatoceles, abscess formations and a loculated effusion. However, the lesion shown here is composed of cystic spaces and contrast-enhancing soft tissue masses, which do not demonstrate aerobronchograms.

b) Pleuropulmonary Blastoma (PPB): Correct! The coronal and axial CT scan demonstrates a multicystic intrapulmonary mass which causes significant mass effect on the mediastinum. The axial T2-weighted and contrast-enhanced T1-weighted axial scans through the lesion show that the lesion contains multiple large, contrast-enhancing soft tissue nodules, in addition to large cystic spaces. These findings in conjunction with the young age of the patient suggest a PPB as the most likely diagnosis. Note that PPB can be associated with a Dicer 1 mutation, which predispose patients to cystic lesions in other organs, including multiloculated cystic nephroma, and other solid malignancies, such as Wilms tumor. PPB can present as cystic, mixed, and solid intrapulmonary or pleural-based masses. The images here show a mixed type PPB.

c) A congenital pulmonary airway malformation (CPAM) can present as a macrocystic, microcystic or apparently solid (microcysts that cannot be resolved by medical imaging techniques) intrathoracic mass which shows mass effect on the mediastinum with displacement of the heart to the opposite side. A PPB can be associated with a co-existing CPAM. The large enhancing soft tissue nodules within the multi-cystic lesion here clearly suggests a PPB.

d) A congenital diaphragmatic hernia (CDH) can present with aur-filled lucencies within the left or right hemithorax, due to herniation of bowel loops into the chest. Intrathoracic herniations of abdominal organs can also be noted. However, the large enhancing soft tissue nodules within the multi-cystic lesion here suggest a different diagnosis.

Patient 35: Newborn baby girl with respiratory distress

Author: Heike E. Daldrup-Link, M.D.

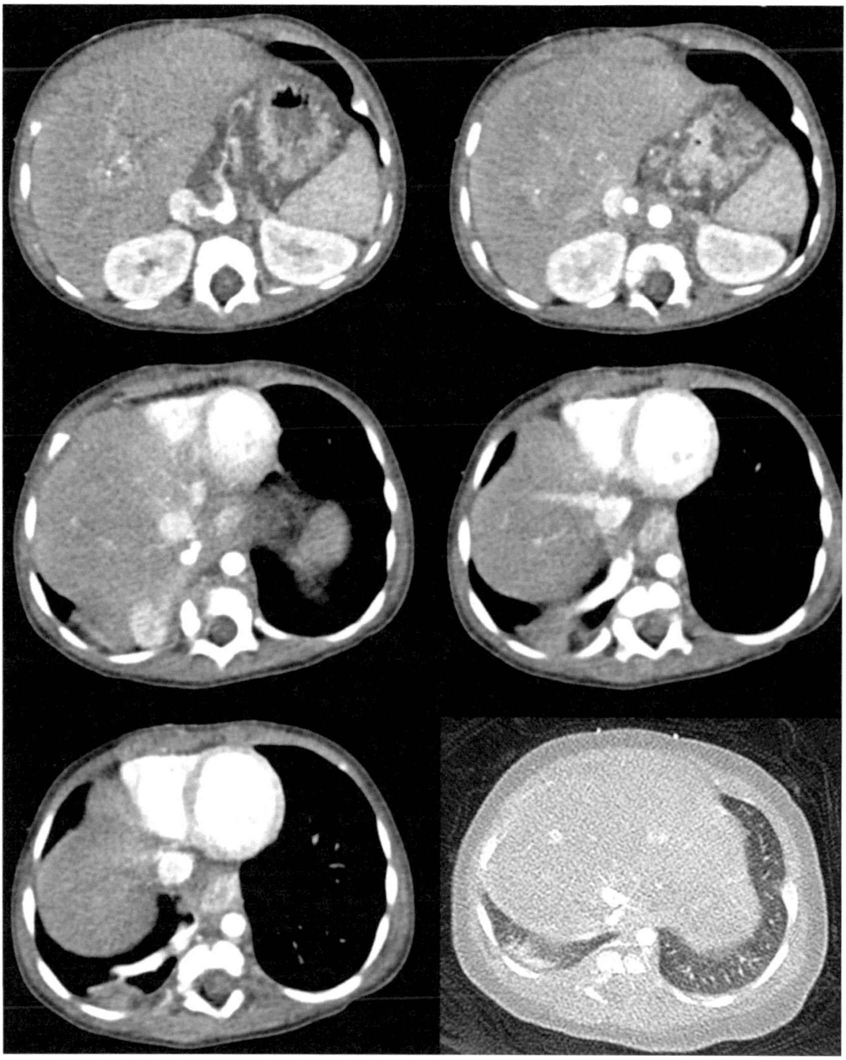

What is the most likely diagnosis:

a) Pulmonary Sequestration
b) Scimitar Syndrome
c) Bronchial Atresia
d) Pulmonary Arteriovenous Malformation

Case 35: Pulmonary Sequestration

a) Pulmonary Sequestration: Correct! A pulmonary sequestration is characterized by an abnormal segment of lung, which is supplied by an abnormal artery that arises directly from the aorta. In this case, the axial CT scans demonstrate an abnormal artery which arises from the abdominal aorta and can be followed to the right lower lung, where it supplies an abnormal lung segment in the right lower lobe. The abnormal lung segment is not connected to the tracheobronchial tree. The extralobar type of pulmonary sequestrations is more common in the neonatal period and most commonly drains into a systemic vein. By comparison, intralobar pulmonary sequestrations are more common, are more commonly diagnosed in older children and typically drain through a pulmonary vein.

b) A Scimitar Syndrome is characterized by a hypoplastic lung and partial anomalous pulmonary venous return, most commonly involving an abnormal vein in the right lower lobe which drains into the inferior vena cava or the right atrium.

c) Bronchial atresia presents with a mucus-filled blind ending bronchus and surrounding oligemia and hyperinflation of the adjacent lung. The serpiginous structure seen here enhances on contrast-enhanced images and connects to the abdominal aorta, consistent with an abnormal artery.

d) A pulmonary arteriovenous malformation is characterized by well-circumscribed, non-calcified pulmonary nodules, which are connected to a serpiginous blood vessel. The lesion is composed of a feeding artery, an aneurysmal connection, and a draining vein.

Patient 36: 18-year-old female with chest pain and dyspnea

Authors: Desiree R. Eshraghi, Soni C. Chawla, M.D.

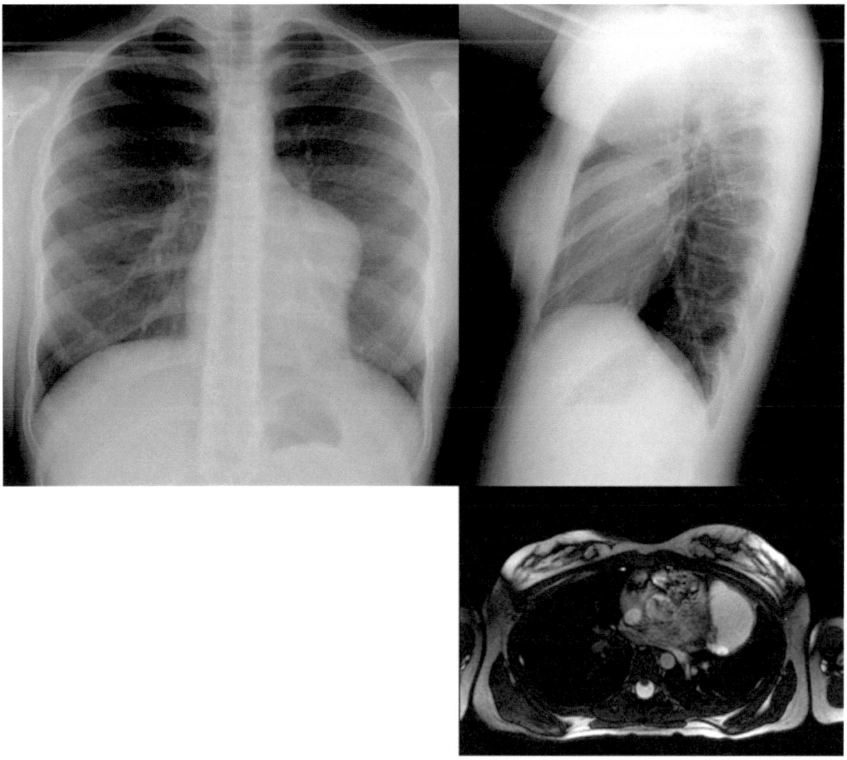

What is the most likely diagnosis:

a) Left atrial enlargement
b) Left atrial appendage aneurysm
c) Mediastinal lymphoma
d) Pericardial cyst

Case 36: Pericardial Cyst

a) A left atrial enlargement (LAE) would demonstrate an enlargement of the left atrium, which is not the case here.

b) An aneurysm of the left atrial appendage (LAAA) would demonstrate a continuity of the lesion with the left atrium, which is not the case here.

c) A Hodgkin lymphoma would typically present as a relatively homogenous soft tissue mass in the mid and anterior mediastinum with limited T2-signal due to a high cell density. A Non-Hodgkin lymphoma could present as a more inhomogeneous soft tissue mass, with areas of necrosis. In both instances, accompanying enlarged lymph nodes are often noted. The lesion seen here, is composed of T2-hyperintense fluid.

d) Pericardial cyst: Correct! Frontal and lateral views of the chest demonstrate a prominence and bulging of the left heart border. Axial T2 haste MRI image through the mid-thorax demonstrates a well-defined cystic lesion, which abuts the left heart border, consistent with a pericardial cyst.

Patient 37: 14-year-old female with shortness of breath

Author: Heike E. Daldrup-Link, M.D.

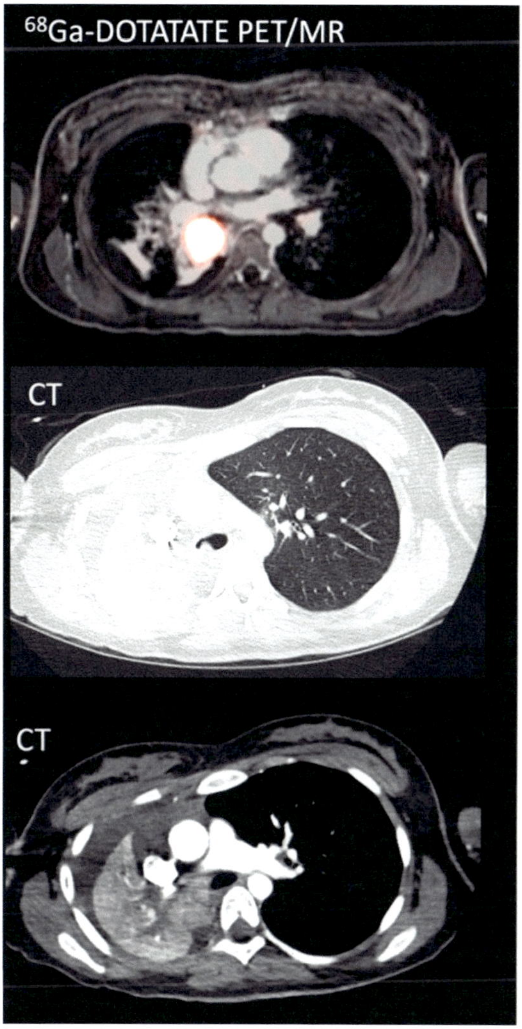

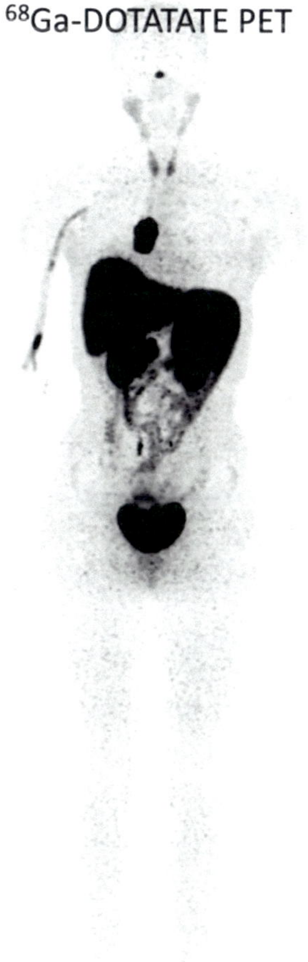

What is the most likely diagnosis:

a) Inflammatory Pseudotumor
b) Neuroendocrine Tumor (NET)
c) Papillomatosis
d) Mucoepidermoid carcinoma

Case 37: Neuroendocrine Tumor (NET)

a) An inflammatory pseudotumor can present as an endobronchial lesion. However, it would not show uptake of 68-Ga DOTATETE radiotracer.

b) Neuroendocrine Tumor (NET). Correct! The CT scan demonstrates an endobronchial lesion, which leads to collapse of the right lung and shift of the mediastinum to the right. The PET/MR shows uptake of 68-Ga DOTATETE radiotracer. The combination of an endobronchial mass and 68-Ga DOTATATE radiotracer uptake suggests the diagnosis of an NET. 68-Ga DOTATATE binds to the somatostatin receptor found in NET.

c) Papillomatosis of the lower respiratory tract in children typically presents with laryngeal, tracheal and/or endobronchial lesions, with or without multiple bilateral pulmonary nodules and thin-walled cysts. The juvenile form is due to an HPV infection before (via the placenta) or during birth. 68-Ga DOTATETE PET would be negative.

d) Mucoepidermoid carcinomas are rare in children. They can present as an endobronchial lesion, but 68-Ga DOTATETE PET would be negative.

Patient 38: Teenager with shortness of breath

Author: Heike E. Daldrup-Link, M.D.

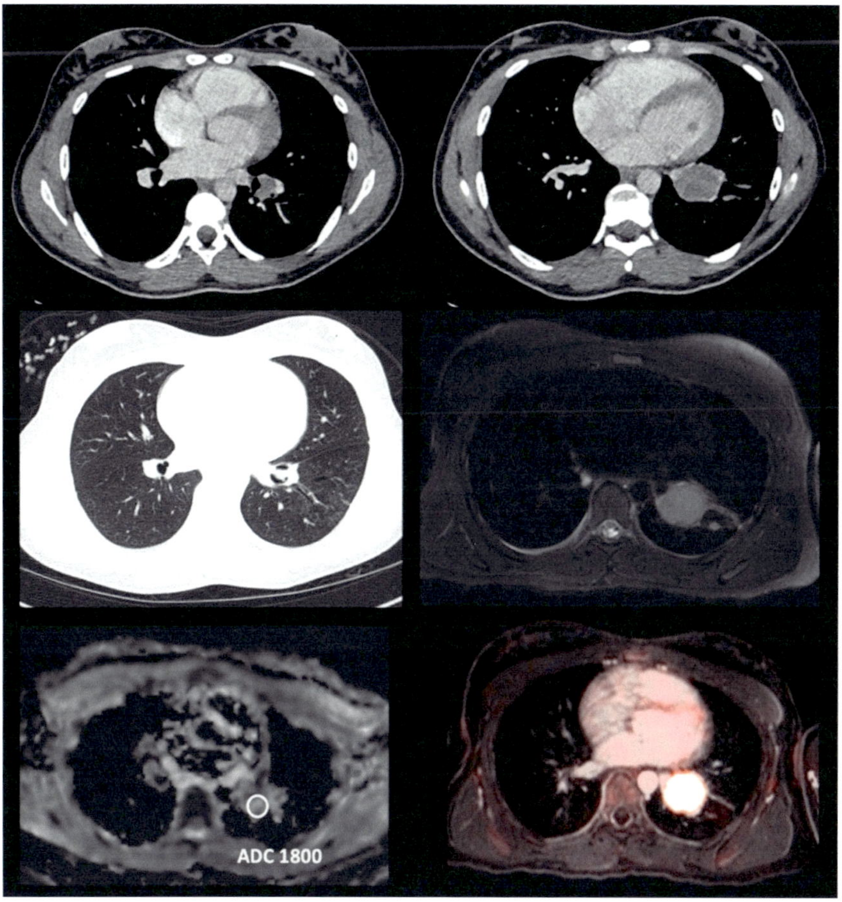

What is the most likely diagnosis:

a) Inflammatory Myofibroblastic Tumor
b) Neuroendocrine Tumor (NET)
c) Papillomatosis
d) Mucoepidermoid carcinoma

Case 38: Inflammatory Myofibroblastic Tumor

a) Inflammatory myofibroblastic tumor (inflammatory pseudotumor): Correct! The CT scan demonstrates a soft tissue lesion below the left hilum, which infiltrates the left main stem bronchus. The lesion demonstrates non-specific hyperintense signal on an axial T2-weighted MRI scan and markedly increased metabolism on an integrated 18F-FDG PET/MR scan. The lesion also demonstrates no significant restricted diffusion on diffusion-weighted MRI, with high ADC values of more than 1000 mm^2/s, suggesting a benign lesion.

b) A Neuroendocrine Tumor (NET) can present as an endobronchial mass with restricted diffusion. An 18F-FDG PET/MR scan would demonstrate non-specific high metabolic activity. A 68-Ga DOTATATE radiotracer uptake can confirm a suspected diagnosis of an NET.

c) Papillomatosis of the lower respiratory tract in children typically presents with small, laryngeal, tracheal and/or endobronchial lesions, with or without multiple bilateral pulmonary nodules and thin-walled cysts.

d) Mucoepidermoid carcinomas are rare in children. They can present as an endobronchial lesion, but would demonstrate markedly restricted diffusion on diffusion-weighted MRI, with ADC values of less than 1000 mm^2/s.

Patient 39: Five-day old female, shortness of breath

Author: Heike E. Daldrup-Link, M.D.

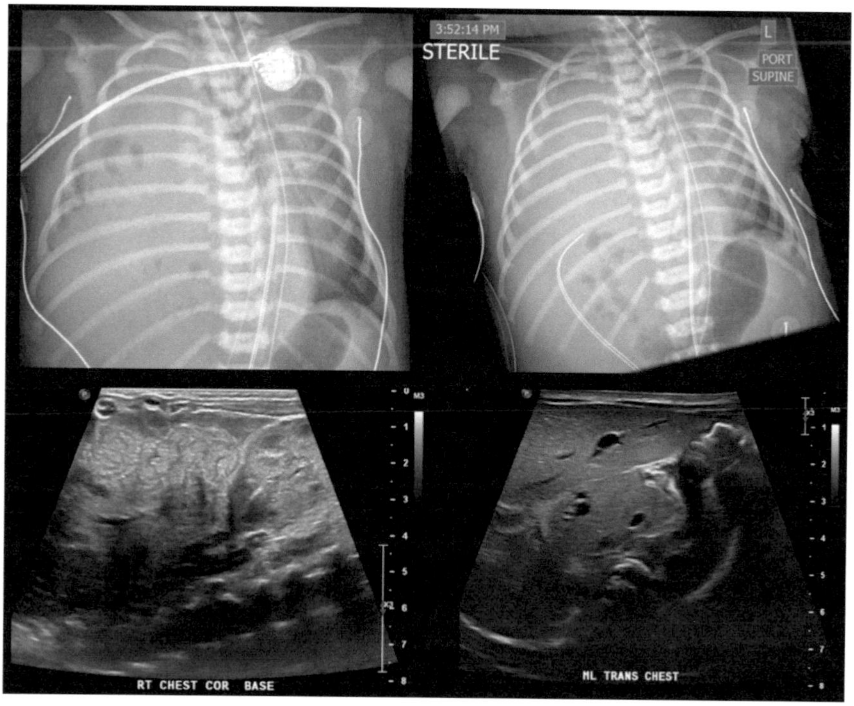

What is the most likely diagnosis:

a) Pneumonia
b) Pleuropulmonary blastoma
c) Congenital pulmonary airway malformation
d) Congenital diaphragmatic hernia

Case 39: Congenital Diaphragmatic Hernia

a) A pneumonia can present with a consolidation of an entire lung. However, there are no aerobronchograms noted here. A large pleural effusion can cause mediastinal shift. But the ultrasound shown here does not support this diagnosis.

b) A pleuropulmonary blastoma present as a cystic or solid intrapulmonary mass which can displace the mediastinum. But the ultrasound shown here does not support this diagnosis.

c) A congenital pulmonary airway malformation can present as a cystic or solid intrathoracic mass which shows mass effect on the mediastinum with displacement of the heart to the opposite side. But the ultrasound shown here does not support this diagnosis.

d) Congenital diaphragmatic hernia (CDH): Correct! The chest x-ray shows a dense mass in the right hemithorax which displaces the mediastinum to the left. There are several focal lucencies projecting on the right mid chest, consistent with air in bowel loops. The umbilical venous catheter demonstrates leftward bowing of the umbilical segment of the portal vein. The ultrasound confirms the presence of bowel loops in the right mid chest and intrathoracic herniation of the liver. Right sided CDHs are much rarer than left sided CDHs and often present later in life because the liver initially covers the defect. Large CDH such as the case shown here have a poor prognosis due to associated pulmonary hypoplasia, pulmonary hypertension, and cardiac dysfunction.

Musculoskeletal, Spine, CNS

1) Brain and skull

Patient 40: Three-year-old female, palpable lump of the head
Author: Heike E. Daldrup-Link, M.D.

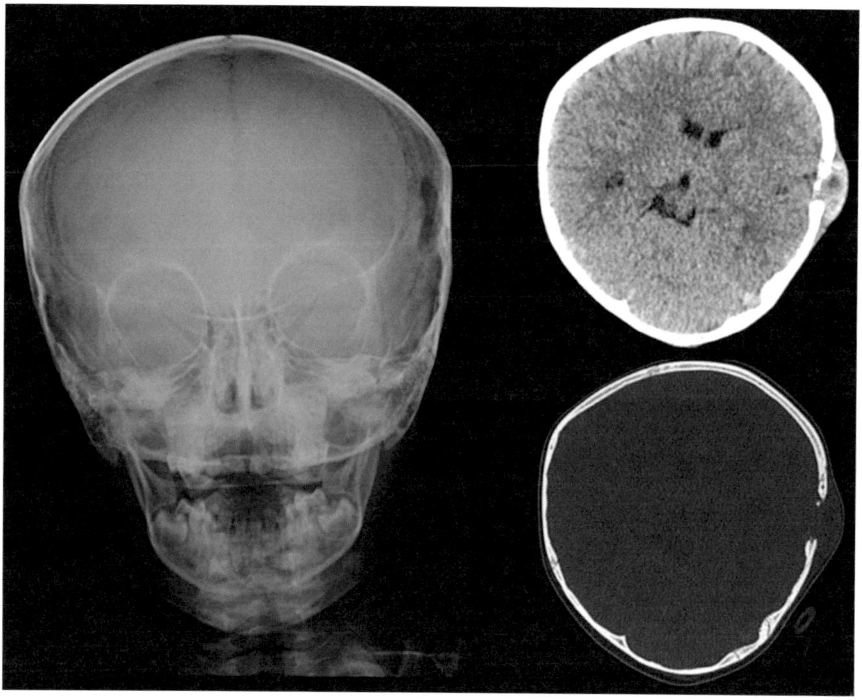

What is the most likely diagnosis:

a) Langerhans Cell Histiocytosis
b) Fibrous dysplasia
c) Epidermoid cyst
d) Cleidocranial dysostosis

Case 40: Langerhans Cell Histiocytosis

a) Langerhans cell histiocytosis: Correct! The radiograph demonstrates a classical "punched out" lytic lesion of the left calvarium with scalloped edges. The CT confirms an osteolytic lesion with characteristic "beveled edge" due to asymmetric involvement of the inner and outer table of the bone. The soft tissue window shows that there is an underlying solid mass lesion, not a cyst.

b) Fibrous dysplasia of the skull demonstrates a typical "ground glass" opacity, which this lesion does not show. The soft tissue component of the lesion shown here would be unusual.

c) Epidermoid cysts are well-demarcated intradiploic osteolytic lesions with homogenous, fluid-equivalent contents. Rarely, the lesions might have homogenously increased attenuation on CT. The thinned inner and outer table of the bone can often be delineated.

d) Cleidocranial dysostosis is associated with an incomplete intra-membranous ossification of midline bones. In the skull, this leads to Wormian bones, islands of bone in the sagittal and lambdoid sutures. The lesion shown here does not have bone attenuation and is not located in a suture.

Patient 41: 6-month-old male, palpable lump of the head

Author: Heike E. Daldrup-Link, M.D.

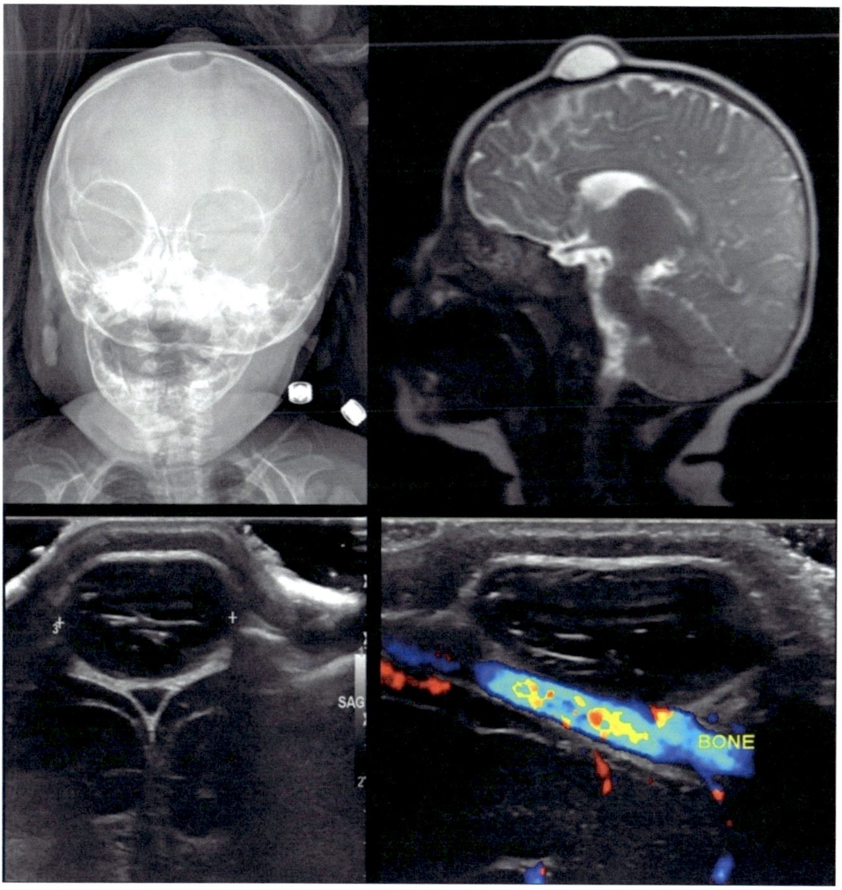

What is the most likely diagnosis:

a) Langerhans Cell Histiocytosis
b) Fibrous dysplasia
c) Epidermoid cyst
d) Cephalhematoma

Case 41: Epidermoid Cyst

a) Langerhans cell histiocytosis can present with a "punched out" lytic lesion of the calvarium However, it is usually associated with a soft tissue mass, which would demonstrate intermediate signal on T2-weighted MRI and internal vascularity on doppler ultrasound.

b) Fibrous dysplasia of the skull demonstrates a typical "ground glass" opacity, which this lesion does not show. The soft tissue component of the lesion shown here would be unusual.

c) Epidermoid cyst: Correct! The frontal radiograph demonstrates are well-demarcated osteolytic lesion of the frontal bone. The sagittal MRI shows that the lesion contains homogenous, fluid-equivalent contents. The doppler ultrasound demonstrates lack of internal vascularity. Diffusion weighted MRI would classically show restricted diffusion of the lesion.

d) A cephalhematoma would not be associated with a lytic lesion of the bone, as noted here.

Patient 42: One day old premature infant, born at 32 weeks gestation, severe metabolic acidosis

Authors: Marcello Chang, Jayne Seekins, D.O.

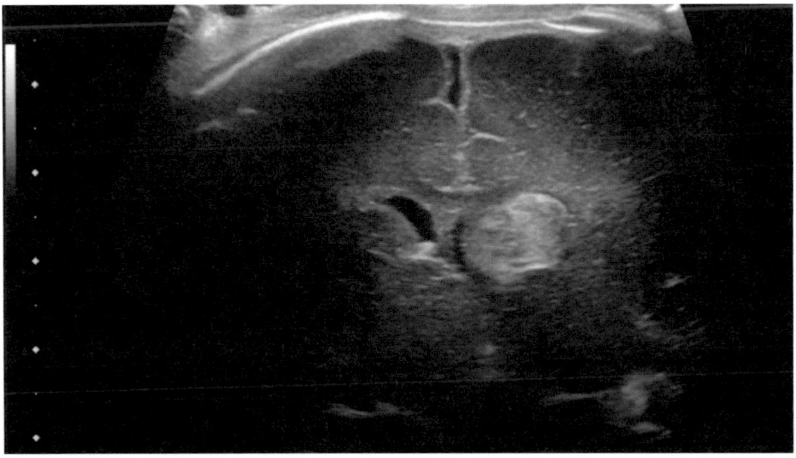

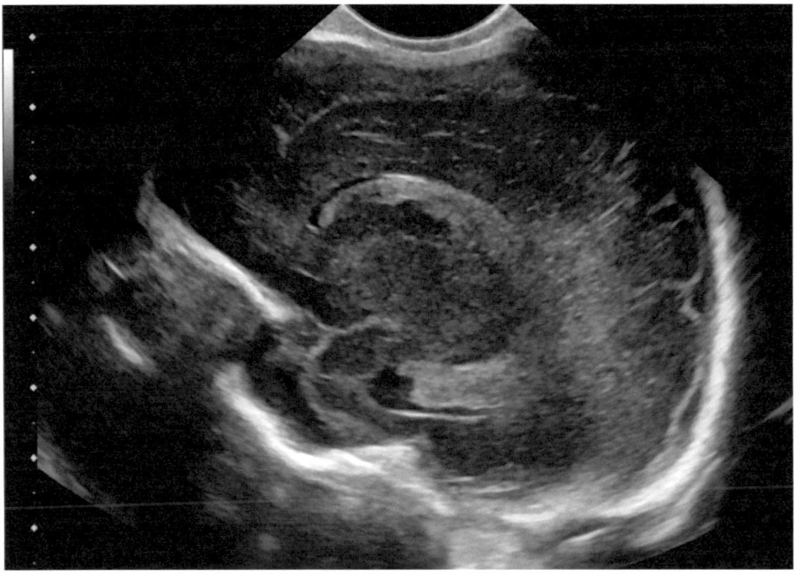

What is the most likely diagnosis:

a) Grade I hemorrhage
b) Grade III hemorrhage
c) Periventricular leukomalacia
d) Hypoxic-ischemic brain injury

Case 42: Grade III Germinal Matrix Hemorrhage

a) A grade I hemorrhage is confined to the caudothalamic groove and does not extend into the ventricular system or lead to a dilation of the lateral ventricles.

b) Grade III germinal matrix hemorrhage: Correct! The coronal and sagittal ultrasound exam of the brain shows an echogenic lesion in the caudothalamic groove which extends into the left lateral ventricle, consistent with an acute intraventricular hemorrhage. This hemorrhage has led to dilation of the left lateral ventricle. There is no extension of the hemorrhage into brain tissue. These features classify this hemorrhage as a grade III hemorrhage.
The germinal matrix is a highly vascular site of neuronal differentiation in the fetal brain. The vascularity reduces slowly and ultimately disappears at around 35 weeks gestation. Since these vessels are highly predisposed to bleeding, the risk of germinal matrix hemorrhage is strongly related to prematurity. Note that the choroid plexus is also echogenic on greyscale ultrasound. However, color doppler ultrasound demonstrates an increased vascularity of the choroid plexus, while a blood clot in the ventricle does not.

c) Periventricular leukomalacia presents with anechoic foci in the periventricular white matter, typically anterior and lateral to the frontal horns. It would not present with hyperechogenic lesions within the ventricles or ventriculomegaly.

d) Hypoxic-ischemic brain injury (HIE) can present with small ventricles, effaced sulci, heterogeneous periventricular white matter and/or increased resistive index of the middle cerebral artery.

Patient 43: 7-year-old male with short stature

Author: Heike E. Daldrup-Link, M.D.

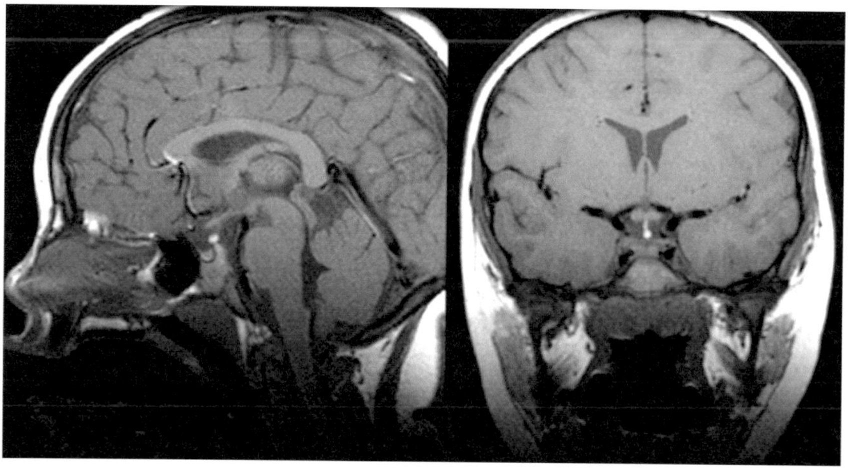

What is the most likely diagnosis:

a) Normal
b) Ectopic posterior pituitary
c) Rathke's cleft cyst
d) Thrombosed aneurysm

Case 43: Ectopic posterior pituitary

a) The MRI scans shown are not normal. There is a T1-hyperintense soft tissue nodule at the floor of the third ventricle.

b) Ectopic posterior pituitary: Correct! The sagittal and coronal T1-weighted MRI scans show a hyperintense soft tissue nodule caudal and posterior to the pituitary stalk, above the pituitary fossa. The usual T1-hyperintense signal of the posterior pituitary is missing.

c) Rathke's cleft cyst is a sellar or suprasellar cyst, which is usually larger than the lesion here. It can be T1-hyperintense or T1-hypointense. The majority of cases show a typical small non-enhancing T1-hyperintense and T2-hypointense intracystic nodule.

d) Thrombosed aneurysm: The lesion shown here is not associated with a vessel. An aneurysm would not be associated with the described clinical presentation of short stature.

Patient 44: A preterm male, gestational age 32 weeks, chronological age 4 weeks.

Author: Wipawee Morakote, M.D.

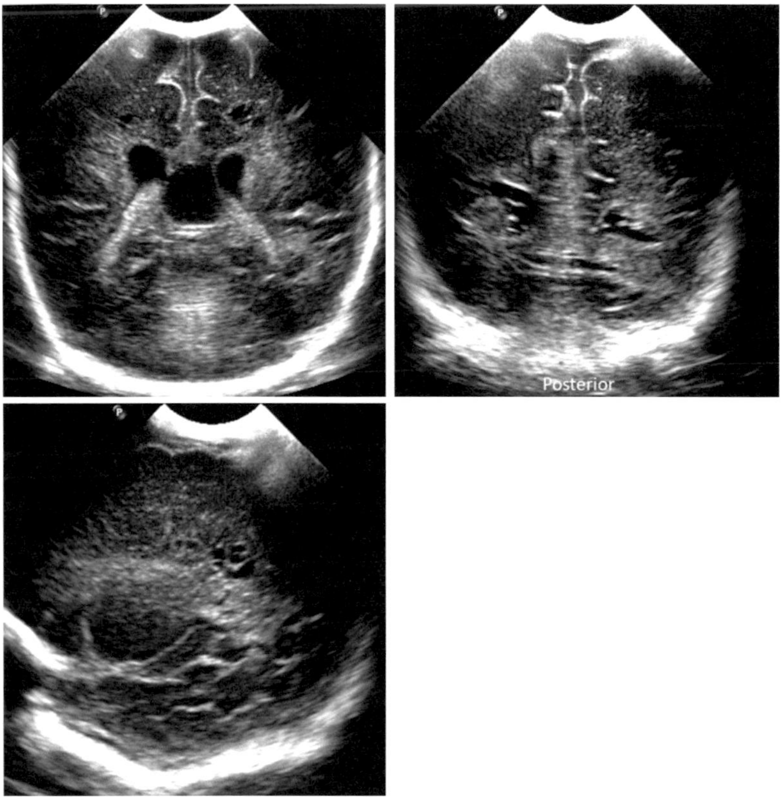

What is the most likely diagnosis:

a) Periventricular leukomalacia
b) Subependymal cyst
c) Intraventricular hemorrhage
d) Connatal cyst

Case 44: Periventricular leukomalacia

a) Correct! Periventricular leukomalacia (PVL) is result of hypoxic-ischemic brain injury. Ischemic injury in premature infant usually involves the bilateral periventricular white matter. Early findings of PVL include an increased echogenicity of the white matter greater than that of the choroid plexus. Cystic changes develop later and are the hallmark of PVL. The ultrasound of the brain here shows multiple small cystic lesions in the periventricular white matter of the bilateral parieto-occipital lobes.

b) A subependymal cyst may be congenital or develop after germinal matrix hemorrhage. It should be located below the external angle of the lateral ventricles.

c) No intraventricular hemorrhage is demonstrated on the ultrasound images here. The most common site of the hemorrhage in the premature infant is the caudothalamic groove where the germinal matrix is located.

d) Connatal cyst, or coarctation of lateral ventricle, is considered a normal variation. It is located at the superolateral margins of the body and frontal horns of the lateral ventricles.

Patient 45: 3-year-old female with hydrocephalus
Author: Heike E. Daldrup-Link, M.D.

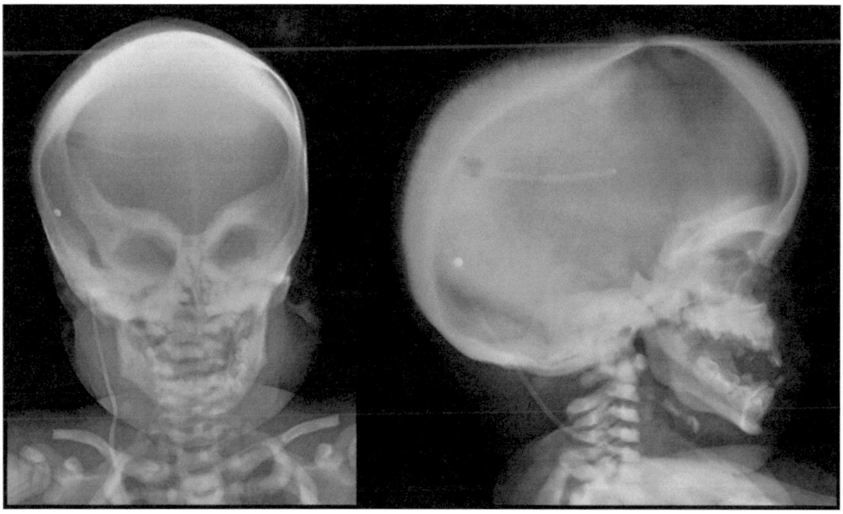

What is the most likely diagnosis:

a) Osteopetrosis
b) Fibrous dysplasia
c) Hypervitaminosis D
d) Lead poisoning

Case 45: Osteopetrosis

a) Osteopetrosis: Correct! The radiograph demonstrates a classical markedly sclerosed and thickened skull base, facial bones, and cranial vault with "hair-on-end" appearance. Osteopetrosis is a sclerosing bone dysplasia where osteoclasts are dysfunctional which leads to unopposed function of osteoblasts. Sclerosis of the orbits and sphenoid wings leads to a "harlequin mask" effect. The "hair-on-end" sign describes long, thin vertical striations in the calvarium that resemble hairs standing on end. The thickened bone decreases the space for hematopoietic bone marrow which expands along the diploic space. The alternating opaque, thickened trabeculae and radiolucent marrow spaces produce the hair-on-end appearance. Note that the "hair-on-end sign" can be also seen in several other conditions, including thalassemia.

b) Fibrous dysplasia of the skull demonstrates a typical "ground glass" opacity, which this lesion does not show. Fibrous dysplasia of the skull can progress to a sclerosed state but does not show the "hair on end" pattern shown here.

c) Hypervitaminosis D can lead to increased sclerosis of bones. However, it is usually not associated with bone expansion. Hypervitaminosis D is often associated with extra-osseous calcifications, such as calcifications along the falx, which are not noted here. Hypervitaminosis D typically requires excessive doses of Vitamin D over a prolonged time.

d) Lead is an osteoclast poison and antagonist of heme formation. Radiographs can demonstrate increased density of bones, which is most typically noted at the metaphyses of long bones. The marked expansion of the calvarium and "hair on end" pattern shown here suggest a different diagnosis.

Musculoskeletal, Spine, CNS

2) Spine

Patient 46: 9-year-old male, history of cerebral palsy
Author: Heike E. Daldrup-Link

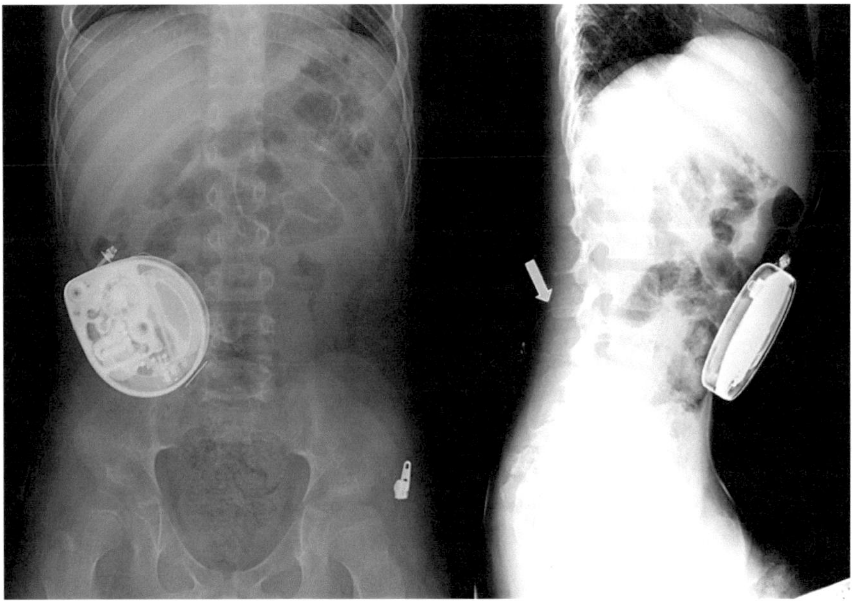

The device in the right lower abdominal quadrant is a:

a) Cardiac pacemaker
b) Vagal nerve stimulator
c) Insulin pump
d) Baclofen pump

Case 46: Baclofen pump

a) A cardiac pacemaker is usually smaller in size and is most commonly implanted in the subcutaneous soft tissues of the chest wall (although it can be also placed in the subcutaneous sift tissues of the upper abdomen). A location in the lower abdomen would be very unusual. A cardiac pacemaker has one or two leads which lead to the right atrium and right ventricle.

b) A vagal nerve stimulator is most commonly implanted in the subcutaneous soft tissues of the left upper chest wall. The leads can be followed to the location of the vagus nerve in the left lower neck. The device sends regular, mild pulses of electrical energy through the vagus nerve to the brainstem for the treatment of epilepsy and severe mood disorders, such as depression and anxiety.

c) An insulin pump is a small battery-operated device, often rectangular in shape, that is adhered to the skin surface of the abdomen. The device provides subcutaneous insulin delivery via a narrow plastic tube that is inserted just under the skin.

d) Baclofen pump: Correct! The frontal and lateral radiograph of the abdomen demonstrates a radiopaque device in the right lower abdomen with a catheter that extends to the posterior soft tissues and from there into the spinal canal. The pump delivers baclofen, a muscle relaxer and antispasmodic agent, into the spinal fluid. It is used in patients with cerebral palsy to reduce muscle spasms.

Patient 47: 6-month-old male infant

Author: Heike E. Daldrup-Link, M.D.

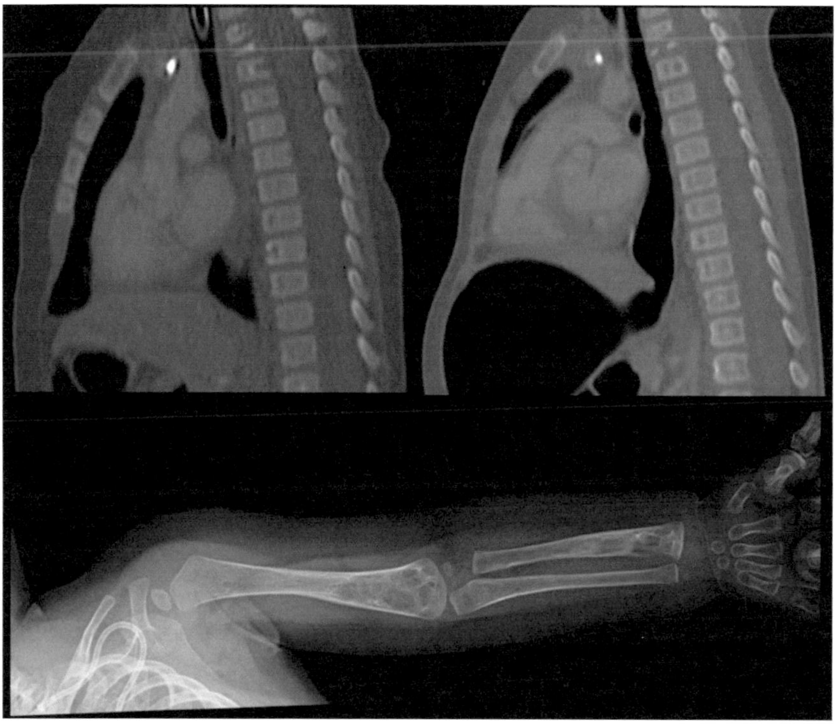

What is the most likely diagnosis:

a) Langerhans Cell Histiocytosis
b) Tuberculous Spondylitis
c) Morquio disease
d) Nonaccidental trauma

Case 47: Langerhans Cell Histiocytosis

a) Langerhans Cell Histiocytosis (LCH): Correct! The sagittal CT scan demonstrates a vertebra plana, a complete collapse of the T3 vertebral body. LCH is the most common cause for vertebra plana in children. In addition, the radiograph of the left arm shows focal osteolytic lesions of the distal humerus and distal radius, in keeping wit multifocal disease. The lesions demonstrate a permeative growth pattern and no sclerotic rim.

b) Tuberculous Spondylitis can lead to a vertebra plana. However, in the typical case, multiple subsequent vertebral bodies are involved, often accompanied by an abscess in front of the infected vertebral bodies. In this case here, the prevertebral soft tissues are not thickened.

c) Morquio disease represents one of the mucopolysaccharidoses (type IV) and can be associated with multiple flattened vertebrae (platyspondyly) and/or anterior vertebral beaking, which is not noted here. Long bones in patients with Morquio disease are short and wide, with metaphyseal flaring. Focal osteolytic lesions would be unusual.

d) Non-accidental trauma can lead to compression fracture(s) of one or more vertebral bodies. However, the lesions noted in the humerus and radius suggest a different diagnosis.

Patient 48: A newborn with a visible mass below the pelvis.
Authors: Wipawee Morakote, M.D., Pannee Visrutaratna, M.D.

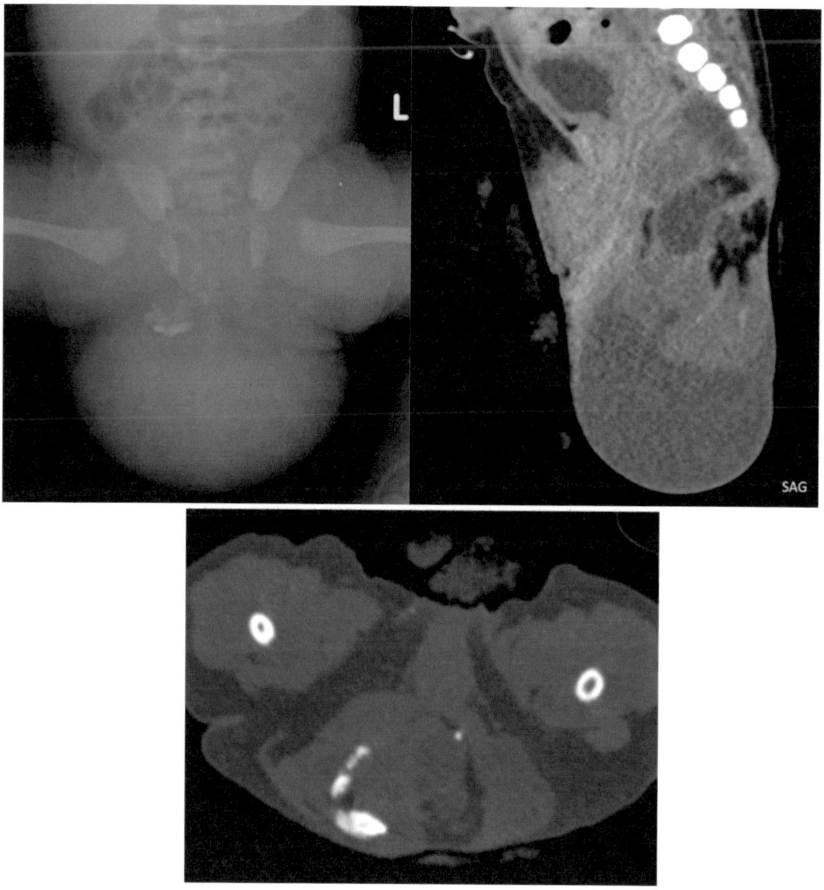

What is the most likely diagnosis:

a) Myelomeningocele
b) Lipoma
c) Sacrococcygeal Teratoma
d) Rhabdomyosarcoma of the urinary bladder

Case 48: Sacrococcygeal Teratoma

a) Myelomeningocele: There is no spinal dysraphism and the mass does not extend from the dural sac.

b) A lipoma should be primarily composed of fatty components.

c) Sacrococcygeal Teratoma: Correct! The radiograph demonstrates widening of the pubic symphysis, a mass below the level of the pelvis and intra-lesional calcifications. The coronal and axial CT scan demonstrates an inhomogeneous mass, which arises from the presacral area and is composed of cystic components, fat, and mature calcifications.

d) Rhabdomyosarcoma of the urinary bladder: The mass shown here does not arise from the urinary bladder. A rhabdomyosarcoma typically presents as an inhomogeneous soft tissue. While areas of cysts and necrosis can be seen within a rhabdomyosarcoma, calcifications would be uncommon.

Patient 49: 4-week-old male infant with a tilted head

Author: Heike E. Daldrup-Link, M.D., Shelby Payne, M.D.

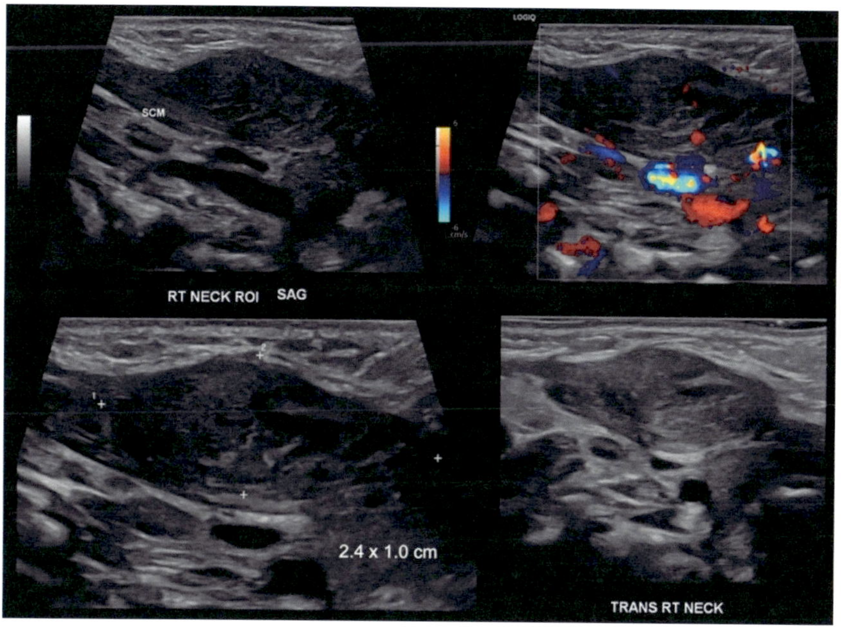

What is the most likely diagnosis:

a) Rhabdomyosarcoma
b) Acquired Torticollis
c) Fibromatosis Colli
d) Ectopic Thymus

Case 49: Fibromatosis Colli

a) Rhabdomyosarcoma: There is no discrete mass noted on the ultrasound images shown here.

b) Torticollis describes a congenital or acquired deformity characterized by rotational deformity of the cervical spine with secondary tilting of the head. Acquired torticollis occurs in older children (beyond infancy) due to trauma, inflammatory disorders (e.g., juvenile rheumatoid arthritis), infection (e.g., meningitis, otitis, spondylitis, diskitis etc.) or neoplasms.

c) Fibromatosis Colli: Correct! In infants, fibromatosis colli represents the most common form of congenital muscular torticollis. Some cases have been linked to birth trauma while other cases were idiopathic. The ultrasound of the neck shown here demonstrates an asymmetrically enlarged sternocleido-mastoid muscle with typical fusiform shape on the sagittal view. The enlarged muscle fibers can be followed into unaffected muscle fibers at the upper and lower end of the lesion. The contralateral muscle is normal. There is little or no vascularity on doppler ultrasound. Small, localized, internal hyper- or hypoechoic foci can be due to internal hemorrhage and/or calcification. The face of the patient is typically turned away from the affected side. The condition is self-limited and usually resolves spontaneously over time.

d) An ectopic thymus can be located in the lower neck, with or without connection to thymus tissue in the mediastinum. It demonstrates a characteristic echotexture on ultrasound images with homogenously low echogenicity and multiple hyperechoic foci, leading to a "starry sky" appearance. The condition is also self-limited as the thymus involutes spontaneously over time.

Patient 50: 10-year-old male patient

Author: Heike E. Daldrup-Link, M.D.

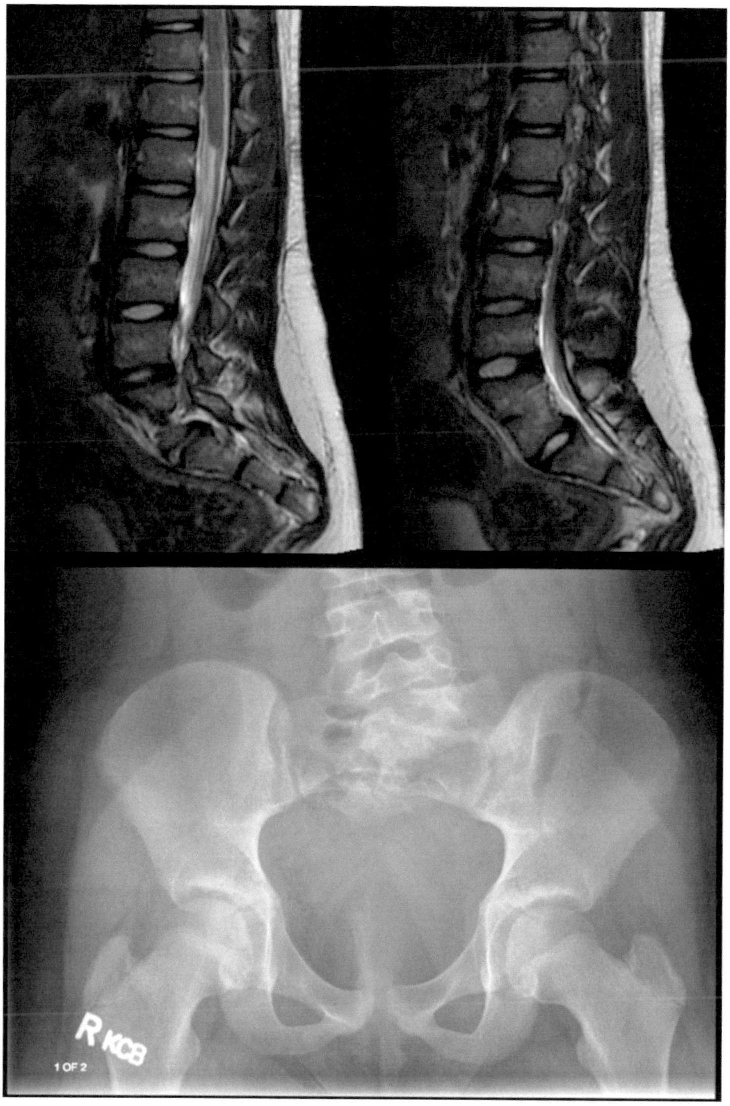

What is the most likely diagnosis:

a) Myelomeningocele
b) Caudal Regression Syndrome
c) Sacrococcygeal Teratoma
d) Sirenomelia

Case 50: Caudal Regression Syndrome

a) A myelomeningocele can be associated with caudal regression syndrome. But it is not noted here.

b) Caudal Regression Syndrome: Correct! The radiograph of the pelvis demonstrates segmentation anomalies of the lower lumbar spine and a hypoplastic sacrum. The sagittal T2-weighted MRI demonstrates partial fusion of the L5 and S1 vertebral body and absent S5 vertebral body and coccyx. The blunted conus medullaris terminated at the L1 level. Findings are consistent with a caudal regression syndrome. There are multiple associated abnormalities, such as renal agenesis, anal atresia, sacral teratoma, meningocele and tethered spinal cord, among others. The conus medullaris can be blunt and terminate above the normal level as shown here. Other patients show an elongated conus below the normal level, tethered by a thickened filum terminale or intraspinal lipoma.

c) A sacrococcygeal teratoma can be associated with caudal regression syndrome. But it is not noted here.

d) Sirenomelia is a rare congenital fetal anomaly with characteristic complete or partial fusion of the lower limbs. Sirenomelia is associated with sacral agenesis. However, in this case here, the bilateral lower limbs appear to be normal.

Patient 51: Female newborn, visible mass over the sacrum.
Author: Heike E. Daldrup-Link, M.D.

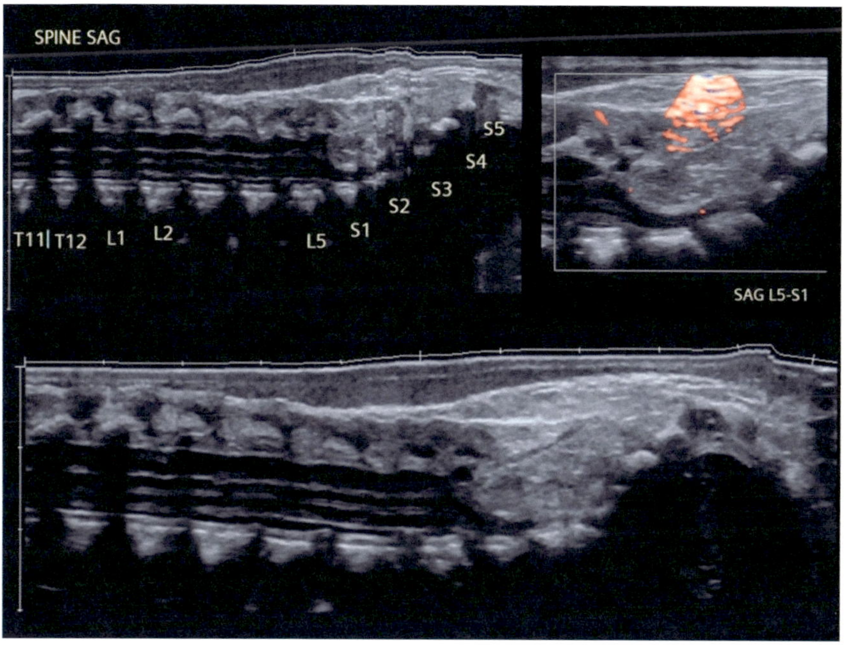

What is the most likely diagnosis:

a) Normal ultrasound of the infant spine
b) Tethered Spinal Cord with Lipomyelocele
c) Sacrococcygeal Teratoma
d) Rhabdomyosarcoma

Case 51: Tethered Spinal Cord with Lipomyelocele

a) Normal scan: The ultrasound shown is not normal.

b) Tethered spinal cord with lipomyelocele: Correct! The sagittal ultrasound demonstrates a low-lying conus medullaris at the level of L5/S1 (normal: at or above L2 vertebral body). The spinal cord extends into a soft tissue mass, which contains fatty and vascularized elements. The MRI from the same day (see below) shows that this is a fibrofatty mass which is attached to the spinal cord and extends through a spina bifida into the subcutaneous soft tissue, consistent with a lipomyelocele.

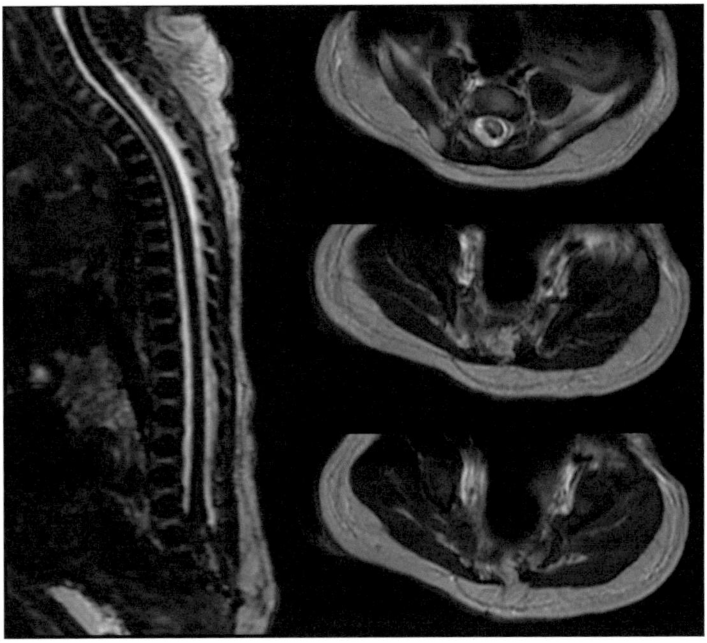

c) A sacrococcygeal teratoma presents as an inhomogeneous soft tissue mass, which is composed of cystic components, fat, and mature calcifications. The lesion can have intraspinal extensions. But the center of the lesion is not usually located in the spinal canal.

d) Pelvic rhabdomyosarcomas in infants most commonly arise from of the urinary bladder, vagina, or prostate gland.

Patient 52: 6-month-old male, fell down the stairs at home

Author: Heike E. Daldrup-Link, M.D.

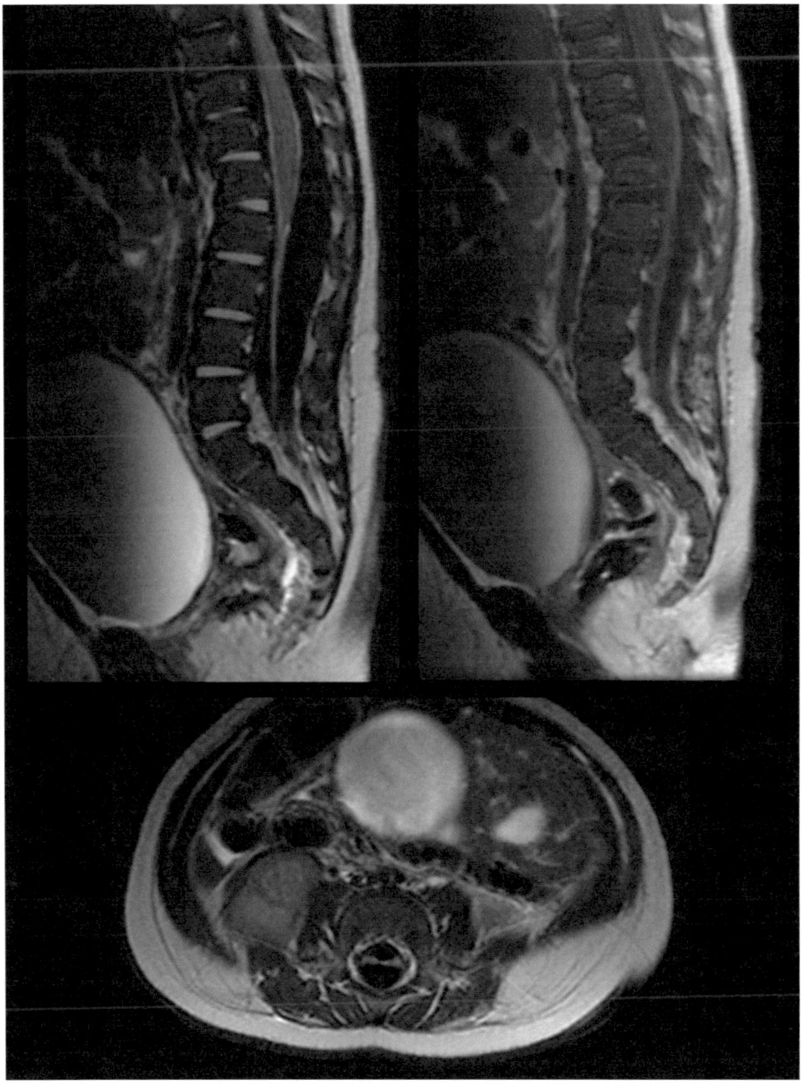

What is the most likely diagnosis:

a) Myelomeningocele
b) Normal MRI of the Spine
c) Sacrococcygeal Teratoma
d) Subdural Hematoma

Case 52: Spinal Subdural Hematoma

a) A myelomeningocele would present with splaying of posterior vertebral elements (spinal dysraphism) and herniation of spinal canal contents.

b) The MRI scans shown here are not normal.

c) A sacrococcygeal teratoma presents as an inhomogeneous soft tissue mass, which is composed of cystic components, fat, and mature calcifications. There is no focal mass noted here.

d) Spinal subdural hematoma: Correct! The sagittal T2-weighted MRI (left) demonstrates abnormally low signal of the entire subdural space, suggesting an extensive subdural hemorrhage which extends caudally to the thecal sac. The sagittal T1-weighted contrast-enhanced MRI (right) demonstrates prominent dural enhancement. The axial T2-weighted MRI shows thecal sac effacement by the hematoma. There is no cord signal abnormality. The patient developed this extensive hematoma due to nonaccidental trauma.

Musculoskeletal, Spine, CNS

3) Musculoskeletal

Patient 53: 8-year-old male with leg pain
Author: Heike E. Daldrup-Link, M.D.

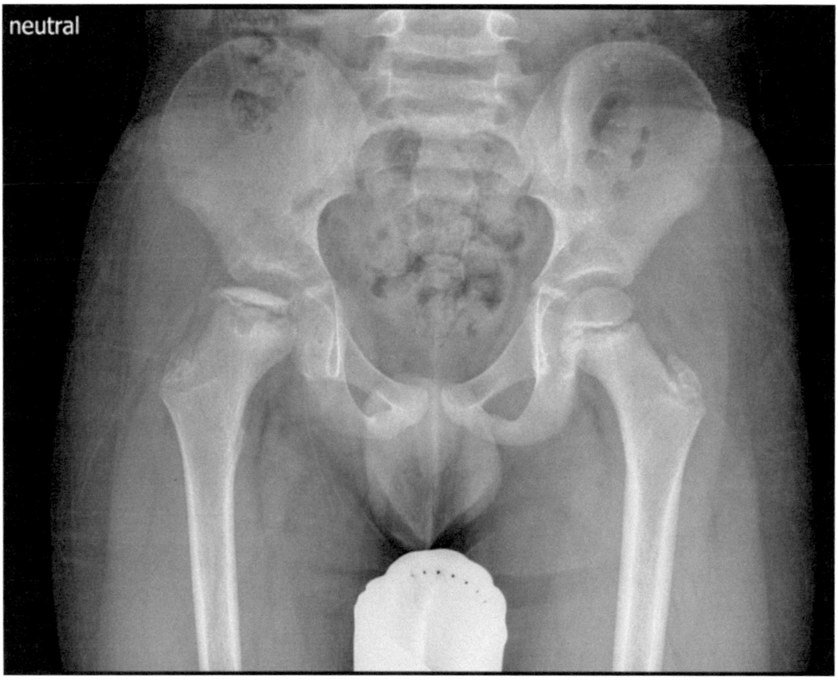

What is the most likely diagnosis:

a) Legg-Calvé Perthes disease
b) Slipped capital femoral epiphysis
c) Osteomyelitis
d) Meyer dysplasia

Case 53: Legg-Calvé Perthes disease

a) Legg-Calvé Perthes disease: Correct! The radiograph demonstrates widening, flattening and sclerosis of the right femoral epiphysis, consistent with an idiopathic osteonecrosis of the right femoral head. There is an associated large metaphyseal defect, which is continuous with the epiphyseal plate.

b) Slipped capital femoral epiphysis: The femoral epiphysis is not posteromedially displaced.

c) Osteomyelitis: There is no periosteal reaction. Fat planes around the hip joint are preserved.

d) Meyer dysplasia refers to a developmental variation which leads to fragmentation and delayed ossification of the femoral capital epiphyses. However, this condition is usually not associated with epiphyseal condensation or collapse.

Patient 54: 5-year-old male with foot pain

Author: Heike E. Daldrup-Link, M.D.

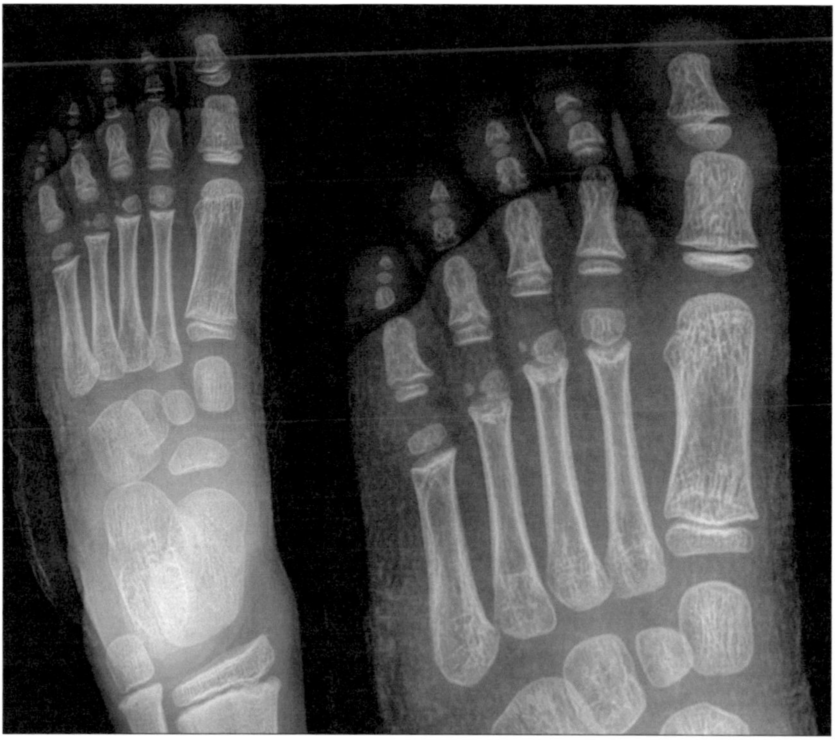

What is the most likely diagnosis:

a) Fracture of the 3rd and 4th metatarsal bone
b) Missing ossification center of the first metatarsal
c) Missing middle phalanx of the first toe
d) Duplicated ossification centers of the 3rd and 4th metatarsal

Case 54: Duplicated Ossification Centers

a) Fracture of the 3rd and 4th metatarsal bone: There is no fracture noted on these foot radiographs

b) Missing ossification center of the first metatarsal: There is no missing ossification center. All metatarsal bones are ossified from two ossification centers, which includes an ossification center for the shaft and the proximal end of the first metatarsal as well as an ossification center for the shaft and the head of each of the other four metatarsals. An epiphysis is frequently present on the tubercle of the base of the fifth metatarsal bone.

c) Missing middle phalanx of the first toe. The first toe has a proximal and end phalanx. The first toe does not have a middle phalanx. All other toes (2-5) have a proximal, middle and end phalanx.

d) Duplicated ossification centers of the 3rd and 4th metatarsal: Correct! The radiographs of the foot show duplicated ossification centers of the 3rd and 4th metatarsal bone, a normal variant.

Patient 55: 11-year-old female with wrist pain

Author: Heike E. Daldrup-Link, M.D.

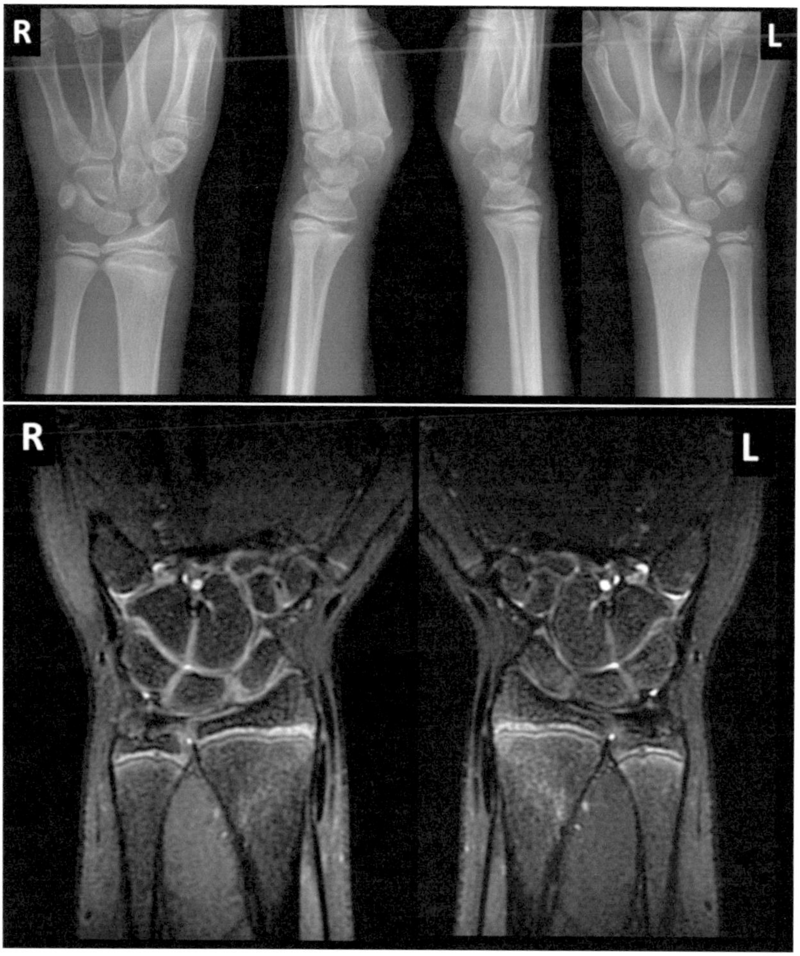

What is the most likely diagnosis:

a) Salter 2 fracture
b) Salter 3 fracture
c) Avascular necrosis
d) Gymnast Wrist

Case 55: Gymnast Wrist

a) A Salter 2 fracture extends through the metaphysis and epiphyseal plate of the affected bone. The findings shown here are consistent with a Salter 1 fracture.

b) A Salter 3 fracture extends through the metaphysis, epiphyseal plate, and epiphysis of the affected bone. The findings shown here are consistent with a Salter 1 fracture.

c) Avascular necrosis: There is evidence of avascular necrosis of the depicted bones.

d) Gymnast Wrist: Correct! The radiographs of the bilateral hands demonstrate widened epiphyseal plates of the distal radius bilaterally, consistent with Salter 1 fractures. The T2-weighted MRI shows widened epiphyseal plates of the distal radius and marrow edema at the metaphyseal side of the physis. The condition is due to repetitive compression injuries of the wrist in patients with immature bones. Complications include physeal bridging and growth arrest.

Patient 56: 12-year-old-male with left hip pain

Author: Marcello Chang, Michael F. Fadell, M.D.

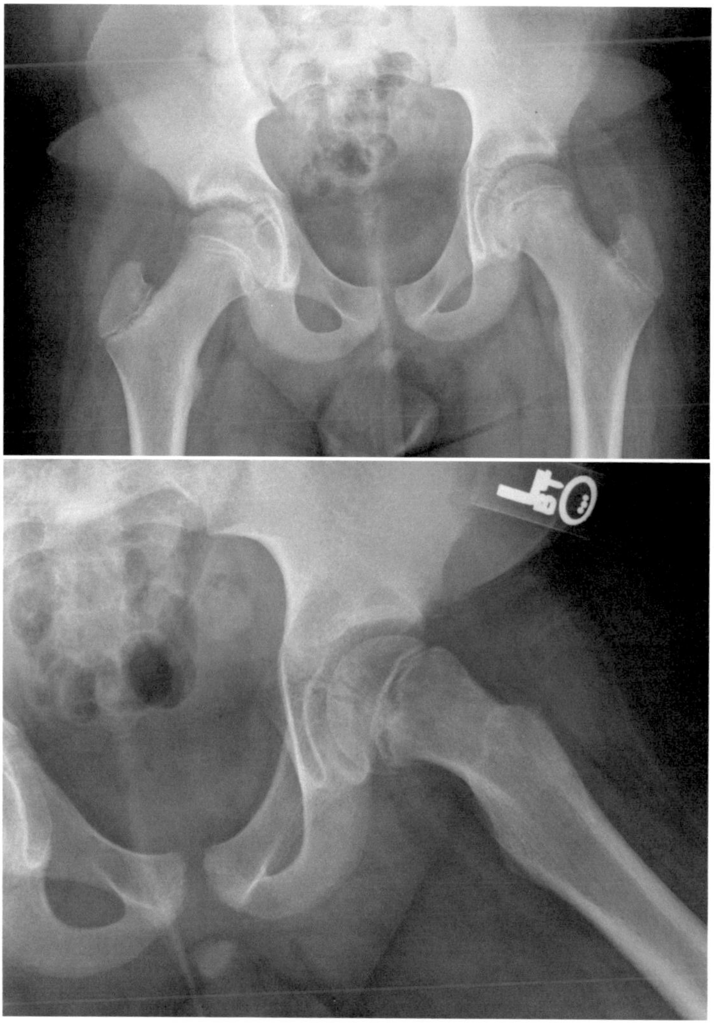

What is the most likely diagnosis:

a) Transient synovitis of the hip
b) Legg-Calve-Perthes Disease
c) Slipped Capital Femoral Epiphysis (SCFE)
d) Developmental dysplasia of the hip

Case 56: Slipped Capital Femoral Epiphysis (SCFE)

b) A transient synovitis represents an acute inflammation of the synovial lining of the hip. Findings on radiographs are nonspecific, such as an increased medial joint space due to a joint effusion.

b) Legg-Calve-Perthes disease or idiopathic osteonecrosis of the femoral epiphysis presents with variable imaging findings which vary from early fragmentation to late destruction of the femoral epiphysis. While late signs could include a displacement or fracture of the epiphysis, there would be other signs such as sclerosis, loss of femoral head height and/or subchondral fractures.

c) Slipped Capital Femoral Epiphysis (SCFE): Correct! The radiograph shows a widening of the proximal epiphyseal plate on the frontal radiograph and slippage of the femoral on the frog-leg view. On the frontal view, a line drawn along the lateral edge of the femoral neck fails to intersect the epiphysis. The displacement of the proximal femoral epiphysis occurs in the posterior medial direction. Therefore, evaluation with a frog leg lateral view, as above, increases the conspicuity. When there is a high clinical suspicion for early SCFE not seen on radiographs, pre-slip SCFE can be diagnosed on MRI as subtle widening of the growth plate, with irregularity and blurring of the physeal edges. SCFE is corrected with pinning. Even with after surgery, SCFE can increase the risk of early osteoarthritis.

d) Developmental dysplasia of the hip presents with a shallow acetabulum and a steep acetabular roof. Additionally, it may involve lateral decentering of the hip and delayed femoral head ossification on the affected side.

Patient 57: Teenager, history withheld

Author: Heike E. Daldrup-Link, M.D.

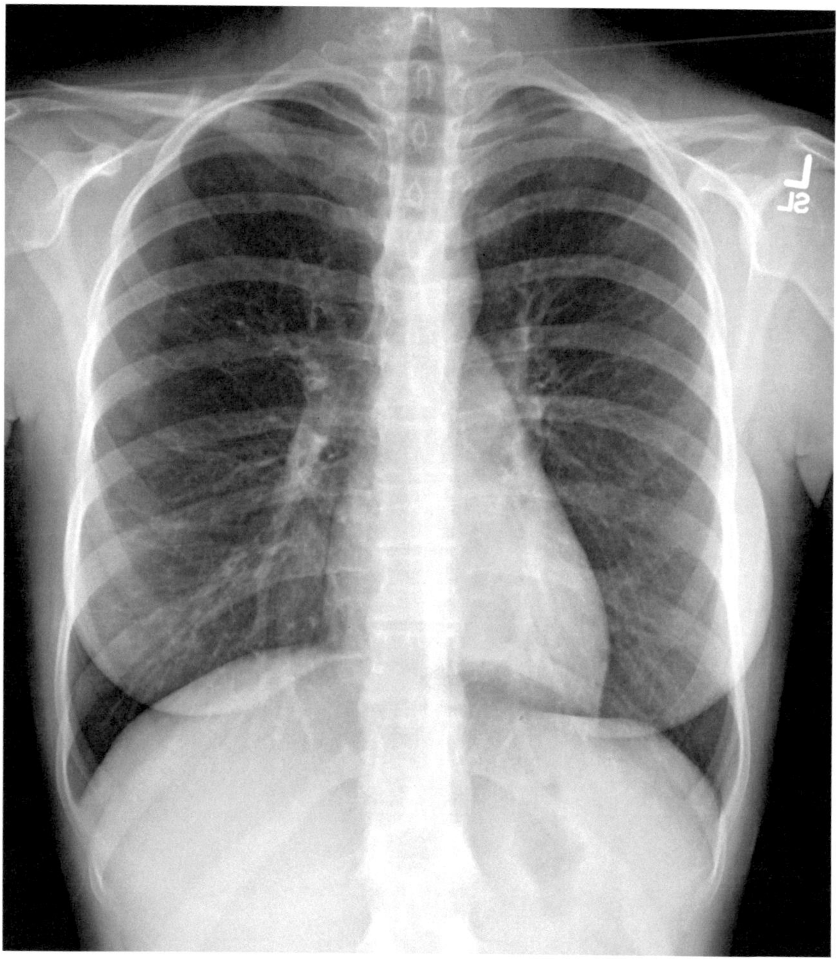

Where is the abnormality:

a) Lungs
b) Mediastinum
c) Soft Tissues
d) Bones

Case 57: Left Clavicular Fracture

a) The lungs are normal.

b) The mediastinum is normal.

c) The soft tissues are normal.

d) Bones: Correct! There is a fracture of the midshaft of the left clavicle with caudal displacement of the distal clavicle. A dedicated radiograph of the left clavicle demonstrates about 1 cm overlap of the proximal and distal clavicle. Shortening of more than 2 cm is often treated with internal fixation.

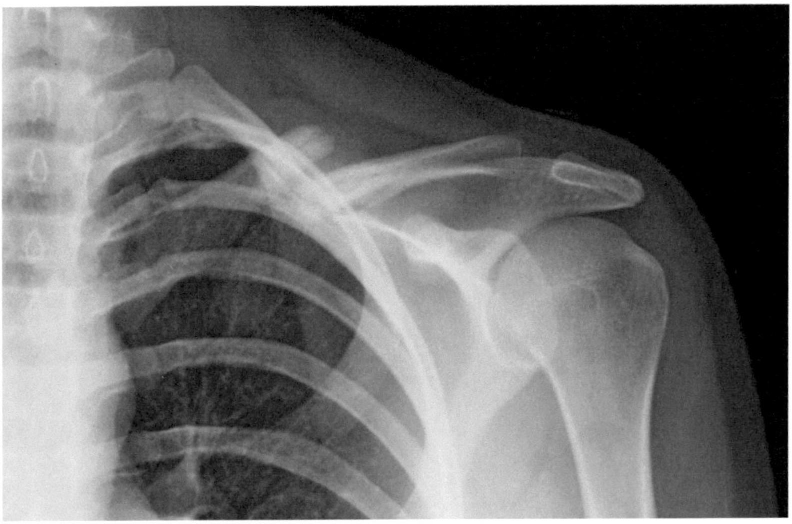

Patient 58: 5-year-old male with knee pain

Author: Heike E. Daldrup-Link, M.D.

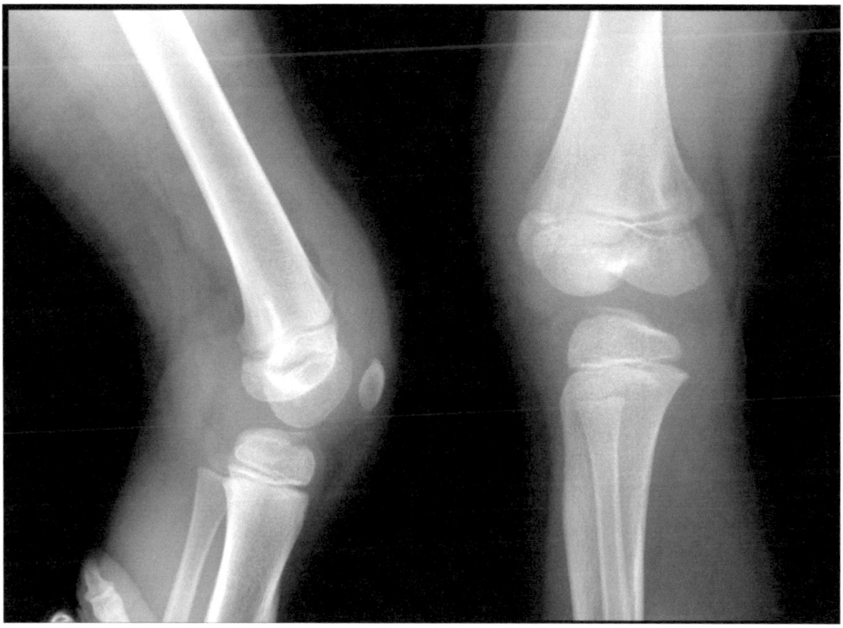

Where is the abnormality:

a) Distal femur
b) Patella
c) Proximal Tibia
d) Proximal Fibula

Case 58: Anterior tibial spine fracture

a) The distal femur does not show any fracture.

b) The patella is normal.

c) Proximal tibia: Correct! The radiograph demonstrates a fracture of the anterior tibial spine with a bone fragment in the joint space. The anterior cruciate ligament has been avulsed from its tibial insertion.

d) The proximal fibula does not show any fracture.

Patient 59: 16-year-old female with knee pain

Author: Heike E. Daldrup-Link, M.D.

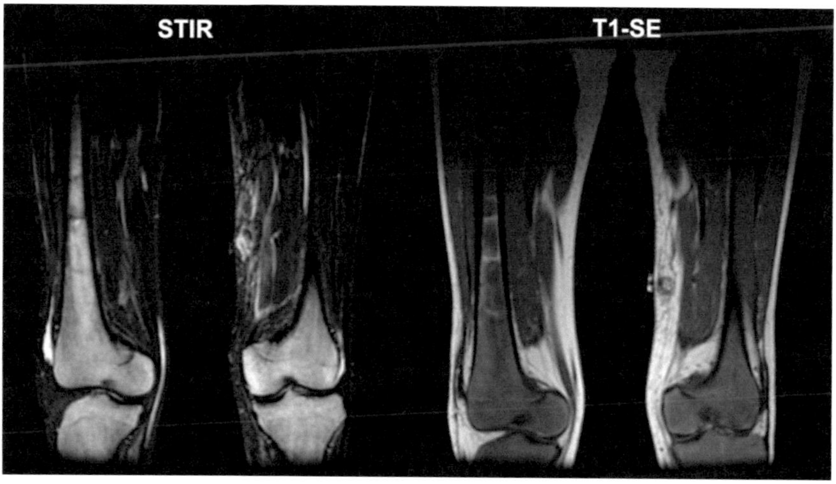

What is the most likely diagnosis:

a) Normal MRI scan of a teenager
b) Acute Lymphocytic Leukemia (ALL)
c) Langerhans Cell Histiocytosis (LCH)
d) Chronic Recurrent Multifocal Osteomyelitis (CRMO)

Case 59: Acute Lymphocytic Leukemia

a) The MRI scan shown here is not normal. At this age, the normal bone marrow should be hypointense on STIR images and hyperintense compared to muscle on plain T1-weighted MR images.

b) Acute Lymphocytic Leukemia (ALL): Correct! The coronal STIR image of the lower legs demonstrates diffusely hyperintense signal of the bone marrow of the bilateral femurs and proximal tibia. The coronal T1-weighted MRI scan demonstrates diffusely hypointense bone marrow signal of all depicted bones. The abnormal bone marrow signal involves the femoral diaphysis, metaphysis, and epiphysis. There is also a small, localized round T2-hyperintense and T1-hypointense soft tissue lesion in the subcutaneous soft tissues of the medial lower thigh (marked with a small marker on the skin, where the patient palpated a nodule), which is most consistent with a chloroma.

c) Langerhans cell histiocytosis would present with unifocal or multi-focal bone marrow lesions. A diffuse bone marrow infiltration would be unusual.

d) Chronic Recurrent Multifocal Osteomyelitis (CRMO) presents with patchy, focal T2-hyperintense and T1-hypointense bone marrow lesions, which are often centered around the metaphyses and epiphyses, rather than the epiphyses. A diffuse bone marrow infiltration would be unusual.

Patient 60: 14-year-old female with leg pain
Author: Heike E. Daldrup-Link, M.D.

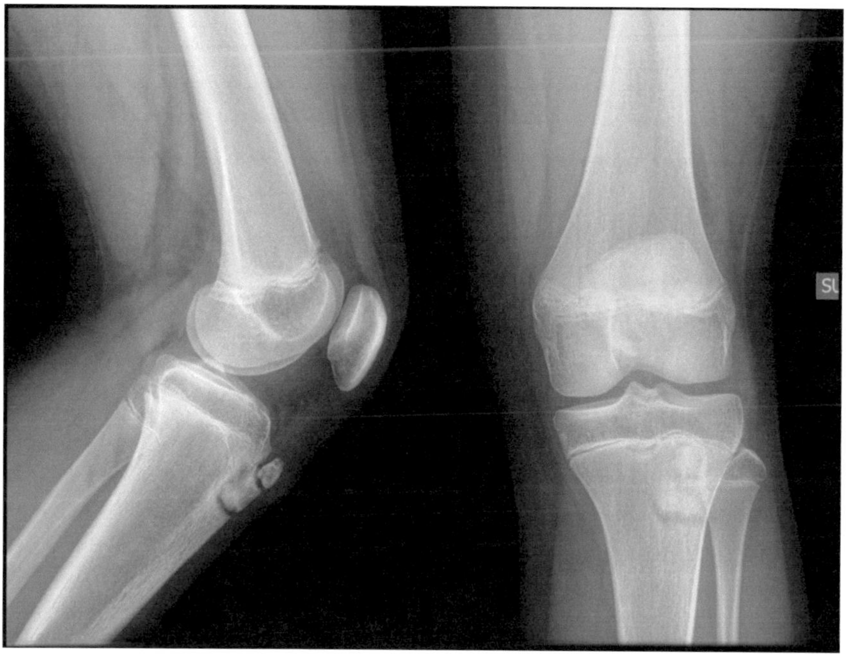

What is the most likely diagnosis:

a) Sinding-Larsen Disease
b) Salter 2 fracture of the proximal tibia
c) Osgood Schlatter Disease
d) Segond Fracture

Case 60: Osgood Schlatter Disease

a) Sinding-Larsen disease represents a chronic fatigue injury of the distal patella and proximal patella tendon.

b) A Salter 2 fracture involves the growth plate and metaphysis of the bone. The pathology shown here represents a chronic fatigue injury of the apophysis of the proximal tibia.

c) Osgood Schlatter: Correct! The radiograph demonstrates a fragmentation of the apophysis of the anterior proximal tibia with associated soft tissue swelling. There is also an edema of the patella tendon, which is thickened and lost its sharp margins.

d) A Segond fracture described an avulsion fracture of the lateral tibial plateau. Radiographs classically show a bone fragment parallel to the lateral aspect of the tibial plateau. It is often associated with a tear of the anterior cruciate ligament.

Patient 61: 8-year-old male with leg pain

Author: Heike E. Daldrup-Link, M.D.

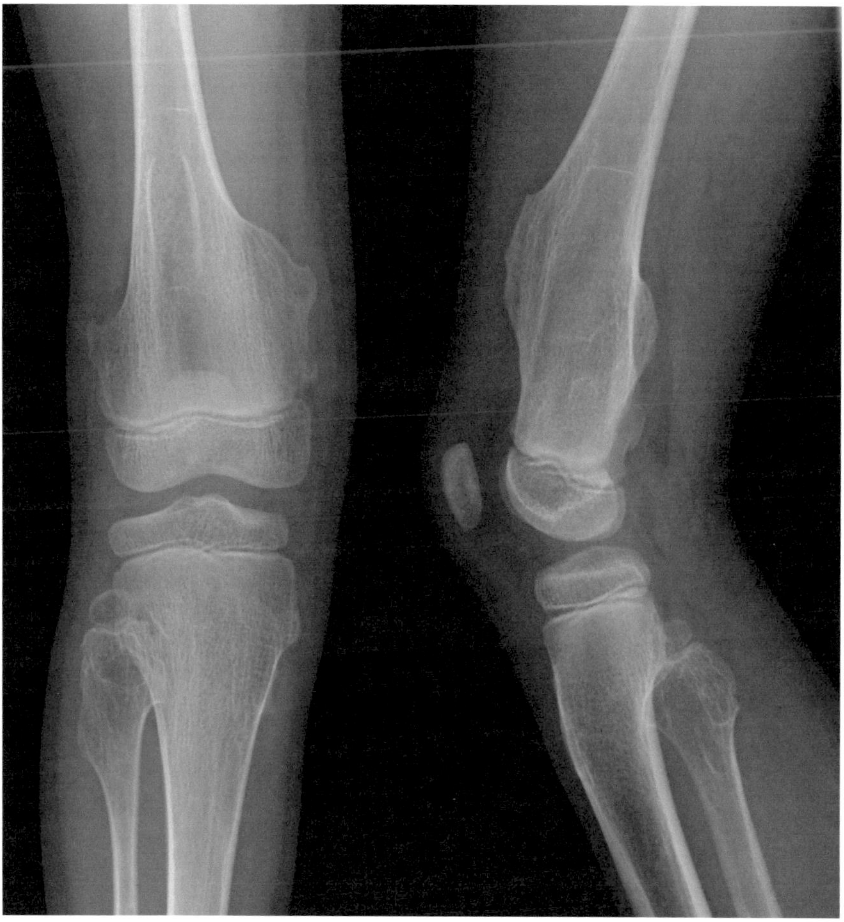

What is the most likely diagnosis:

a) Solitary osteochondroma
b) Multiple hereditary exostoses
c) Trevor disease
d) Ollier disease

Case 61: Multiple Hereditary Exostoses

a) Solitary osteochondroma refers to a single osteochondroma. There are multiple osteochondromas noted in this case.

b) Multiple hereditary exostoses: Correct! The radiograph demonstrates bilateral symmetric sessile and lobulated outgrowths of bone, which extend from the metaphysis outwards and are pointing away from the joint. The lesions are covered by a cartilage cap, which can have a thickness of 1 to 3 cm in children due to the ongoing growth process. Cap thickness exceeding 2 cm in an adult should raise suspicion for malignancy.

c) Trevor disease represents osteochondromas of the epiphyses, which grow towards the joint. It is due to asymmetric overgrowth of cartilage in the epiphyses.

d) Ollier disease refers to multiple enchondromas.

Patient 62: 10-year-old female, tennis injury

Author: Heike E. Daldrup-Link, M.D.

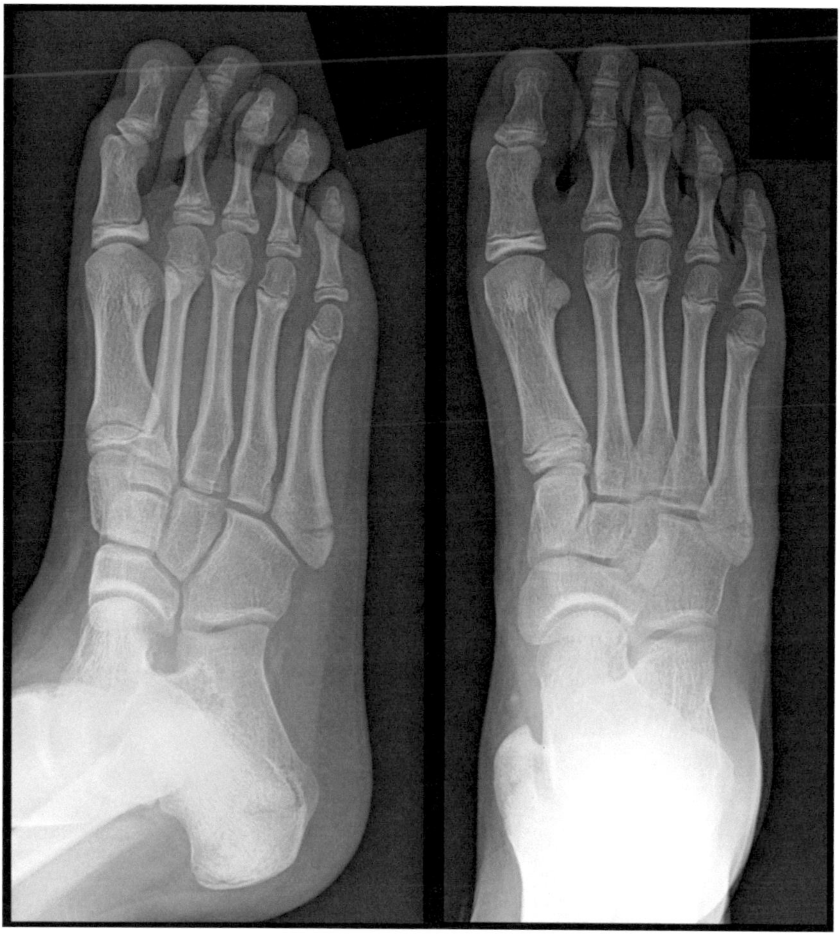

What is the most likely diagnosis:

a) Jones fracture
b) Avulsion fracture of the proximal 5th metatarsal bone
c) Normal apophysis of the 5th metatarsal bone
d) Iselin disease

Case 62: Avulsion fracture of the proximal 5th metatarsal bone

a) A Jones fracture is a fracture of the 5th metatarsal bone at the metadiaphyseal junction, approximately 1.5 to 3 cm distal to the proximal tuberosity. The fracture here is closer to the proximal end of the bone. These fractures are prone to non-union.

b) Avulsion fracture of the proximal 5th metatarsal bone: Correct! This is a transverse fracture of the proximal end of the 5th metatarsal bone, at the insertion site of the peroneus brevis muscle.

c) The normal apophysis of the 5th metatarsal bone is oriented longitudinally, parallel to the shaft of the bone.

d) Iselin disease refers to an obliquely oriented small bony lesion at the base of the 5th metatarsal bone, which is due to repetitive traction of the peroneus brevis tendon with resulting apophysitis.

Patient 63: 12-year-old male, basketball injury
Author: Heike E. Daldrup-Link, M.D.

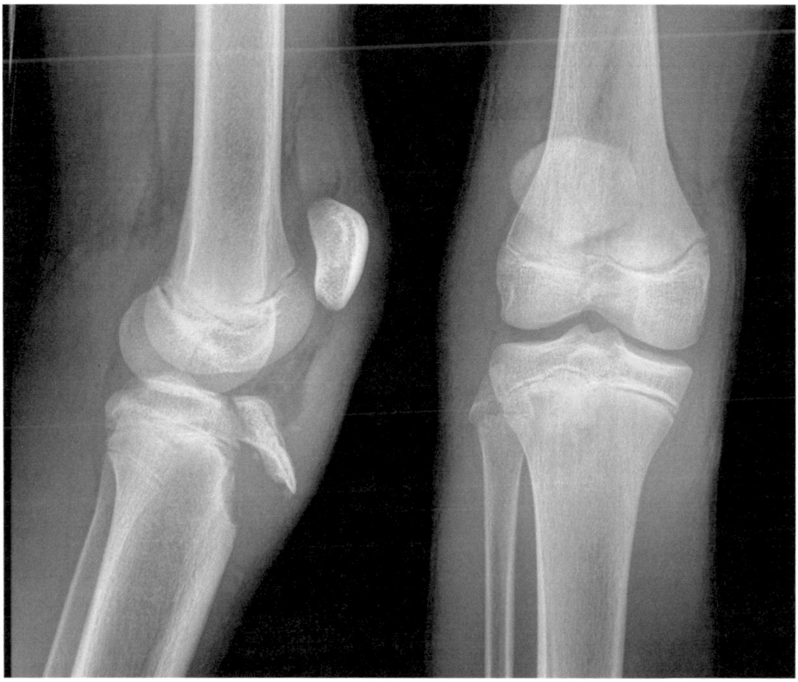

What is the most likely diagnosis:

a) Osgood Schlatter disease
b) Sinding Larsen disease
c) Patellar sleeve fracture
d) Tibial tuberosity avulsion fracture

Case 63: Tibial Tuberosity Avulsion Fracture

a) Osgood Schlatter disease is due to chronic repetitive stress on the patella tendon, which leads to bone fragmentation and soft tissue swelling at the tibial tuberosity.

b) Sinding Larsen disease is due to a chronic traction injury and thickening of the proximal patella tendon, at the inferior pole of the patella.

c) Patellar sleeve fracture refers to an acute chondral or osteochondral avulsion fracture of the inferior pole of the patella.

d) Tibial tuberosity avulsion fracture: Correct! The radiograph shows superior displacement of the apophysis and proximal base of the epiphysis with the fracture line extending into the joint. There is an associated patella alta. Note that patients can develop a compartment syndrome if the recurrent branch of the anterior tibial artery is injured.

Patient 64: 9-year-old female, pain on dorsiflexion

Author: Heike E. Daldrup-Link, M.D.

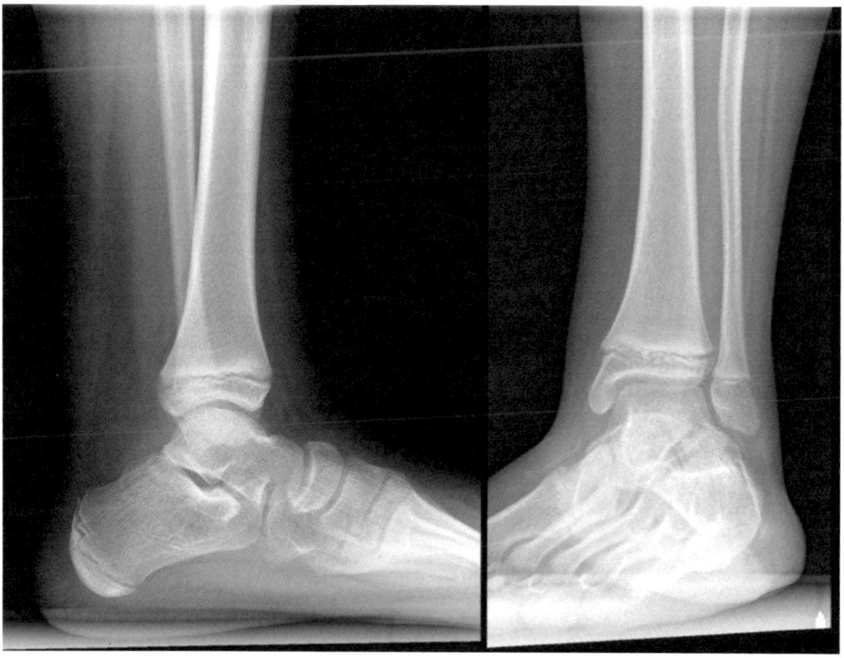

What is the most likely diagnosis:

a) Two-plane fracture
b) Ankle joint effusion
c) Severs disease
d) Achilles Tendinosis

Case 64: Achilles Tendinosis

a) A two-plane fracture or Tilleaux fracture of the distal tibia occurs in teenagers with partially closed growth plate, where the medial aspect of the growth plate is closed, and the lateral aspect of the growth plate is still open. The fracture line extends through the open anterolateral physis. When it hits the closed part of the growth plate, it extends downwards into the epiphysis.

b) There is no effusion noted in the ankle joint.

c) Severs disease or apophysitis of the calcaneus represents an osteochondrosis of the calcaneal apophysis, typically due to repetitive stress of the heel. Radiographic signs include sclerosis and fragmentation of the calcaneal apophysis.

d) Achilles Tendinosis: Correct! The lateral radiograph shows a thickening of the Achilles tendon 5 cm above the calcaneus. The Achilles tendon forms from the fusion of the aponeuroses of the medial and lateral heads of the gastrocnemius and the soleus muscles. The most common abnormality involving the Achilles tendon mid-substance is tendinosis. In adolescent athletes, the most common cause is chronic overuse.

Patient 65: 2-year-old male, knee pain

Author: Heike E. Daldrup-Link, M.D.

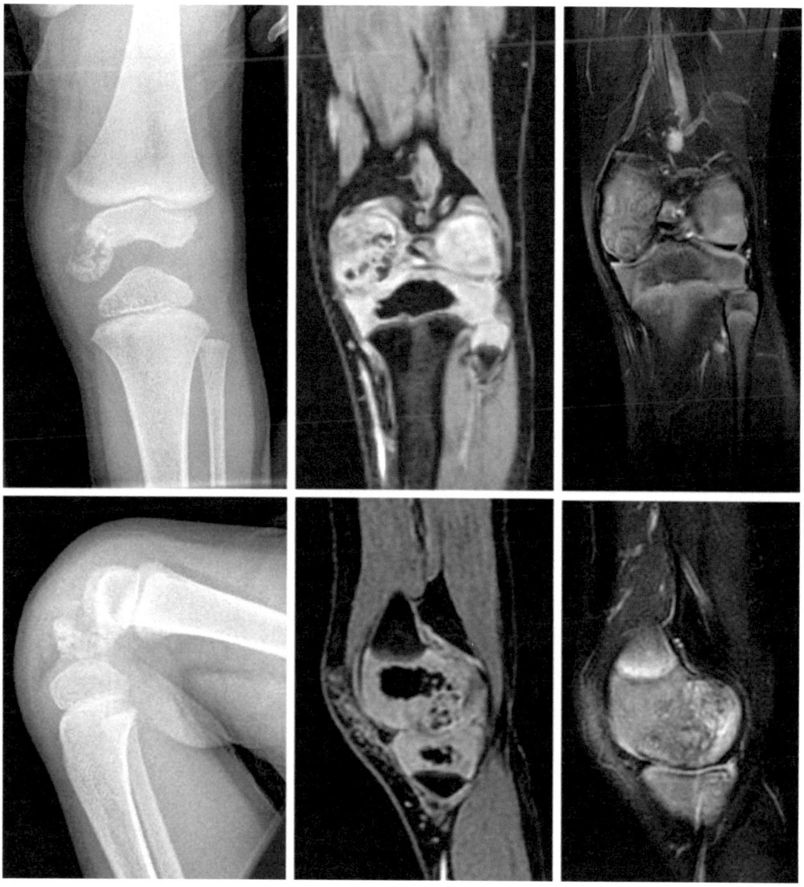

What is the most likely diagnosis:

a) Solitary osteochondroma
b) Multiple hereditary exostoses
c) Trevor's disease
d) Ollier disease

Case 65: Trevor's disease

a) A solitary osteochondroma represents a sessile or lobulated outgrowth of bone, which extends from the metaphysis outwards and is pointing away from the joint.

b) Multiple hereditary exostoses represent multiple outgrowths of bone, which extend from the metaphysis towards the diaphysis of the bone, i.e., away from the joint.

c) Trevor's disease: Correct! Trevor disease is a rare, sporadic, non-hereditary bone dysplasia which can affect a single epiphysis, more than one epiphysis in the same limb or multiple bones throughout the body, including the spine. The radiograph here demonstrates a typical, well defined lobulated irregular bony lesion in the medial distal femoral epiphysis, which extends into the joint. The MRI shows that the lesion contains cartilaginous components, consistent with an osteochondral lesion. These lesions grow with the patient and are usually resected to restore the integrity and function of the joint. The MRI can demonstrate the relation between the lesion and the growth plate, which can be helpful for surgical planning.

d) Ollier disease refers to multiple enchondromas.

Patient 66: 12-year-old male, tennis injury

Author: Heike E. Daldrup-Link, M.D.

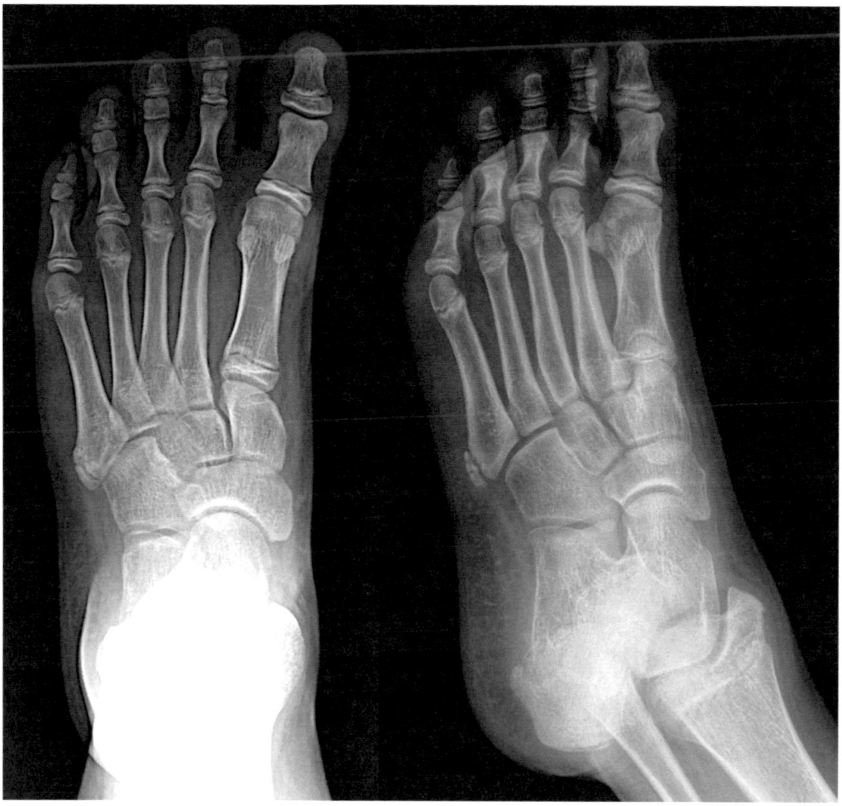

What is the most likely diagnosis:

a) Jones fracture
b) Avulsion fracture of the proximal 5th metatarsal bone
c) Normal apophysis of the 5th metatarsal bone
d) Iselin disease

Case 66: Normal apophysis of the proximal 5th metatarsal bone

a) A Jones fracture is a fracture of the 5th metatarsal bone at the metadiaphyseal junction, approximately 1.5 to 3 cm distal to the proximal tuberosity. Jones fractures are prone to non-union.

b) An avulsion fracture of the proximal 5th metatarsal bone has a transverse orientation, close to the insertion site of the peroneus brevis muscle.

c) Normal apophysis of the proximal 5th metatarsal bone: Correct! The normal apophysis of the 5th metatarsal bone is oriented longitudinally, parallel to the shaft of the bone.

d) Iselin disease refers to an obliquely oriented small bony lesion at the base of the 5th metatarsal bone, which is due to repetitive traction of the peroneus brevis tendon with resulting apophysitis.

Patient 67: 9-year-old male

Author: Heike E. Daldrup-Link, M.D.

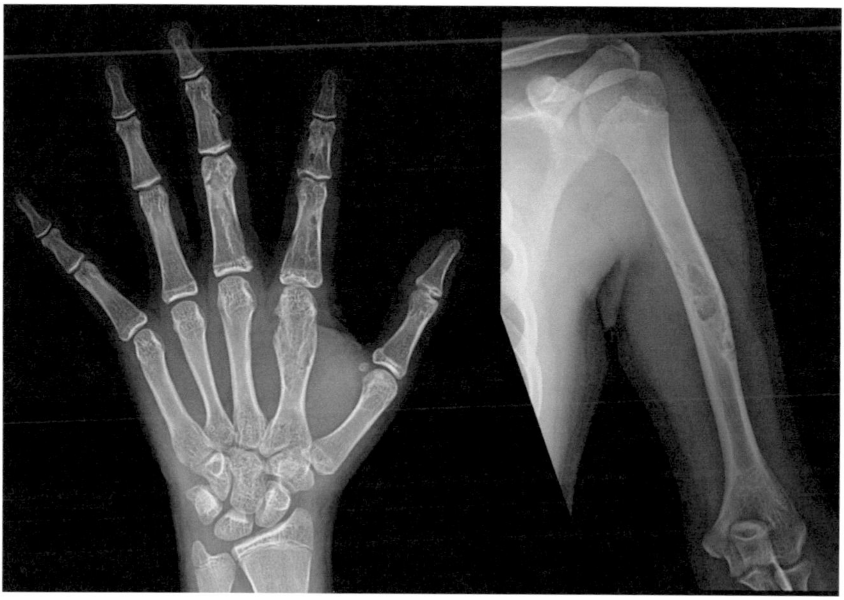

What is the most likely diagnosis:

a) Maffuci syndrome
b) Multiple hereditary exostoses
c) Trevor's disease
d) Ollier disease

Case 67: Ollier disease

a) Maffuci syndrome is characterized by multiple enchondromas and hemangiomas, which present as soft tissue nodules with round calcifications (phleboliths). There are no hemangiomas noted on the images here.

b) Multiple hereditary exostoses represent multiple outgrowths of bone, which extend from the metaphysis towards the diaphysis of the bone, i.e., away from the joint.

c) Trevor's disease is a rare, sporadic bone dysplasia, characterized by osteochondral lesion(s) which originate in the epiphysis and grow towards the joint. The lesions can affect a single epiphysis, more than one epiphysis in the same limb or multiple bones throughout the body, including the spine.

d) Ollier disease: Correct! The radiograph of the right hand demonstrates well defined, expansile lucent lesions in the 2nd metacarpal bone, 2nd and 3rd proximal phalanx, and 2nd and 3rd mid phalanx. Some of the lesions cause cortical thinning or breach of the cortex. The radiographs of the right right proximal humerus demonstrate a well-defined lucent lesion in the mid diaphysis with a narrow zone of transition and internal "ring and arc" calcifications, suggesting a chondroid matrix. The findings are consistent with multiple enchondromas.

Musculoskeletal, Spine, CNS

4) Congenital anomalies and variants

Patient 68: 16-year-old male with chest pain

Authors: Desiree R. Eshraghi, Soni C. Chawla , M.D.

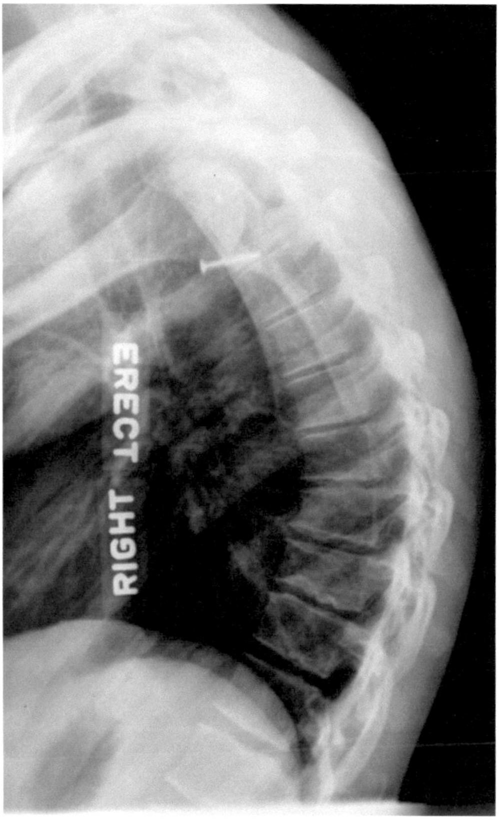

What is the most likely diagnosis:

a) Scheuermann disease
b) Osteoporotic vertebral compression
c) Osteoid Osteoma
d) Osteoblastoma

Case 68: Scheuermann Disease

a) Scheuermann disease: Correct! Scheuermann disease or juvenile kyphosis is defined by an anterior wedging of greater than or equal to 5 degrees in three or more adjacent vertebral bodies, with an associated rigid hyperkyphosis greater than 40 degrees. The lateral radiograph shows endplate irregularities in the mid and lower thoracic spine with multiple Schmorl's nodes, herniations of the cartilage of the intervertebral disc into the adjacent vertebral endplate. There is also an exaggerated kyphosis of the thoracic spine. There are two types of Scheuermann disease: Type 1 involves the thoracic spine, whereas type 2 involves both the thoracic and lumbar spine. There is a strong genetic predisposition for Scheuermann kyphosis, although the specific gene locus has not been identified. Some familial cases have been linked to specific genes on chromosome 5. Both Scheuermann disease and idiopathic scoliosis have a genetic component and can be associated.

b) Osteoporotic vertebral compression fractures are noted in the setting of generalized osteopenia as anterior compression deformities of the vertebral bodies, with more than 20% decreased height of the anterior vertebral body compared to the posterior vertebral body.

c) An osteoid osteoma presents as a focal lucent lesion with a thin central sclerotic nidus.

d) An osteoblastoma typically presents as an expansile lytic lesion in the posterior elements of the vertebral body.

Patient 69: 2-year-old female, palpable lump
Author: Heike E. Daldrup-Link, M.D.

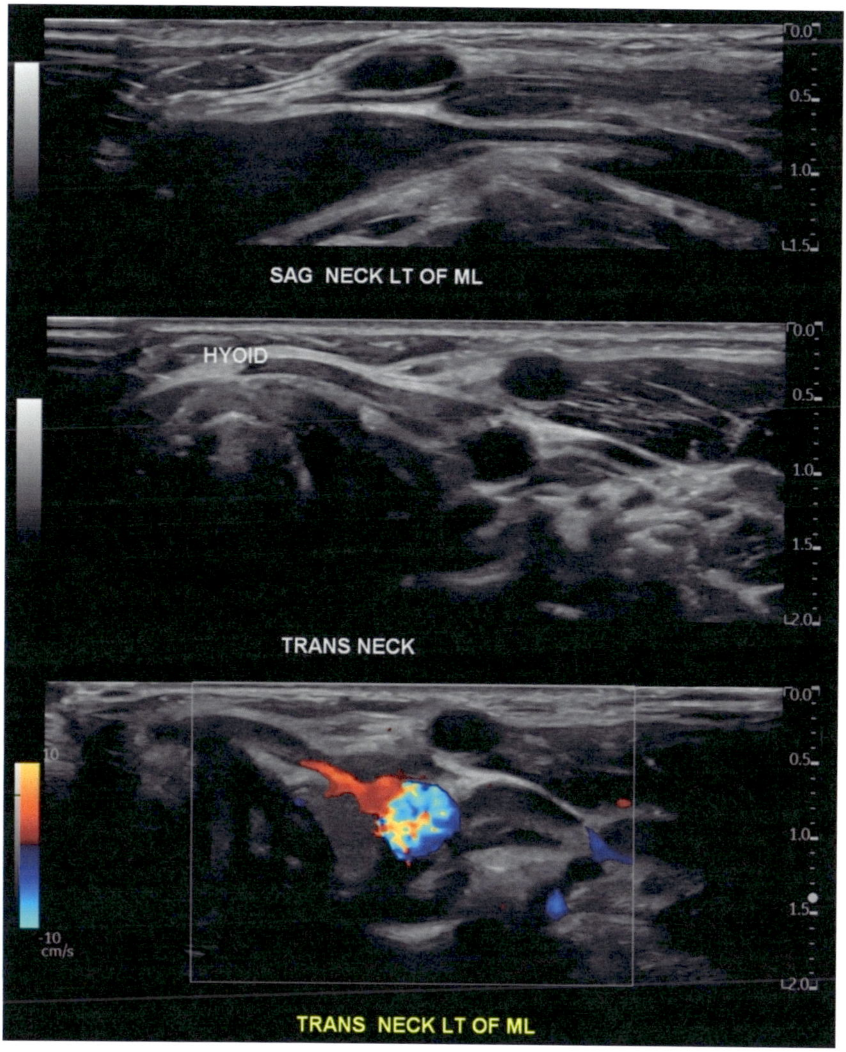

What is the most likely diagnosis:

a) Thyroglossal duct cyst
b) First branchial cleft cyst
c) Second branchial cleft cyst
d) Third branchial cleft cyst

Case 69: Second Branchial Cleft Cyst

a) Thyroglossal duct cysts are typically located near the hyoid bone, in the midline or within 2 cm of the midline.

b) First branchial cleft cysts comprise about 7% of all branchial cleft cysts and are typically located along the external auditory canal (type 1) or within, deep to or superficial to the parotid gland (type 2).

c) Second branchial cleft cyst. Correct! The ultrasound shows a well delineated cystic lesion lateral to the carotid space, deep to the sternocleidomastoid muscle, consistent with the most common presentation of a second branchial cleft cyst (type 2). Other locations include cysts anterior to the sternocleidomastoid muscle (type 1), between internal and external carotid artery (type 3) and in the pharyngeal mucosa space (type 4).

d) Third branchial cleft cysts are located posterior to the carotid arteries, deep to the sternocleidomastoid muscle, often terminating deep to the pyriform sinus. They are most commonly found on the left side.

Patient 70: 16-year-old male with chest pain

Authors: Desiree R. Eshraghi, Soni C. Chawla , M.D.

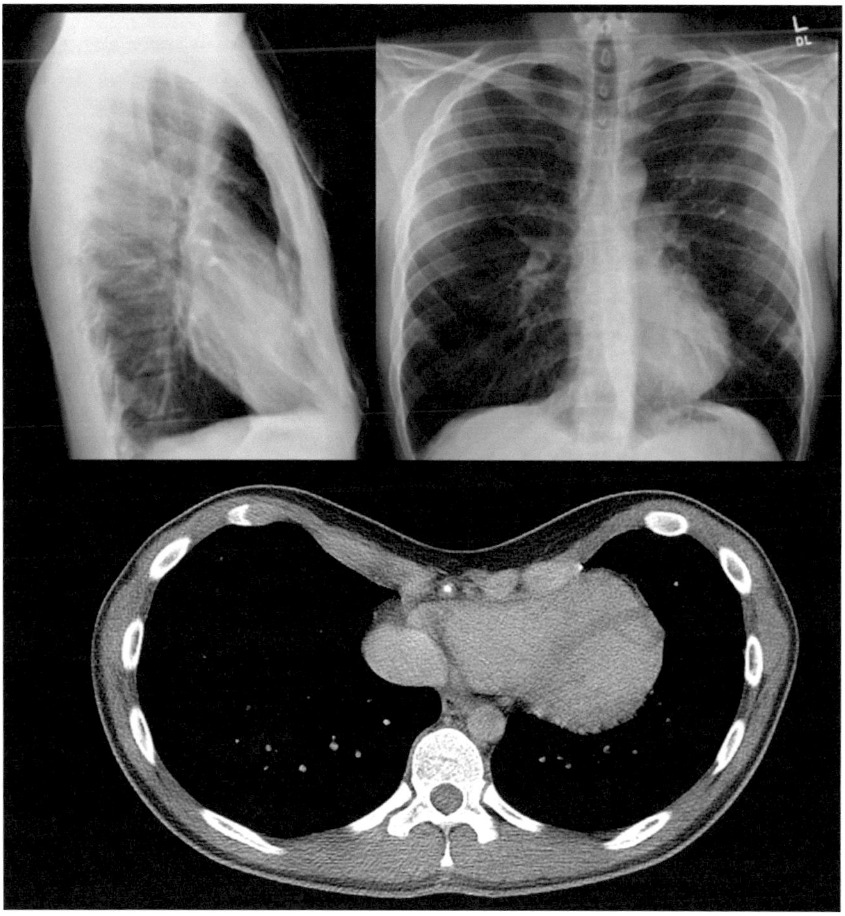

What is the most likely diagnosis:

a) Viral pneumonia
b) Sternal fracture
c) Pectus carinatum
d) Pectus excavatum

Case 70: Pectus excavatum

a) A viral pneumonia can lead to bronchial wall thickening, perihilar pulmonary opacities, peripheral air trapping and peripheral ground glass opacities of the lungs. These findings are not shown here. The radiograph demonstrates a right middle lobe atelectasis. The frontal chest radiograph demonstrates patchy opacities to the right of the right heart border. On the lateral view, there is an opacity projecting over the cardiac silhouette.

b) The radiographs shown here do not demonstrate a sternal fracture. A fracture would be associated with soft tissue swelling and a hematoma in the mediastinum. A pleural effusion might also be noted. There is no history of trauma in this case.

a) A pectus carinatum deformity is characterized by an externally protruding sternum.

b) Pectus excavatum: Correct! The chest x-ray demonstrates a concave appearance of the sternum, which sinks into the chest. Associated imaging findings include heart shaped configuration of the anterior ribs, horizontal configuration of posterior ribs, blurring of the right heart border due to sternal compression, opacity in the right medial lower lung zone due to atelectasis and obliteration of the descending thoracic aorta.

Patient 71: 32-year-old pregnant patient with third trimester fetal MRI

Author: Praveen Jayapal, M.D.

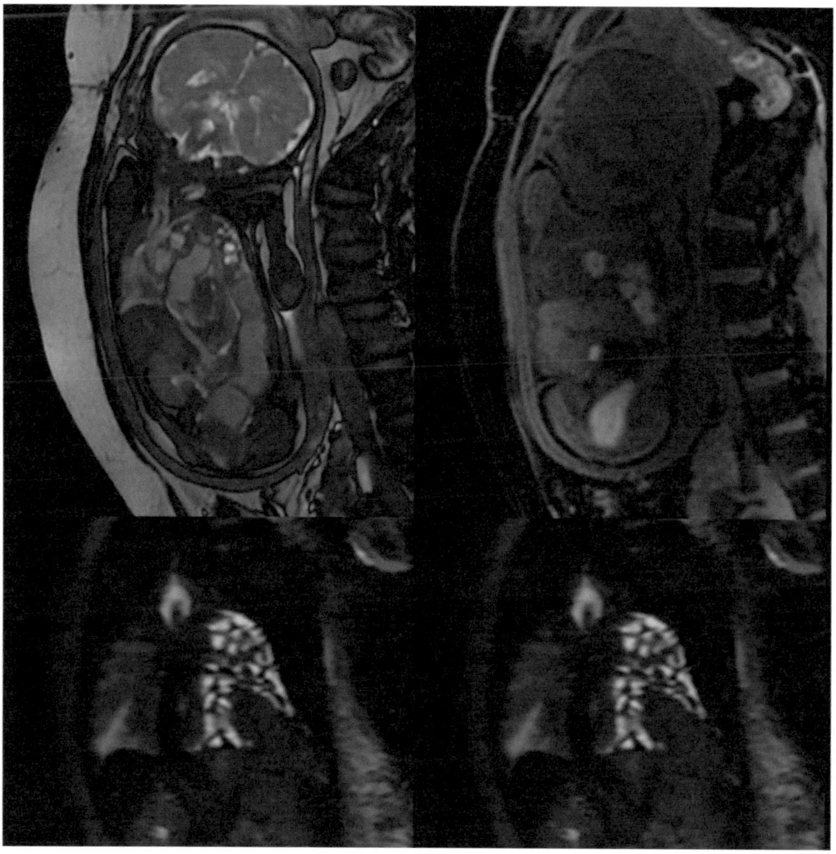

What is the most likely diagnosis:

a) Congenital Pulmonary Airway Malformation (CPAM)
b) Mediastinal Teratoma
c) Bronchial Atresia
d) Congenital Diaphragmatic Hernia (CDH)

Case 71: Congenital Diaphragmatic Hernia

a) Although a Congenital Pulmonary Airway Malformation (CPAM) can present as T2 hyperintense cystic lung mass and cause mass effect, the characteristic tubular morphology of the fluid filled small bowel and the presence of meconium filled colon within the chest suggest a different diagnosis.

b) A mediastinal teratoma usually presents as a large cystic and solid mass, and it would be atypical to have tubular high T1 signal (meconium).

c) On the fetal MRI, Bronchial atresia usually presents as a homogeneous T2 hyperintense wedge shaped lesion. Usually, a mucoid impacted atretic bronchus can be clearly seen in the cases of bronchial atresia.

d) Congenital Diaphragmatic hernia (CDH): Correct! The Coronal FIESTA MRI demonstrates presence of small bowel (high signal fluid filled structure) and colon (Intermediate signal) within the left hemithorax. The herniated contents exert a significant mass effect on the adjacent structures resulting in mediastinal shift towards the right. The coronal T1-weighted LAVA image demonstrates meconium filled colon (T1-hyperintense) within the left hemithorax. Of note, meconium exhibits high T1 signal, low T2 signal and intermediate signal on FIESTA images. The coronal T2-weighted image demonstrates fluid filled small bowel loops in the left hemithorax. The findings are characteristic features of CDH. There is a large defect in the left hemidiaphragm with herniation of small bowel loops into the left hemithorax. The large hernia caused significant mass effect with mediastinal shift towards the right and mass effect on the contralateral right lung. Fetal lung volumes can be calculated using MRI and standard nomograms with expected fetal weights are available for estimating observed vs expected fetal lung volume.

Patient 72: Newborn baby with swollen hand

Author: Heike E. Daldrup-Link, M.D.

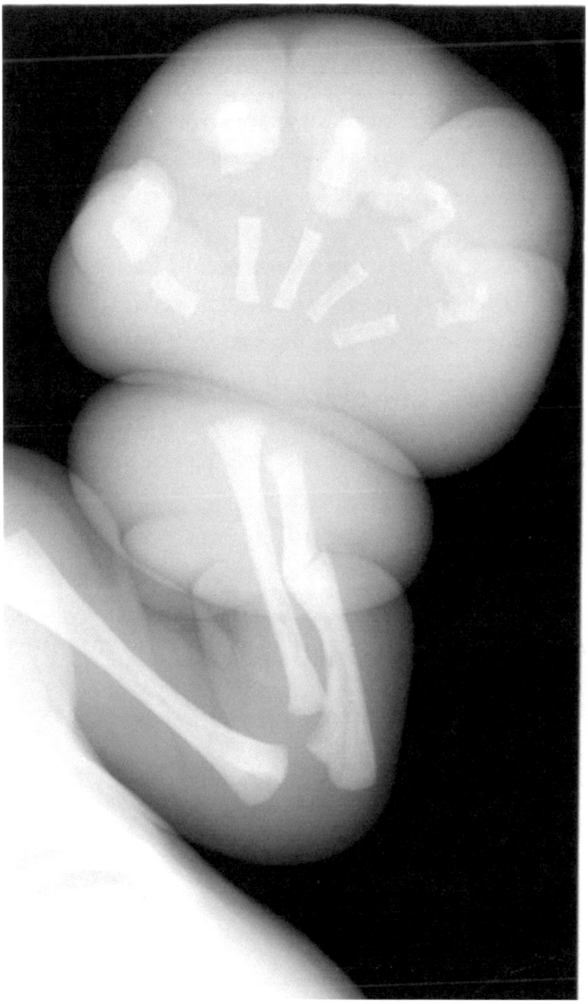

What is the most likely diagnosis:

a) Birth Trauma
b) Rhabdomyosarcoma
c) Amniotic Band Syndrome
d) Lymphatic Malformation

Case 72: Amniotic Band Syndrome

a) A birth trauma would not explain the massive lymphedema of the hand or the band-like soft tissues incisions along the lower arm and wrist.

b) A rhabdomyosarcoma would cause a more localized mass rather than swelling of the hand and all fingers. Band-like soft tissue incisions and an ulnar fracture would not be expected.

c) Amniotic band syndrome: Correct! The radiograph shows multiple band-like soft tissue incisions around the wrist, likely caused by entrapment of the hand in fibrous strands of the amniotic membrane. The hand is markedly swollen, likely due to lymphedema distal to the obstruction. There is also a fracture of the ulna underneath one of the soft tissue incisions. Amniotic band syndrome is a rare congenital disorder which is due to fetal entrapment in strands of amniotic tissue.

d) A lymphatic malformation could cause a similar swelling of the hand and fingers. However, the band-like soft tissue incisions and ulnar fracture would not be expected.

Patient 73: 9-year-old female with foot pain

Author: Heike E. Daldrup-Link, M.D.

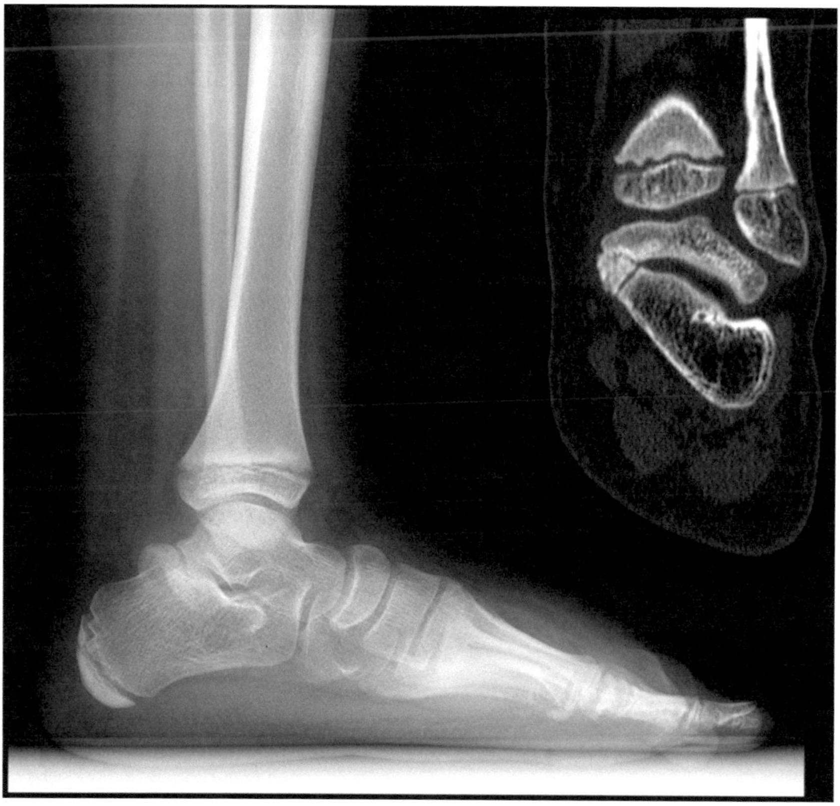

What is the most likely diagnosis:

a) Calcaneonavicular coalition
b) Anterior facet talocalcaneal coalition
c) Middle facet talocalcaneal coalition
d) Posterior facet talocalcaneal coalition

Case 73: Posterior Facet Talocalcaneal Coalition

a) A calcaneonavicular coalition would involve a connection between the calcaneus and the navicular bone, which is not noted here. The talar "beak sign", an elongated anterior process of the calcaneus, may be seen in either calcaneonavicular or talocalcaneal coalition, but it is more commonly seen with talocalcaneal coalitions.

b) An anterior facet talocalcaneal coalition would be located more anteriorly.

c) A middle facet talocalcaneal coalition would be also located more anteriorly. A lateral radiograph of the ankle would typically demonstrate the "C sign" and failure to visualize the middle facet.

d) Posterior facet talocalcaneal coalition: Correct! The radiograph and coronal CT scan demonstrate a posterior facet coalition with an accessory ossicle at the medial and inferior aspect of the talus and superior aspect of the calcaneus.

Patient 74: 7-month-old female, developmental delay

Authors: Shakthi Kumaran Ramasamy, M.D., Wipawee Morakote, M.D.

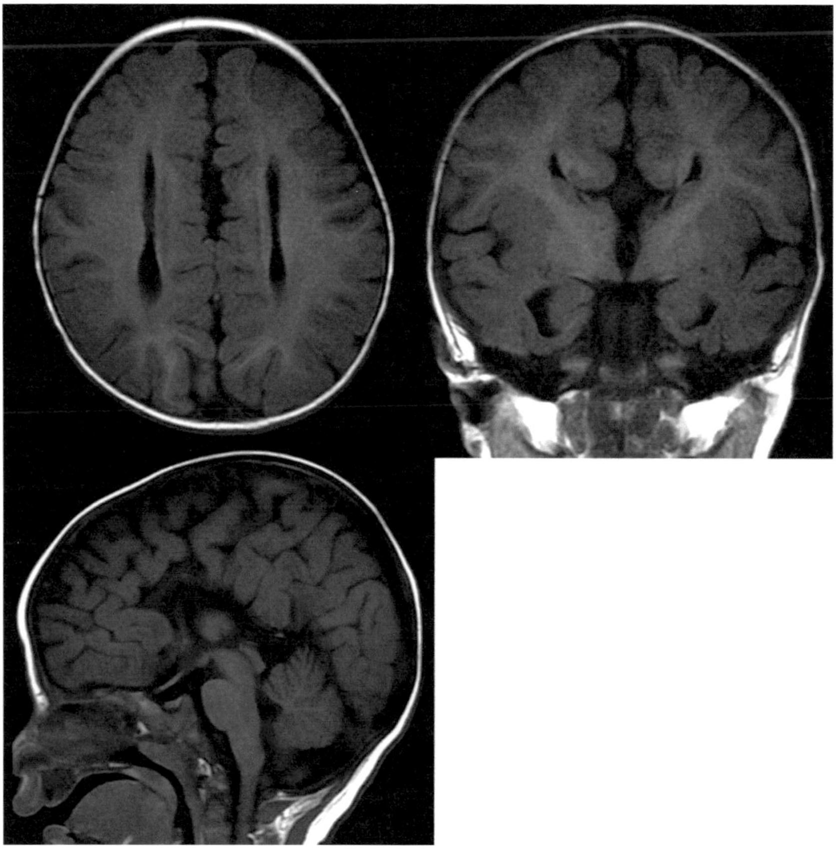

What is the most likely diagnosis:

a) Cavum Septum Pellucidum
b) Cavum Velum Interpositi
c) Corpus Callosum Agenesis
d) Interhemispheric Arachnoid Cyst

Case 74: Corpus Callosum Agenesis

a) Cavum septum pellucidum is a cerebrospinal fluid filled cavity between the two leaflets of the septum pellucidum, between the lateral ventricles. It is considered a normal anatomical variant in the fetus and newborn infant. The two leaflets of the septum pellucidum usually fuse by the age of 6 months.

b) Cavum velum interpositi is characterized by a dilatation of the normal cistern of the velum interpositum. It is a normal anatomic variant in the space below the splenium of the corpus callosum. When is has a transverse diameter of more than 1 cm, it is called a cyst of the velum interpositum and can cause an obstructive hydrocephalus.

c) Corpus Callosum Agenesis: Correct! The axial T1-weighted MR image demonstrates an absent corpus callosum with separation and parallel orientation of the bilateral lateral ventricles (racing car sign). The coronal view demonstrates a high riding third ventricle which is interposed between the bodies of the lateral ventricles. The frontal horns of the lateral ventricles are widely separated (moose head or viking helmet appearance). The sagittal MRI demonstrates an absent corpus callosum and a radiating sulcal pattern toward the roof of the third ventricle.

d) There is no arachnoid cyst located on the images shown here. Arachnoid cysts are benign, asymptomatic cystic lesions located in the subarachnoid space. Gradual expansion of these cysts can cause mass effect, obstruction and/or neurological dysfunction.

Patient 75: 15-year-old male with pectus excavatum

Author: Heike E. Daldrup-Link, M.D.

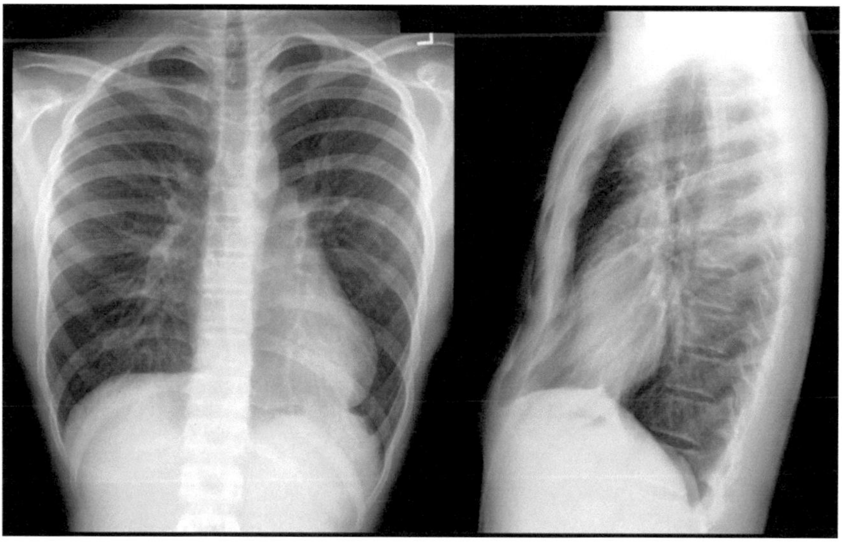

The Haller Index is calculated as:

a) ratio of thoracic anterior-posterior distance divided by the medio-lateral distance at the same level
b) ratio of minimum thoracic anterior-posterior distance divided by the minimum medio-lateral distance
c) ratio of thoracic medio-lateral distance divided by the anterior-posterior distance at the same level
d) ratio of minimum thoracic medio-lateral distance divided by the minimum anterior-posterior distance

Case 75: Pectus excavatum

a) The Haller index is calculated as the ratio of thoracic width and depth.

b) The Haller index is calculated as the ratio of thoracic width and depth.

c) Correct! The Haller index is measured as the inner width of the chest at the lowest level of the pectus deformity and dividing it by the anterior-posterior distance at the same level (between the posterior sternum and the anterior spine). A normal chest has a Haller index of ≤ 2.5. A Haller index of 2.5 - 3.2 represents a mild deformity, a Haller index of 3.2-3.5, represents a moderate deformity; a Haller index of ≥ 3.5 represents a severe deformity. Moderate and severe deformities can be referred to corrective surgery. Recent studies show that simple chest x-rays are just as effective as CT scans for calculating the Haller index and recommend replacing CT scans with chest x-ray to reduce radiation exposure.

d) The Haller index is calculated as the ratio of thoracic width and depth.

Patient 76: Teenage male with chronic foot pain

Author: Heike E. Daldrup-Link, M.D.

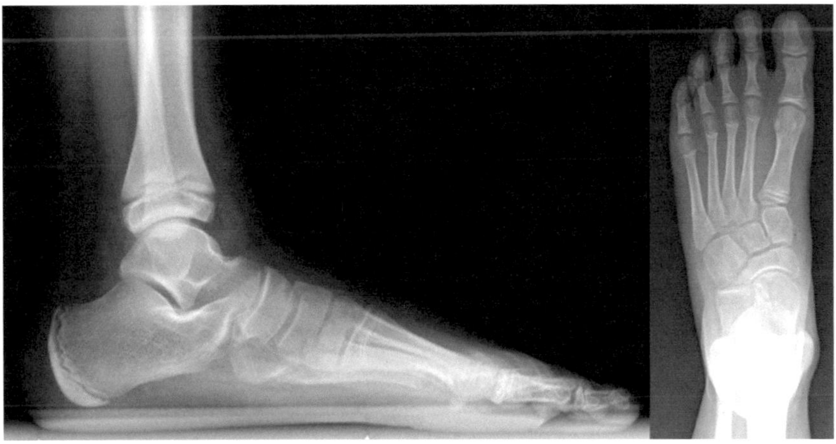

What is the most likely diagnosis:

a) Congenital vertical talus
b) Calcaneovalgus foot
c) Talo-calcaneal coalition
d) Calcaneo-navicular coalition

Case 76: Calcaneo-Navicular Coalition

a) A congenital vertical talus presents with with a vertical orientation of the talus and rocker-bottom foot deformity on radiographs.

b) A calcaneovalgus foot represents an acquired flat foot deformity in infants and young children as a result of intra-uterine positioning with hindfoot dorsiflexion and eversion. There is no underlying coalition.

c) A talo-calcaneal coalition is an osseous or non-osseous connection between the talus and calcaneus. On lateral radiographs of the foot or ankle, it can be diagnosed based on a prominent beak at the anterior aspect of the talus and the C-sign, a posterior continuity between the talus and sustentaculum tali.

d) Calcaneo-navicular coalition: Correct! The lateral radiograph of the foot demonstrates an elongated anterior process of the calcaneus. The ap radiograph demonstrates an elongated proximal surface and lateral tapering of the navicular bone, which connects with the calcaneus. The coalition can be fibrous (syndesmosis), cartilaginous (synchondrosis), or bony (synostosis). A CT confirmed the diagnosis. Tarsal coalitions cause gradual flattening of the medial longitudinal arch resulting in a flat foot deformity.

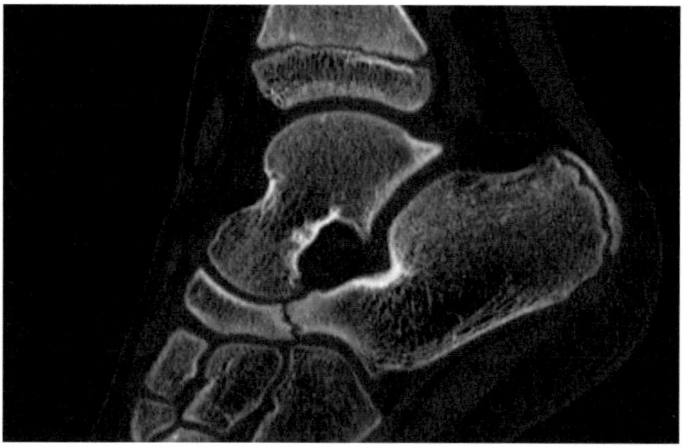

Patient 77: 17-year-old woman, knee pain after soccer injury
Author: Heike E. Daldrup-Link, M.D.

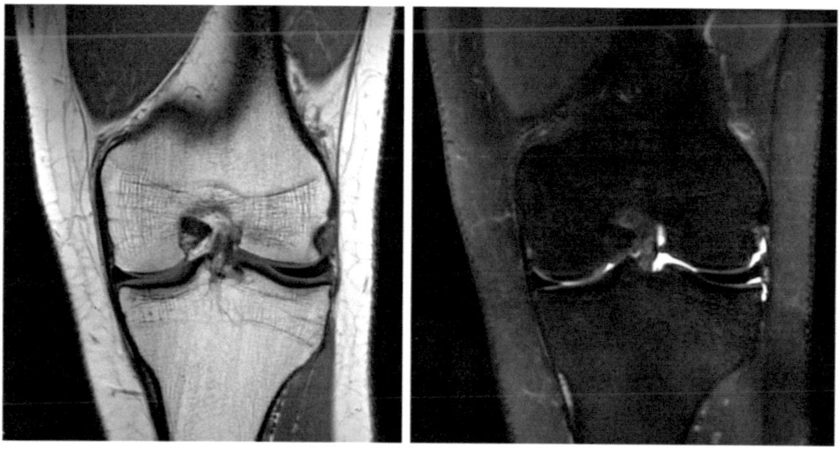

A discoid lateral meniscus is present if:

a) the meniscal body is seen on three or more coronal MR slices
b) the meniscal body width is more than 15 mm on coronal MR images
c) the ratio of the minimal meniscal width to the maximal tibial width is more than 50%
d) the tibia plateau is more than 50% covered by a complete discoid meniscus.

Case 77: Discoid lateral meniscus

a) A discoid meniscus is present if the meniscal body is seen on three or more standard sagittal slices.

b) Correct! A discoid meniscus is present if the meniscal body width is more than 15 mm on coronal MR images.

c) A discoid meniscus is present if the ratio of the minimal meniscal width to the maximal tibial width is more than 20%.

d) A complete discoid meniscus covers more than 80% of the tibial plateau.

Patient 78: 11-year-old male, radiograph for scoliosis workup

Author: Heike E. Daldrup-Link, M.D.

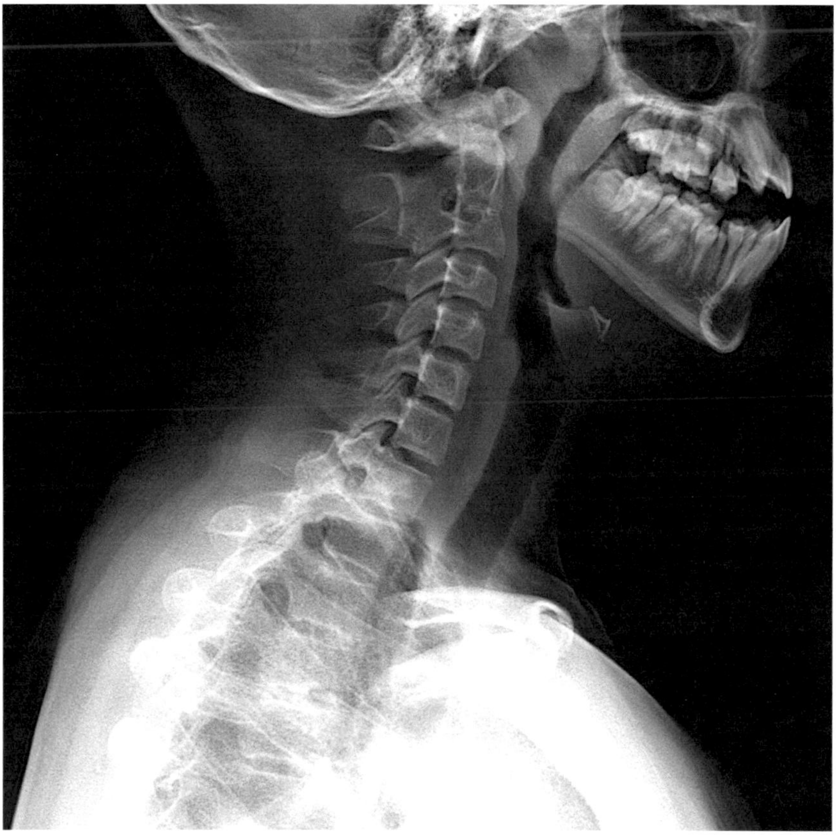

Which incidental finding is noted here:

a) Juvenile idiopathic arthritis
b) Ankylosing spondylitis
c) Sprengel's deformity
d) Klippel Feil Syndrome.

Case 78: Klippel Feil Syndrome

a) Juvenile idiopathic arthritis would present with osteopenia, odontoid erosions, loss of intervertebral disk spaces, facet joint ankylosis and atlantoaxial dislocation.

b) Ankylosing spondylitis would involve multiple vertebral bodies and present at an older age.

c) Sprengel's deformity is characterized by congenital elevation of the scapula, with or without an omovertebral bone. Sprengel's deformity occurs in about 15 to 30% of patients with Klippel Feil Syndrome but is not shown here.

d) Klippel Feil Syndrome. Correct! The radiograph demonstrates fusion of the second and third cervical vertebral body. There is a horizontal lucent line noted through the dens axis, indicating an associated persistent C2 synchondrosis. Klippel Feil Syndrome represents a congenital sporadic or inherited segmentation anomaly of one or multiple cervical vertebrae, most commonly C2/3 as shown here. The original definition described a clinical triad of a short neck, low posterior hairline and restricted cervical motion. Associations with other vertebral anomalies of the thoracic and lumbar spine, scapula anomalies and rib anomalies can be observed.

Patient 79: 12-year-old male, pain at medial aspect of the foot
Author: Heike E. Daldrup-Link, M.D.

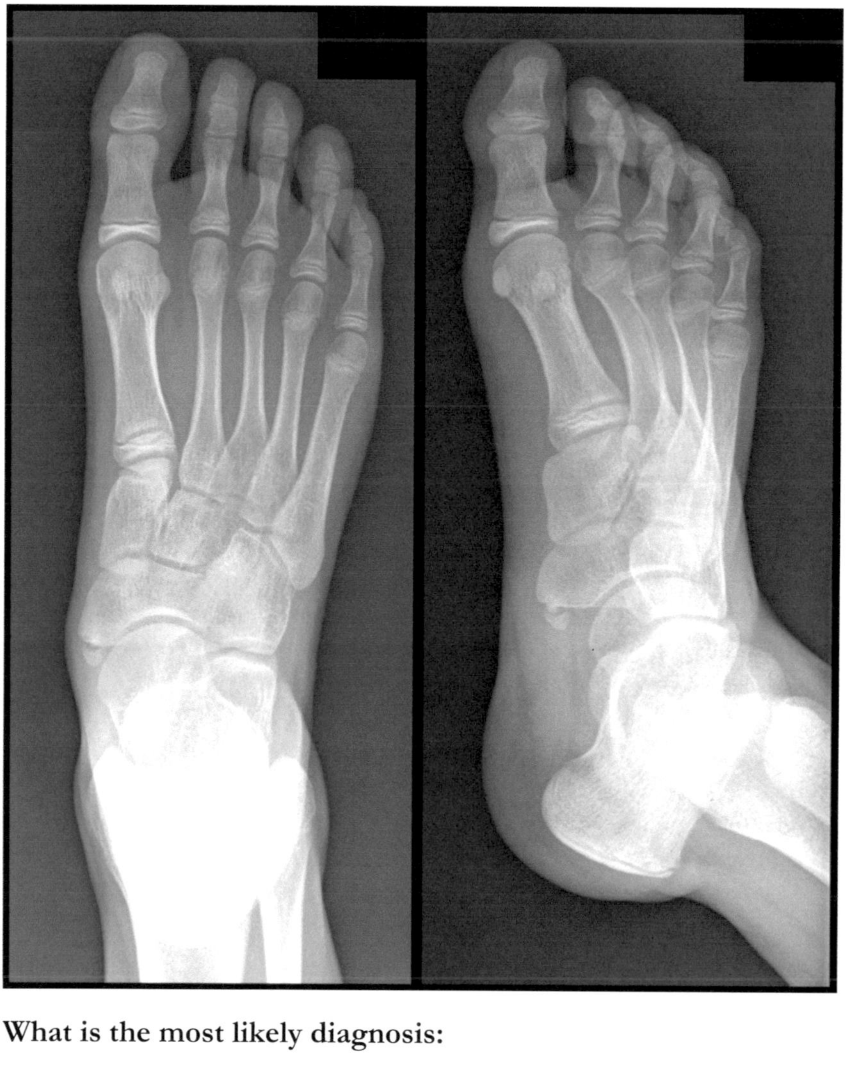

What is the most likely diagnosis:

a) Fracture of the navicular bone
b) Os subtibiale
c) Accessory navicular
d) Os trigonum

Case 79: Accessory Navicular Bone

a) The smooth border, typical location and absence of adjacent soft tissue swelling suggest a different diagnosis.

b) An os subtibiale is an accessory ossicle that is located below the medial malleolus of the tibia.

c) Accessory navicular bone: Correct! The radiograph shows an accessory ossicle medical to the navicular bone. The posterior tibialis tendon often inserts at this ossicle, which can lead to a painful tendinosis

d) An os trigonum is an accessory ossicle that is located posterior to the talus.

Patient 80: 1-day-old female

Author: Heike E. Daldrup-Link, M.D.

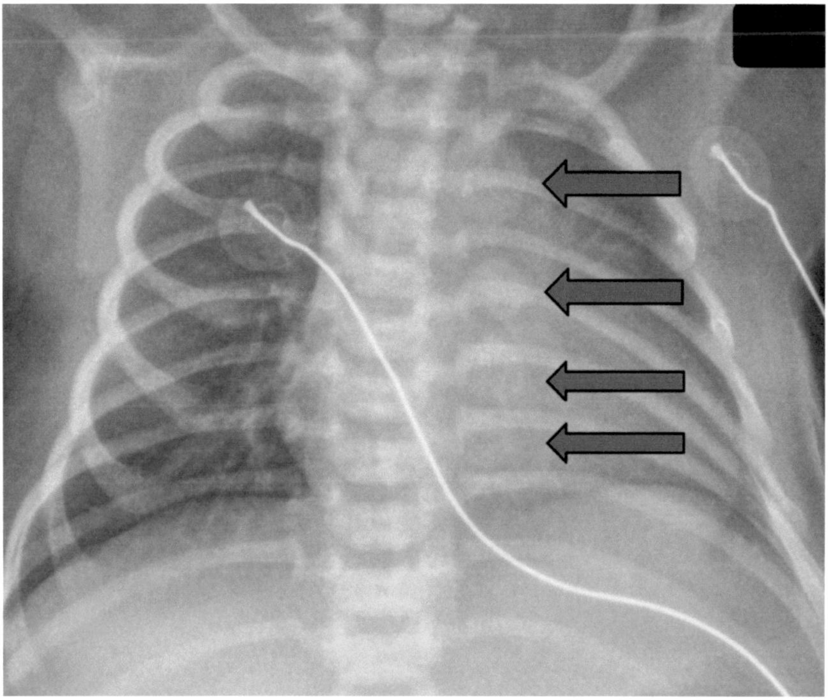

What do the arrows point out:

a) Swallowed foreign bodies
b) Normal anatomy
c) Rib fractures
d) Vertebral segmentation anomalies

Case 80: Normal Ossification Centers of the Sternum

a) There are no ingested foreign bodies noted here. The vast majority of foreign body ingestions occur in children around 3 months to 6 years of age, who can move around and actively grab and swallow foreign bodies.

b) Normal anatomy: Correct! The radiograph shows the four ossification centers of the sternum. While the number of ossification centers can vary, most children have 4 ossification centers at birth (1 segment of the manubrium and 3 mesosternal segments). A fifth inferior mesosternal and a sixth xiphoid segment may ossify later. Note that the sternal ossification centers can ossify at different times. Particularly the second ossification center from above can demonstrate a delayed ossification, which should not be mistaken for pathology.

c) Rib fractures: There are no rib fractures noted here. The ribs are intact.

d) Vertebral segmentation anomalies are not noted here. The vertebral bodies are normal.

Patient 81: 10-year-old female, inversion injury

Author: Heike E. Daldrup-Link, M.D.

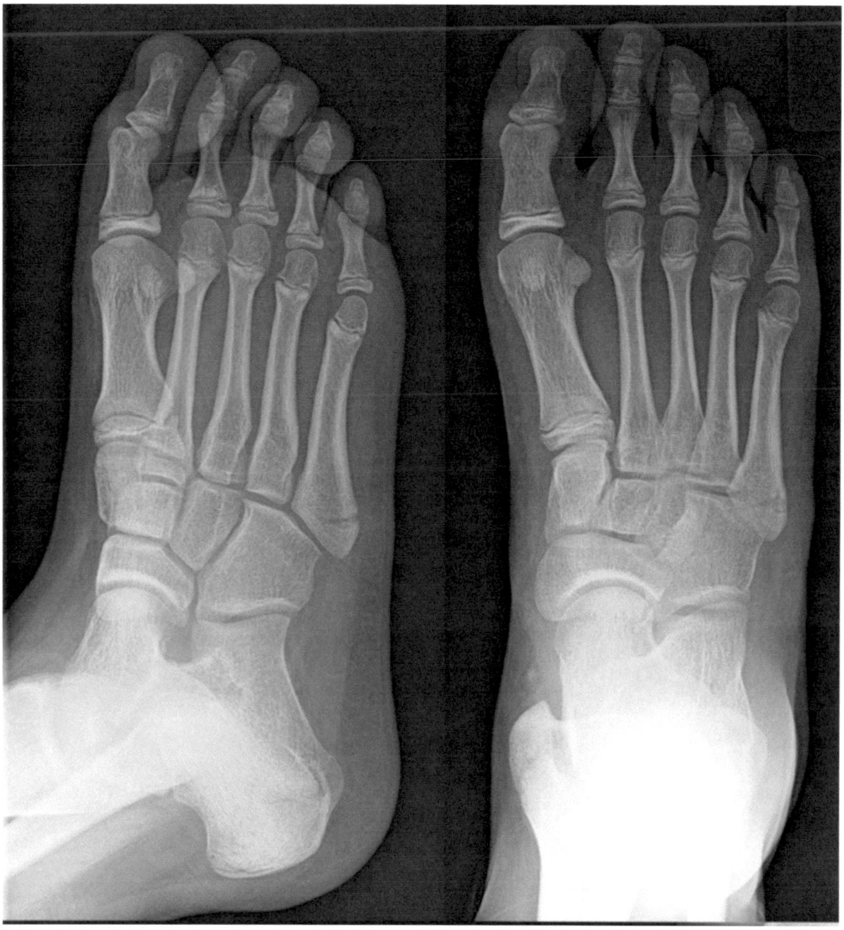

What is the most likely diagnosis:

a) Fracture of the medical cuboid bone
b) Normal apophysis
c) Fracture of the 5th metatarsal bone
d) Os vasalianum

Case 81: Fracture of the 5th metatarsal bone

a) The medial cuboid bone is normal.

b) The finding noted here is not normal. The normal apophysis of the 5th metatarsal bone is classically oriented parallel to the long axis of the 5th metatarsal bone.

c) Fracture of the 5th metatarsal bone: Correct! The radiograph shows a transverse fracture through the base of the proximal 5th metatarsal bone, at the insertion site of the peroneus brevis muscle.

d) An os vesalianum is an accessory ossicle that is located proximal to the base of the 5th metatarsal, in the distal tendon of the peroneus brevis muscle.

Musculoskeletal, Spine, CNS

5) Infection

Patient 82: Teenager with severe back pain
Author: Heike E. Daldrup-Link, M.D.

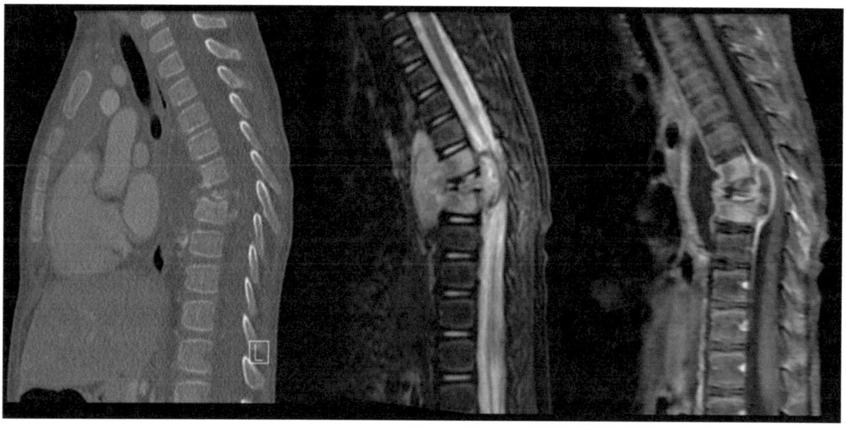

What is the most likely diagnosis:

a) Langerhans Cell Histiocytosis
b) Tuberculous Spondylitis
c) Cat scratch disease
d) Chance fracture

Case 82: Tuberculous Spondylitis

a) Langerhans Cell Histiocytosis (LCH) can lead to collapse of one or more vertebral bodies. However, LCH would not be associated with an abscess.

b) Tuberculous Spondylitis: Correct! The CT scan demonstrates destruction of a mid-thoracic vertebral body. On the MRI, three subsequent vertebral bodies are involved. The abnormal vertebral bodies demonstrate hyperintense signal on T2-weighted images and contrast-enhanced T1-weighted images. The intervertebral discs are relatively spared. The infection has spread beneath the anterior longitudinal ligament, causing a large abscess in front of the infected vertebral bodies. There is also an abscess posteriorly, which compresses the spinal cord.

c) Cat scratch disease can lead to a spondylitis. However, this extensive abscess would be unusual. Patients often also have a lymphadenopathy

d) A chance fracture is an anterior wedge fracture of the vertebral body with a horizontal fracture through posterior elements. It most commonly involves the upper lumbar spine.

Patient 83: 10-year-old female, soft tissue mass of the forearm

Author: Heike E. Daldrup-Link, M.D.

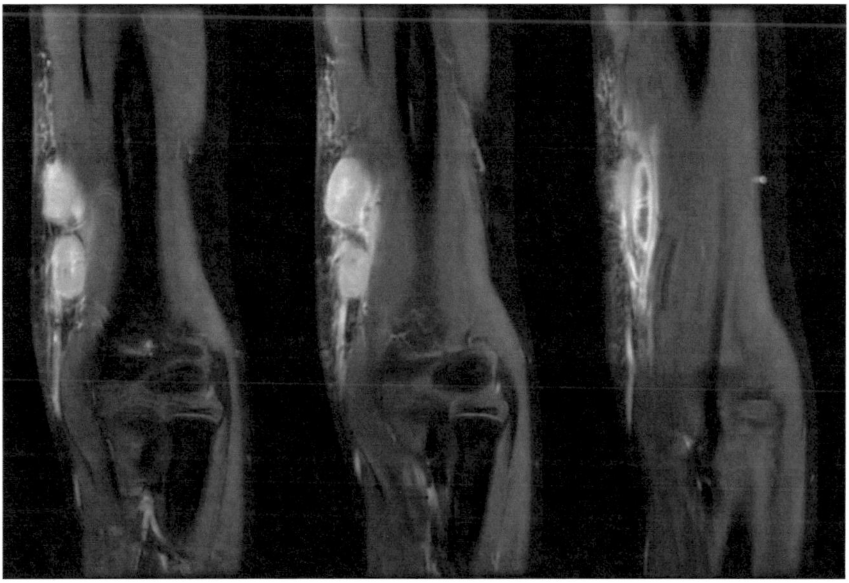

What is the most likely diagnosis:

a) Langerhans Cell Histiocytosis
b) Rhabdomyosarcoma
c) Cat Scratch Disease
d) Vascular Malformation

Case 83: Cat Scratch Disease

a) Langerhans Cell histiocytosis (LCH) can lead to lymphadenopathy. However, the location of these lymph nodes here suggests a different diagnosis.

b) A rhabdomyosarcoma presents as an ill defined, homogenous soft tissue mass. The lesions here are oval and show an enhancing hilum, characteristic of enlarged lymph nodes.

c) Cat scratch disease: Correct! The contrast-enhanced T1-weighted MRI of the forearm demonstrates enlarged lymph nodes with surrounding edema in the subcutaneous soft tissues of the elbow. Upon further questioning the patient reported that she was repeatedly scratched by a cat pet at home. The disease is due to a bacterial infection with Bartonella henselae.

d) A vascular malformation would present as a well-defined, lobulated, contrast-enhancing mass. The lesions here are oval in shape and show an enhancing hilum, characteristic of enlarged lymph nodes.

Patient 84: Teenage patient, knee pain

Author: Heike E. Daldrup-Link, M.D.

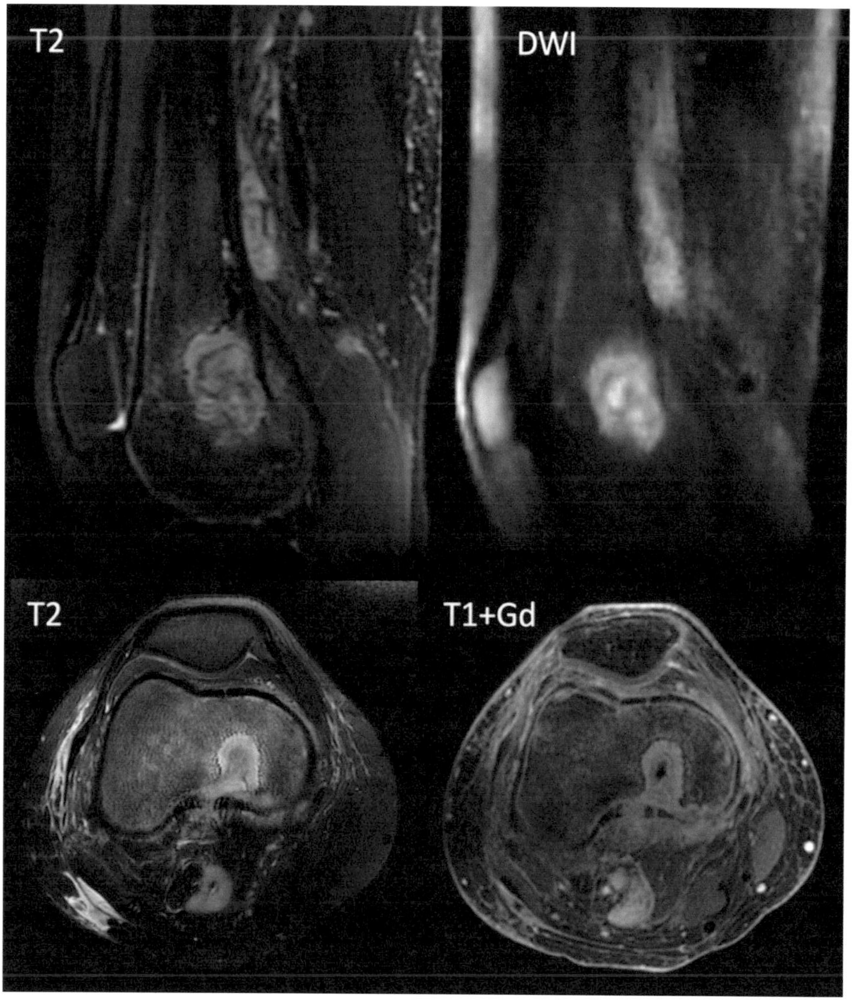

What is the most likely diagnosis:

a) Langerhans Cell Histiocytosis
b) Osteosarcoma
c) Brodie Abscess
d) Vascular Malformation

Case 84: Brodie Abscess

a) Langerhans cell histiocytosis (LCH) is a great mimicker and can have many presentations. Most bone lesions in patients with LCH are well defined and do not demonstrate a large extra-osseous soft tissue component or extensive perosseous edema. The penumbra sign and fistula through the cortex, seen here, would be unusual.

b) An osteosarcoma typically presents as a highly aggressive, ill-defined inhomogeneous intraosseous soft tissue mass with a wide zone of transition. A location in the metaphysis of long bones is often seen. However, osteosarcomas typically cause aggressive cortical destruction and are often associated with a large soft tissue mass. The penumbra sign, seen here, would be unusual.

c) Brodie abscess: Correct! The T2-weighted MRI scans demonstrate a focal intramedullary lesion in the distal posterior femur with a typical "penumbra sign", a central abscess cavity surrounded by a layer of granulation tissue and a layer of perilesional edema. The diffusion-weighted MRI (DWI) demonstrates restricted diffusion of the lesion. The contrast-enhanced T1-weighted MRI demonstrates lack of enhancement of the central abscess and marked enhancement of the surrounding granulation tissue. There is erosion of the lesion through the posterior cortex with formation of a fistula and extension of the abscess into the adjacent soft tissues. The findings are consistent with a Brodie abscess, an intraosseous abscess related to a focus of subacute or chronic pyogenic osteomyelitis.

d) A vascular malformation would present as a well-defined, lobulated, contrast-enhancing mass. The penumbra sign, seen here, is not consistent with this diagnosis.

Patient 85: A newborn with limited motion of the lower legs

Authors: Wipawee Morakote, M.D., Pannee Visrutaratna, M.D.

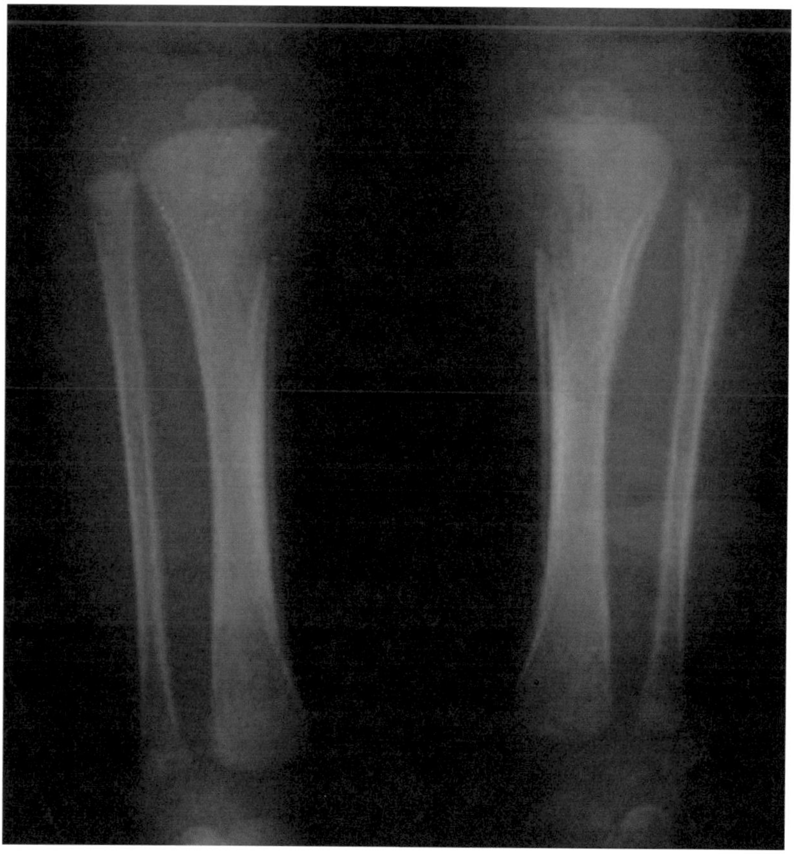

What is the most likely diagnosis:

a) Congenital rubella
b) Congenital CMV
c) Congenital Syphilis
d) Congenital Toxoplasmosis

Case 85: Congenital Syphilis

a) Congenital rubella can cause chronic osteomyelitis of the long bones, with alternating radiodense and radiolucent vertical lines of the metaphyses (celery stalk appearance). In addition, patients can present with a microcephalus, deafness, and cataract. A CT or MRI of the brain may show enlarged ventricles, periventricular calcifications, and white matter lesions. Congenital cardiac abnormalities, such as ventricular septal defects or tetralogy of Fallot may be also seen.

b) Congenital cytomegalovirus (CMV) infection is often asymptomatic at birth. Patients can present with hepatosplenomegaly, microcephaly, hydrocephalus, intracranial calcifications, and skin lesions. CMV can also cause a chronic osteomyelitis with the celery stalk appearance.

c) Congenital Syphilis: Correct! The radiograph of the lower legs demonstrates a periosteal reaction of the long bones and a typical destruction at the medial metaphyses of the bilateral proximal tibia. This Wimberger sign is pathognomonic for congenital syphilis. However, it is not seen in all cases. Below is another case, which does not show it. The radiographs of both legs and the left forearm rather show a diffuse periostitis and transverse radiolucent metaphyseal bands.

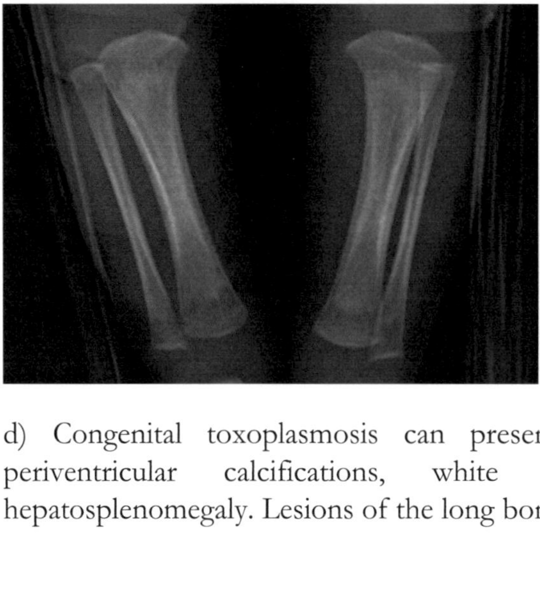
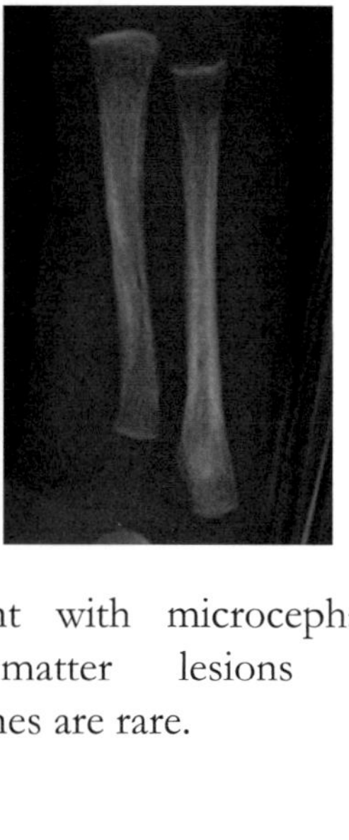

d) Congenital toxoplasmosis can present with microcephalus, periventricular calcifications, white matter lesions and hepatosplenomegaly. Lesions of the long bones are rare.

Musculoskeletal, Spine, CNS

6) Neoplasms - bone, soft tissue

Patient 86: 11-year-old male with hip pain
Author: Heike E. Daldrup-Link, M.D.

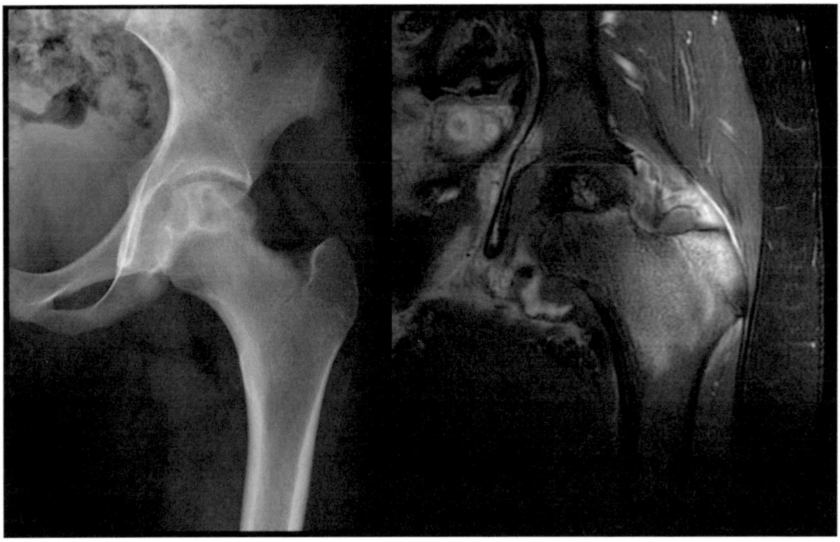

What is the most likely diagnosis:

a) Aneurysmal Bone Cyst
b) Giant Cell tumor
c) Chondroblastoma
d) Langerhans Cell Histiocytosis

Case 86: Chondroblastoma

a) An aneurysmal bone cyst (ABC) would have predominantly fluid-equivalent signal and would demonstrate fluid-fluid levels (which can be also noted in chondroblastoma). The epiphyseal location and the extensive edema are rather unusual for an ABC.

b) A giant cell tumor would be more common older patients with closed growth plates. Giant cell tumors do not usually have a sclerotic rim (although few cases with sclerotic rim have been described).

c) Chondroblastoma: Correct! The radiograph shows a well-defined lytic bone lesion in the proximal femur with thin sclerotic margins and a narrow zone of transition. There is no associated periosteal reaction. The MRI scan shows a well-defined T2-hyperintense, heterogenous lesion with characteristic extensive associated bone marrow edema.

d) Langerhans cell histiocytosis. While this would be a potential differential diagnosis, the sclerotic rim and extensive bone marrow edema would be unusual.

Patient 87: 10-year-old male with osteoblastic osteosarcoma
Author: Heike E. Daldrup-Link, M.D.

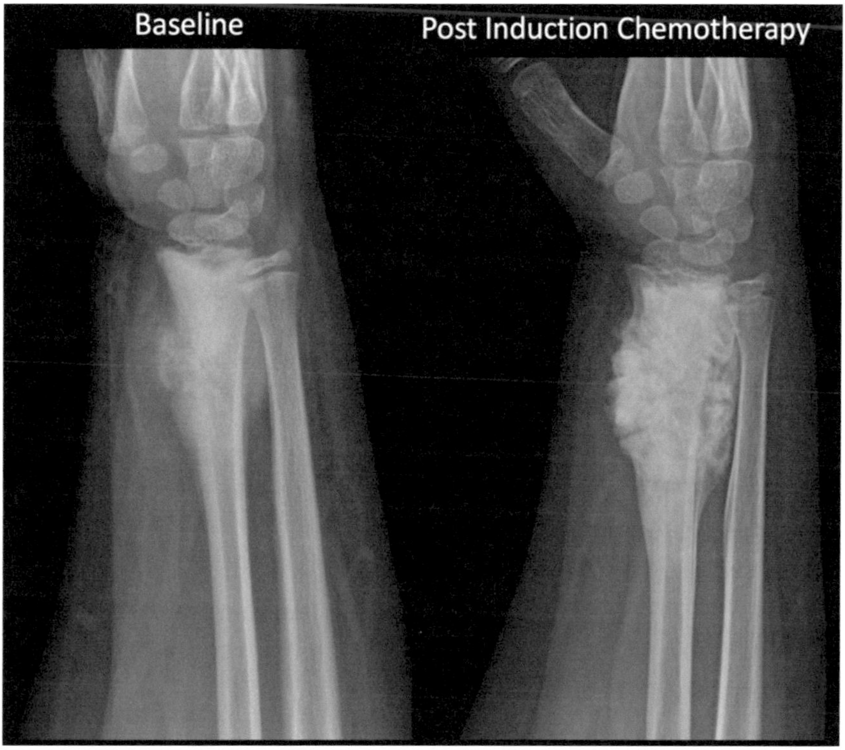

The radiograph after induction chemotherapy shows:

a) Tumor progression
b) Extraskeletal disease
c) Tumor response
d) Therapy complication

Case 87: Osteogenic Osteosarcoma

a) Tumor progression: Tumor progression during induction chemotherapy is rare in osteoblastic osteosarcomas. It would be associated with an increased tumor size.

b) Extraskeletal disease is located outside of the bone. The lesion here is centered in the distal radius and has an associated soft tissue component.

c) Tumor response to induction chemotherapy: Correct! The baseline radiograph demonstrates an aggressive lesion in the distal metaphysis of the right radius, which disrupts the adjacent cortex and infiltrates the adjacent soft tissues. The lesion demonstrates an osteogenic matrix with new bone formation and a sunburst periosteal reaction. The findings are characteristic of an osteogenic sarcoma. After induction therapy, there is an increased sclerosis of the tumor tissue, consistent with response to chemotherapy. Bone forming osteosarcomas often do not decrease much in size in response to chemotherapy. This tumor was resected after the second radiograph shown here and histology demonstrated 100% necrosis of the tumor tissue.

d) There is no therapy complication shown here.

Patient 88: 13-year-old male with left posterior neck mass

Author: Heike E. Daldrup-Link, M.D.

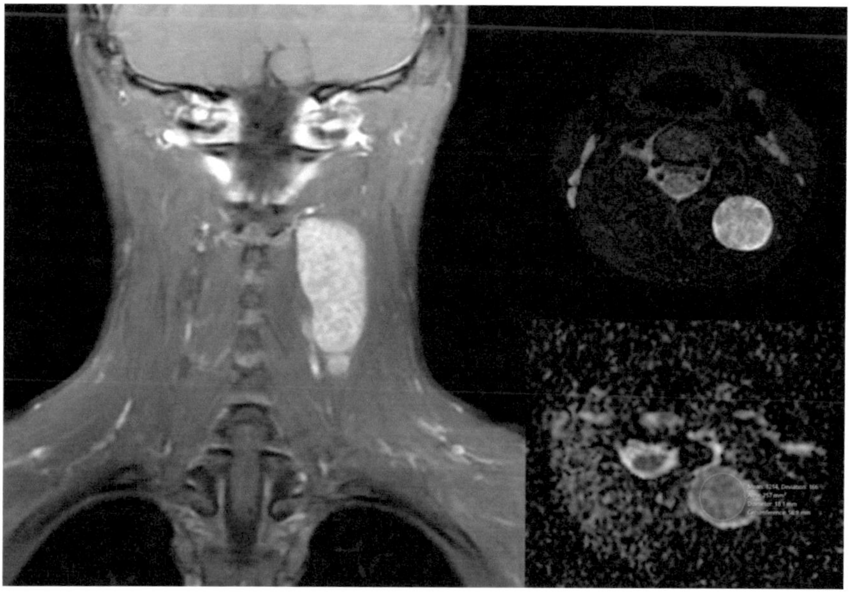

Which criteria favors a benign peripheral nerve sheath tumor:

a) SUVmax > 4.5
b) Longest diameter > 4.5 cm
c) Central necrosis > 25%
d) ADC value > 1.0×10^{-3} mm^2/s

Case 88: Peripheral Nerve Sheath Tumor

a) A benign peripheral nerve sheath tumor would demonstrate limited 18F-FDG radiotracer uptake on a positron emission tomography (PET) scan. A standardized uptake value (SUV) of more than 4.5 on an 18F-FDG PET scan would be concerning for a malignant peripheral nerve sheath tumor (MPNST). Increasing 18F-FDG tumor accumulation on delayed PET scan could further confirm a concern for malignant degeneration.

b) A diameter of more than 4.5 cm is concerning for malignant degeneration and formation of a MPNST.

c) Benign peripheral nerve sheath tumors are relatively homogenous. Development of a central necrosis which comprises more than 25% of the tumor tissue is concerning for malignant degeneration and formation of a MPNST.

d) ADC value > 1.0 × 10^{-3} mm^2/s. Correct! The MRI demonstrates a well-defined T2-hyperintense, intensely enhancing lesion in the soft tissues of the left posterior neck. The relatively small size, the absence of necrosis and the lack of restricted diffusion all favor a benign peripheral nerve sheath tumor. Limited restricted diffusion of the mass with an ADC value of 1.2 × 10^{-3} mm^2/s is in favor of a benign lesion. Restricted diffusion with an ADC value of less than 1.0 × 10^{-3} mm^2/s would be concerning for malignant degeneration.

Patient 89: Young woman, incidental finding

Author: Heike E. Daldrup-Link, M.D.

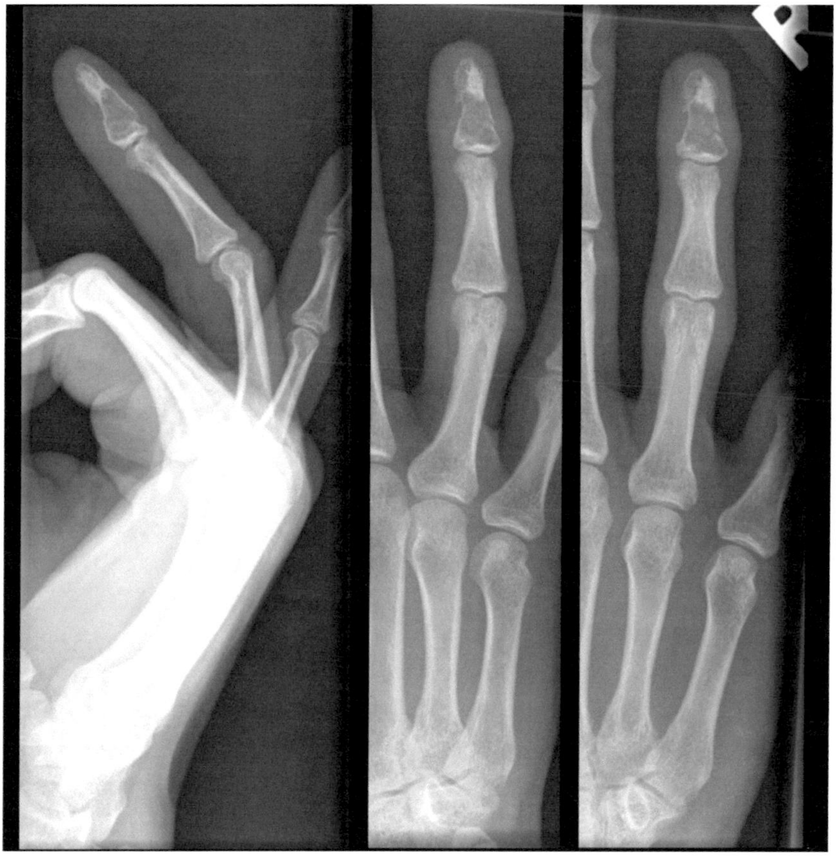

What is the most likely diagnosis:

a) Osteomyelitis
b) Giant Cell tumor
c) Enchondroma
d) Langerhans Cell Histiocytosis

Case 89: Enchondroma

a) An osteomyelitis would present with cortical destruction, an associated periosteal reaction and more severe soft tissue swelling.

b) A giant cell tumor (GCT) typically occurs in long bones of the extremity in patients with closed growth plates. Less than 2% of GCT are found in the bones of the hand. A GCT does not usually have a sclerotic rim (although few cases have been described).

c) Enchondroma: Correct! An enchondroma is a benign cartilaginous neoplasm of the medullary cavity and the most common benign tumor of the hand in children. The x-ray shows a well-defined, expansile lytic bone lesion in the distal phalanx of the fourth finger with thin sclerotic margins and a narrow zone of transition. There are thin ring and arc like calcifications, which are characteristic of the underlying chondroid matrix of the lesion. The lesion involves the area of the growth plate, where these lesions often arise. There is no associated bone destruction and no periosteal reaction. A pathologic fracture is seen, traversing the lesion.

d) Langerhans cell histiocytosis. While this would be a potential differential diagnosis, the location, sclerotic rim and arc-like internal calcifications would be unusual.

<u>Mnemonic for lytic bone lesions</u>: FOG MACHINES
Fibrous dysplasia
Osteoblastoma
GCT (giant cell tumor)
Metastases
ABC (aneurysmal bone cyst)
Chondroblastoma
Hyperparathyroidism
Infection/Osteomyelitis
NOF (non-ossifying fibroma)
Enchondroma and Eosinophilic granuloma
Simple (unicameral) bone cyst

Patient 90: 14-year-old male, palpable lump at third toe

Author: Heike E. Daldrup-Link, M.D.

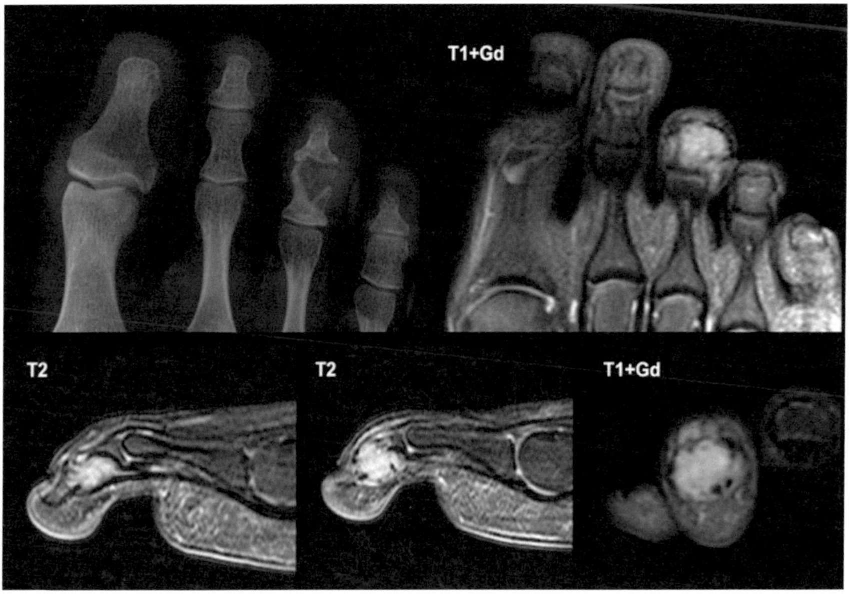

What is the most likely diagnosis:

a) Osteomyelitis
b) Giant Cell Tumor
c) Enchondroma
d) Langerhans Cell Histiocytosis

Case 90: Giant Cell Tumor of the Tendon Sheath

a) An osteomyelitis would present with cortical destruction, an associated periosteal reaction and edema. A localized soft tissue mass as shown here would be unusual.

b) Giant cell tumor (GCT) of the tendon sheath. Correct! The radiograph demonstrates a well-defined lytic lesion in the distal mid phalanx of the third toe. The MRI demonstrates a lobulated soft tissue lesion surrounding the flexor tendon at the level of the third distal interphalangeal joint. The lesion has solid components which enhance on contrast-enhanced scans. The lesion causes scalloping of the adjacent bone.

c) An enchondroma is a benign cartilaginous neoplasm of the medullary cavity which presents as a well-defined, expansile lytic bone lesion with thin sclerotic margins and a narrow zone of transition. It can contain thin ring and arc like calcifications. There is usually no associated bone destruction, no associated soft tissue mass, and no periosteal reaction.

d) Langerhans cell histiocytosis. While this would be a potential differential diagnosis, the location, sharp rim, and connection to the flexor tendon would be unusual.

Patient 91: 15-year-old female, several months of leg pain

Authors: Shakthi Kumaran Ramasamy, M.D., Joe B. Baker, M.D.

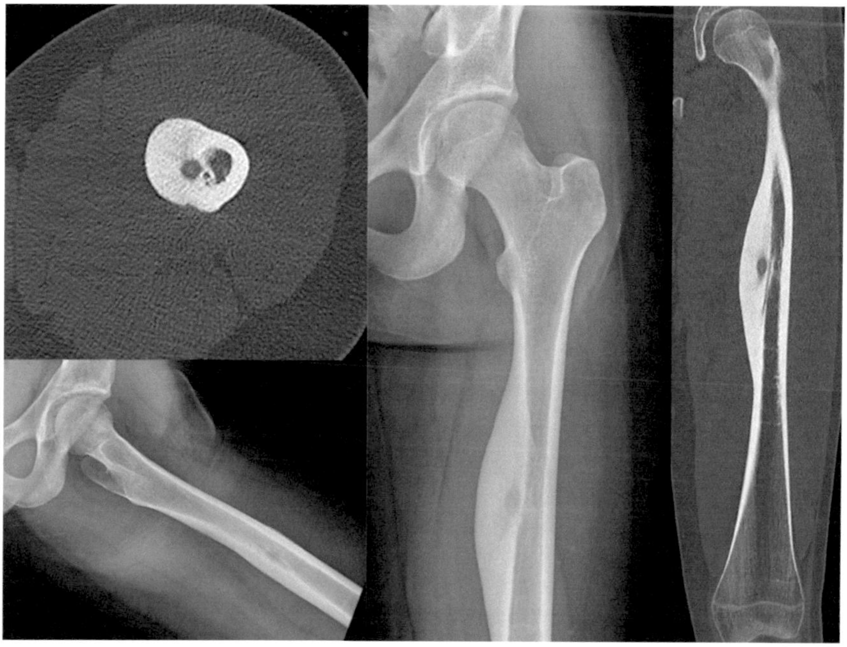

What is the most likely diagnosis:

a) Brodie Abscess
b) Osteoid Osteoma
c) Osteoblastoma
d) Periosteal Osteosarcoma

Case 91: Osteoid Osteoma

a) A Brodie abscess is a focus of osteomyelitis that presents as an intramedullary focal lucent lesion with a surrounding sclerotic rim. It is most commonly found in children with open growth plates and typically located in the metaphyses of long bones. A periosteal reaction may be present, but the degree of cortical thickening shown here would be unusual.

b) Osteoid Osteoma: Correct! The radiographs demonstrate a typical oval lucent lesion in the medial cortex of the left femur, consistent with a nidus, and extensive associated cortical thickening. The CT images demonstrate a faint central sclerotic dot within the nidus. The lesion is benign and can be treated with radiofrequency ablation.

c) Osteoblastoma presents as a well-defined expansile lytic bone lesion with a size of more than 1.5-2 cm, which is most commonly located in the axial skeleton, although it can be also found in long bones. Osteoblastomas usually have a surrounding rim of reactive sclerosis and a narrow zone of transition.

d) A Periosteal Osteosarcoma is a malignant bone tumor which presents as a broad-based soft tissue mass of the bone cortex. It is most commonly found along the diaphysis of long bones and often associated with cortical destruction and an aggressive periosteal reaction, such as a sunburst phenomenon or Codman triangle.

Patient 92: 18-year-old female, leg pain

Authors: Shakthi Kumaran Ramasamy, M.D., Joe B. Baker, M.D.

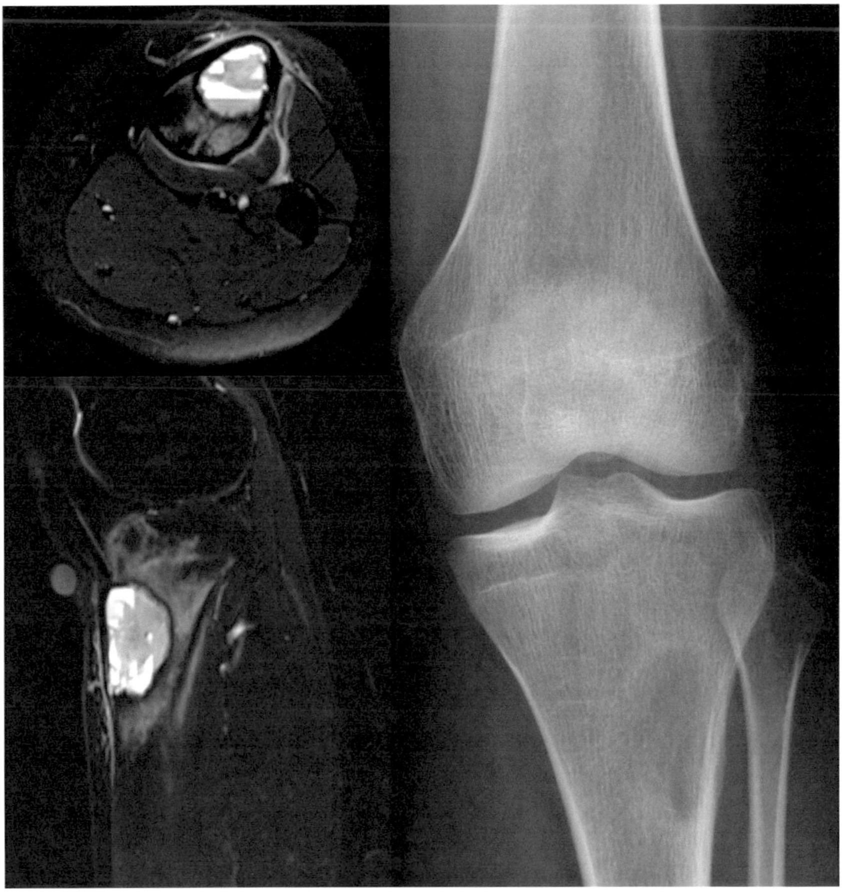

What is the most likely diagnosis:

a) Giant Cell Tumor
b) Chondroblastoma
c) Aneurysmal Bone Cyst
d) Telangiectatic Osteosarcoma

Case 92: Aneurysmal Bone Cyst (ABC)

a) A giant cell tumor usually presents in patients with closed growth plates. Radiographs demonstrate a well circumscribed lytic bone lesion, which often extends into the epiphysis. The lesion usually has a well defined, non-sclerotic margin and can show fluid-fluid levels on T2-weighted MRI scans.

b) A chondroblastoma presents as a well-defined lytic bone lesion in radiographs with thin sclerotic margin and narrow zone of transition. It is most commonly found in the epiphysis of long bones. On T2-weighted MRI scans, the lesion can be T2-hyperintense or demonstrate fluid-fluid levels. It has a characteristic extensive associated bone marrow edema.

c) Aneurysmal Bone Cyst (ABC): Correct! The radiograph demonstrates a well-defined, solitary, eccentric oval lucent lesion in the proximal tibia metaphysis. The axial and sagittal T2-weighted MRI demonstrates multiple fluid-fluid levels. There is no definite soft tissue component of the lesion. The findings are most consistent with an ABC.

d) A telangiectatic osteosarcoma presents as an ill-defined, mostly lytic bone lesion on radiographs, which has a wide zone of transition and destructs the adjacent bone cortex. On MRI scans, it presents as an aggressive intramedullary mass with a substantial associated extraosseous soft tissue component. The lesion can show extensive fluid-fluid levels on T2-weighted MRI, but it also shows extensive soft tissue components.

<u>Mnemonic for bone lesions with fluid-fluid levels:</u>
G – Giant Cell Tumor
O – Osteoblastoma
A – Aneurysmal Bone Cyst
T – Telangiectatic Osteosarcoma
C – Chondroblastoma
S – Simple bone cyst after trauma
F – Fibroxanthoma

Patient 93: 12-year-old female with palpable lump

Author: Heike E. Daldrup-Link, M.D.

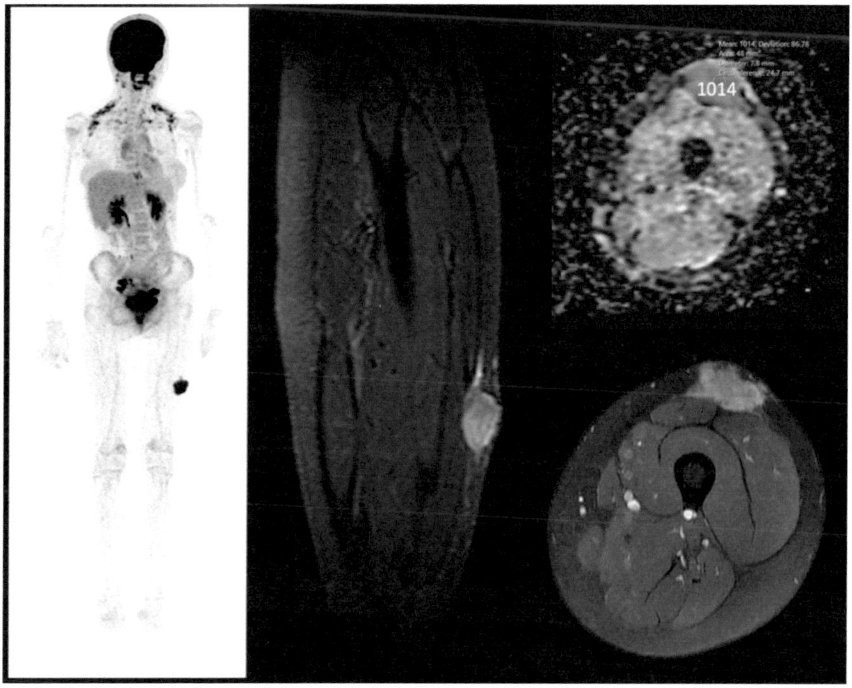

What is the most likely diagnosis:

a) Hemangioma
b) Fat Necrosis
c) Morel-Lavallée lesion
d) Soft Tissue Sarcoma

Case 93: Soft Tissue Sarcoma

a) Hemangiomas of the subcutaneous soft tissue would typically demonstrate a lobulated shape with visible flow voids and/or vessels on T1- and T2-weighted MRI scans. They would show high ADC values and moderate-low metabolic activity on 18F-FDG PET.

b) A fat necrosis of the thigh would present after a trauma as a localized lesion with fluid-equivalent signal on T2-weighted MRI, and multiple areas of fat-equivalent signal on fat-sensitive sequences. The lesion can demonstrate high metabolic activity on 18F-FDG PET but would not show restricted diffusion on DWI.

c) A Morel-Lavallée lesion is a post-traumatic fluid collection in the subcutaneous tissues composed of blood products, lymphatic fluid, and fat. It would not show contrast enhancement on contrast enhanced scans, and it would not show restricted diffusion on DWI.

d) Soft Tissue Sarcoma: Correct! The sagittal T2-weighted MRI and the axial contrast-enhanced T1-weighted MRI demonstrate a soft tissue mass in the subcutaneous soft tissues of the left thigh, which demonstrates ill defined borders with superior and inferior extensions and marked contrast enhancement. The lesion shows restricted diffusion with an ADC value around 1000 mm^2/s, which is indicative of a malignant tumor. The lesion also demonstrates marked 18F-FDG uptake on the positron emission tomography (PET) scan. In an adolescent patient, the most common diagnosis would be a soft tissue sarcoma. The histological diagnosis revealed a spindle cell sarcoma.

Patient 94: Seven-year-old with right ankle pain
Author: Marcello Chang, Michael F. Fadell, M.D.

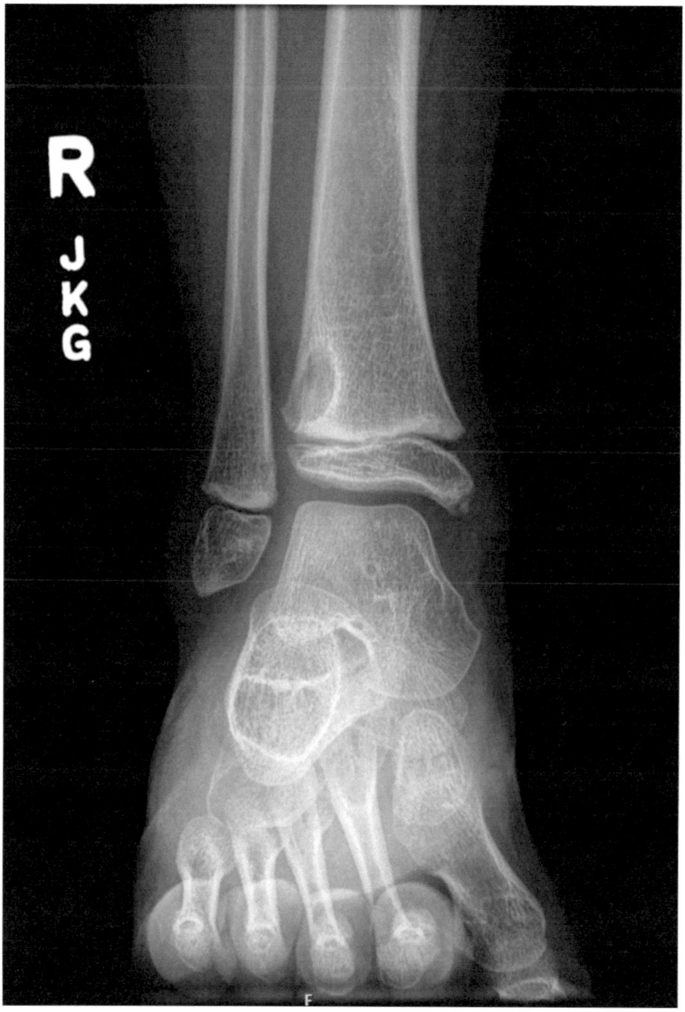

What is the most likely diagnosis:

a) Fibrous Dysplasia
b) Giant Cell Tumor
c) Aneurysmal Bone Cyst
d) Non-Ossifying Fibroma

Case 94: Non-Ossifying Fibroma (NOF)

a) Fibrous dysplasia may also contain hypo-intense fibrous tissue with well-defined borders but typically has a "ground glass" appearance and does not have the well-defined sclerotic border seen here. It may also become sclerotic over time.

b) A giant cell tumor (GCT) may present as a well-defined, eccentric radiolucent lesion. However, GCT typically do not have a sclerotic margin. They occur in patients with closed growth plates and extend into the epiphysis. They also may involve cortical breakthroughs and periosteal reactions.

c) An aneurysmal bone cyst typically presents as a single expansile, well-defined lucent bone lesion with thin sclerotic margin. A pathologic fracture is not uncommon.

d) Non-ossifying fibroma (NOF): Correct! The radiograph demonstrates a classical well-defined cortically based lucent lesion with thin sclerotic rim in the lateral aspect of the distal tibia. Additional supporting features include location in the metaphysis near the physis and long axis of the lesion parallel to the long axis of the bone. Note that NOFs may be polycyclic and multiloculated as well.
Non-ossifying fibromas are benign and generally self-limiting bone lesions estimated to occur in 30-40% of all normal children with a peak in the second decade. While the patient reported pain in the ankle region, the NOF is unlikely to be the cause. Be careful to look for other causes of pain. Note that NOFs are biologically active and can grow initially and become more polycyclic over time before beginning to regress. NOFs will usually remain in the same location, so they seem to migrate away from the physis over time in the growing bone.
NOFs are usually not seen beyond the age of 30 as they heal spontaneously after puberty and ossify gradually.

Patient 95: 10-year-old female with pain in the right leg

Authors: Marcello Chang, Michael F. Fadell, M.D.

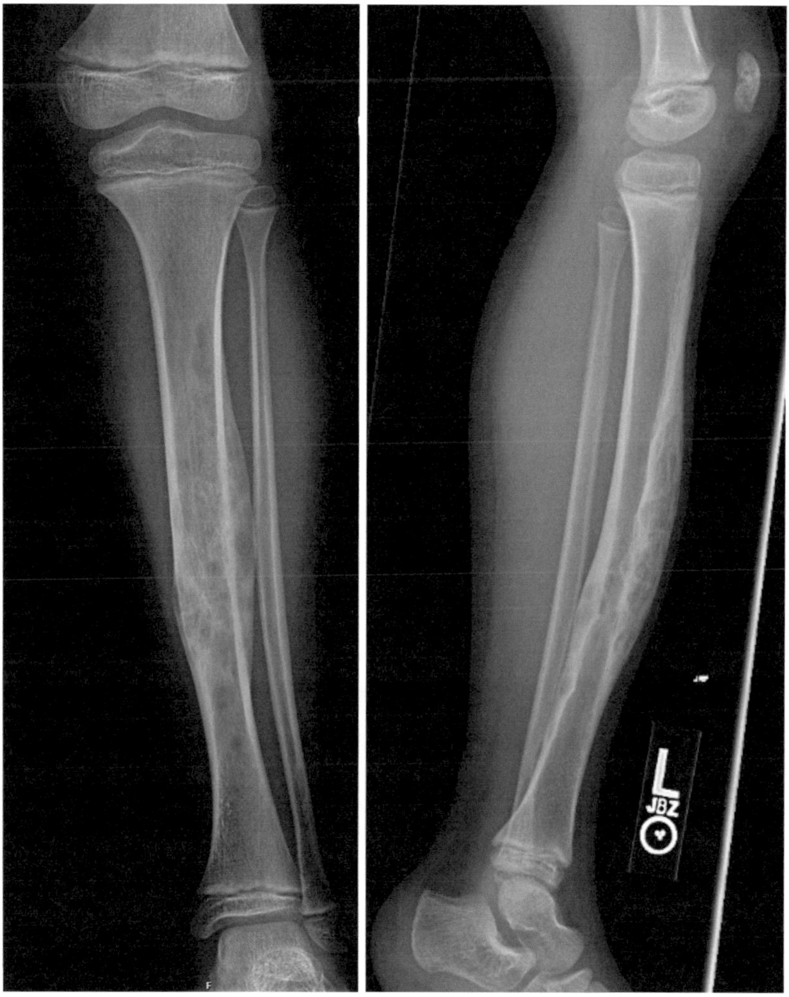

What is the most likely diagnosis:

a) Non-Ossifying Fibroma
b) Adamantinoma
c) Osteofibrous Dysplasia
d) Periosteal Osteosarcoma

Case 95: Osteofibrous Dysplasia

a) A non-ossifying fibroma is a cortically based eccentric lucent lesion with thin sclerotic rim in skeletally immature patients

b) An adamantinoma can demonstrate similar imaging features of an osteolytic cortical lesion in the tibial diaphysis which may have interspersed sclerosis. Compared to osteofibrous dysplasia, adamantinomas tend to be larger (>10 cm), have less distinct margins, and are more likely to involve the medullary cavity. Adamantinomas also tend to occur in patients in their 20s or 30s while osteofibrous dysplasia usually occurs before the age of ten. MRI can elicit additional information and serial radiographs can be obtained to evaluate for development of aggressive features, though biopsy may be required for definitive diagnosis in some cases.

c) Osteofibrous dysplasia: Correct! The radiographs demonstrate a lytic lesion which is centered in the cortex of the mid-diaphysis of the tibia. The proximal and distal ends of the lesion are centered in the cortex. The lesion demonstrates interspersed sclerosis and benign periosteal thickening without periosteal disruption. Note that an osteofibrous dysplasia may have a bubbly, ground glass or lucent internal matrix. Osteofibrous dysplasia is a benign fibrous bone lesion classically seen in the mid-diaphysis of the tibia. While the most common location is in the tibia, osteofibrous dysplasia may also occur in other long bones such as the fibula, humerus, radius, and ulna. Most cases will stop growing or regress with increasing age and can therefore be managed conservatively. However, larger, or symptomatic lesions may be managed with surgery.

d) A periosteal osteosarcoma arises from the periosteum and presents on radiographs as a broad-based lesion which causes extrinsic erosion and thickening of the underlying diaphyseal cortex. An associated periosteal reaction is common and typically demonstrates aggressive features such as a Codman triangle or a sunburst phenomenon.

Patient 96: 15-year-old patient with foot pain

Authors: Marcello Chang, Michael F. Fadell, M.D.

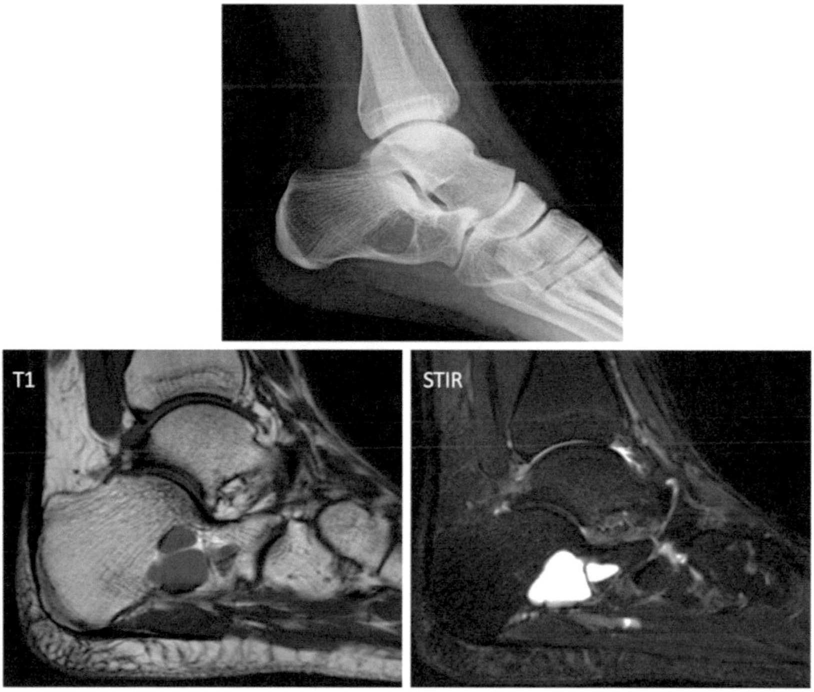

What is the most likely diagnosis:

a) Unicameral bone cyst
b) Intraosseous lipoma
c) Fibrous dysplasia
d) Giant Cell Tumor

Case 96: Unicameral Bone Cyst

a) Unicameral bone cyst: Correct! The radiograph shows a lytic lesion in the anterior body of the calcaneus with a narrow zone of transition and no appreciable matrix. There is no soft tissue involvement or periosteal reaction. The MRI of the ankle shows a well-defined homogeneous lesion with content that is hypointense to skeletal muscle on a T1 and hyperintense to muscle on a STIR sequence which is compatible with fluid. Additionally, fluid-fluid levels are present. Unicameral bone cysts are often asymptomatic, but they can also present with pain. They are typically found in the medullary space of the metaphysis of long bones, especially the humerus and the femur, however, may also occur in other bones like the calcaneus. Unicameral means "one chamber" and describes the single fluid-filled chamber in each cyst. There can be several cysts per lesion. Active cysts that are next to the growth plate, can expand over time and lead to pathological fractures. As the child grows the cysts tend to move away from the growth plate. Latent cysts located away from the growth plate are no longer growing and fill in with bone over time.

b) An intraosseous lipoma could show similar findings on ankle x-ray. However, the MRI would show fat equivalent T1-hyperintense and STIR hypointense signal, which is not seen here.

c) Fibrous dysplasia classically has a ground-glass appearance with cortical thinning due to the expansive nature of the lesion. Note that though ground-glass appearance is most common, cystic, or sclerotic appearances are also possible. The MR would show heterogeneous intermediate T1-signal and low T2-signal.

d) A giant cell tumor could appear similar on radiographs but would have solid components on MRI, potentially with surrounding bone marrow edema, soft tissue extension and hemorrhagic components.

Patient 97: 1-year old male, palpable mass in the left axillary
Author: Heike E. Daldrup-Link, M.D.

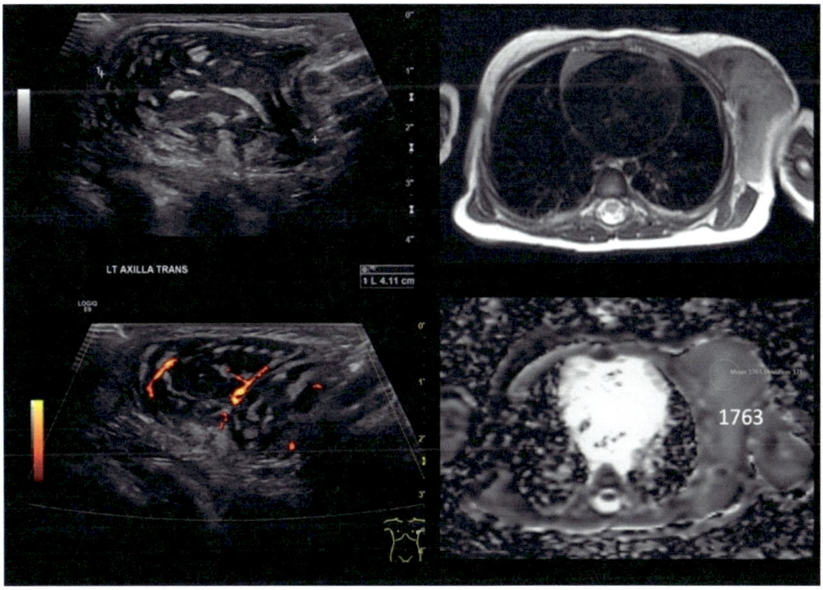

What is the most likely diagnosis:

a) Abscess
b) Rhabdomyosarcoma
c) Lymphoma
d) Fibrous Hamartoma of Infancy

Case 97: Fibrous Hamartoma of Infancy

a) An abscess would present as a fluid collection with a vascularized rim of granulation tissue. The lesion here is a soft tissue mass with internal flow on Doppler exam.

b) A rhabdomyosarcoma would typically present with markedly restricted diffusion and an ADC value of less than 1000 mm^2/second.

c) Lymphoma: A lymphoma would typically present at an older age. Lesions in the axillary would present as a lymph node conglomerate with markedly restricted diffusion and an ADC value of less than 1000 mm^2/second.

d) Fibrous Hamartoma of Infancy (FHI): Correct! The ultrasound shows a well-defined mass in the subcutaneous soft tissues of the left axillary with characteristic texture of serpentine hypoechoic and hyperechoic bands. Doppler ultrasound demonstrated minimal internal vascularity. The MRI demonstrates moderate signal of the lesion on T2-weighted MR images with limited restricted diffusion and a relatively high ADC value of 1763 mm^2/second, suggesting a benign lesion. Typical features of FHI include a single, solitary mass with internal components of macroscopic fat and serpentine bands of fibrous tissue. 20% of lesions can be congenital.

Patient 98: 2-year-old girl with palpable mass

Author: Heike E. Daldrup-Link, M.D.

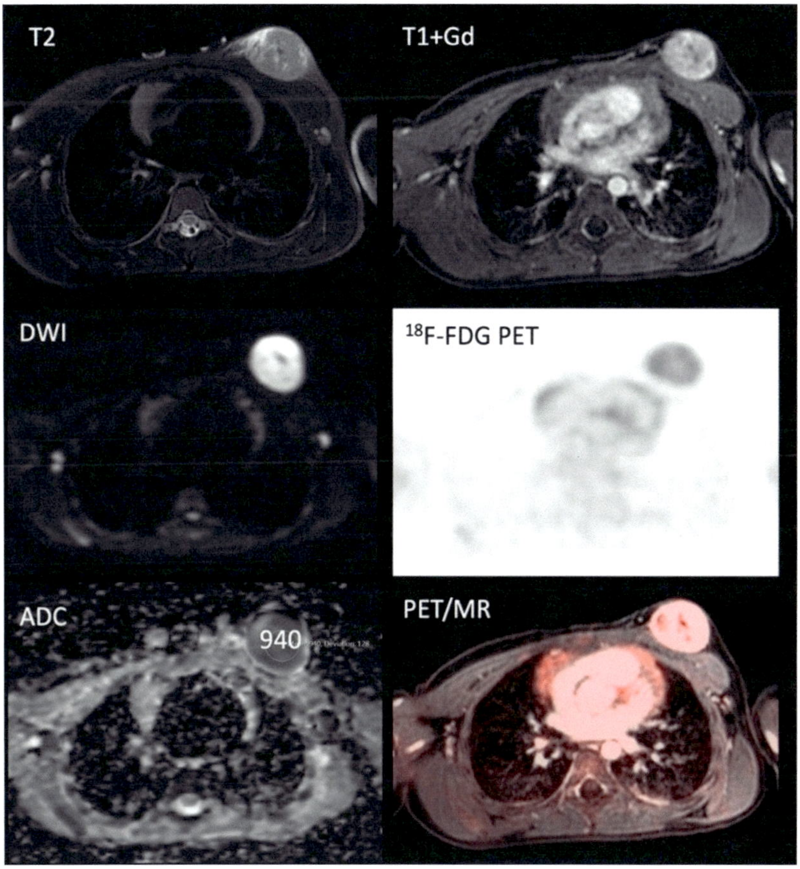

What is the most likely diagnosis:

a) Abscess
b) Rhabdomyosarcoma
c) Vascular Malformation
d) Fibrous Hamartoma of Infancy

Case 98: Rhabdomyosarcoma

a) An abscess would present as a fluid collection with high signal on T2-weighted images and a vascularized rim of granulation tissue on contrast-enhanced images. The lesion would only demonstrate peripheral uptake of 18F-FDG radiotracer on the PET scan.

b) Rhabdomyosarcoma: Correct! The MRI demonstrates a soft tissue mass in the subcutaneous soft tissues of the left breast with relatively low signal on T2-weighted images and restricted diffusion on diffusion-weighted MRI (DWI), suggesting a high cell density of the lesion. The ADC value is less than 1000 mm^2/second, suggesting a malignant tumor. This is further confirmed by uptake of 18F-FDG radiotracer on the PET scan.

c) A vascular malformation would demonstrate fluid-equivalent signal intensity on T2-weighted MR images and no restricted diffusion.

d) A fibrous hamartoma of infancy (FHI) would present as a subcutaneous mass with a relatively high ADC value of more than 1000 mm^2/second. Typical features of FHI include internal components of macroscopic fat and serpentine bands of fibrous tissue.

Patient 99: 17-year-old female with palpable mass
Author: Heike E. Daldrup-Link, M.D.

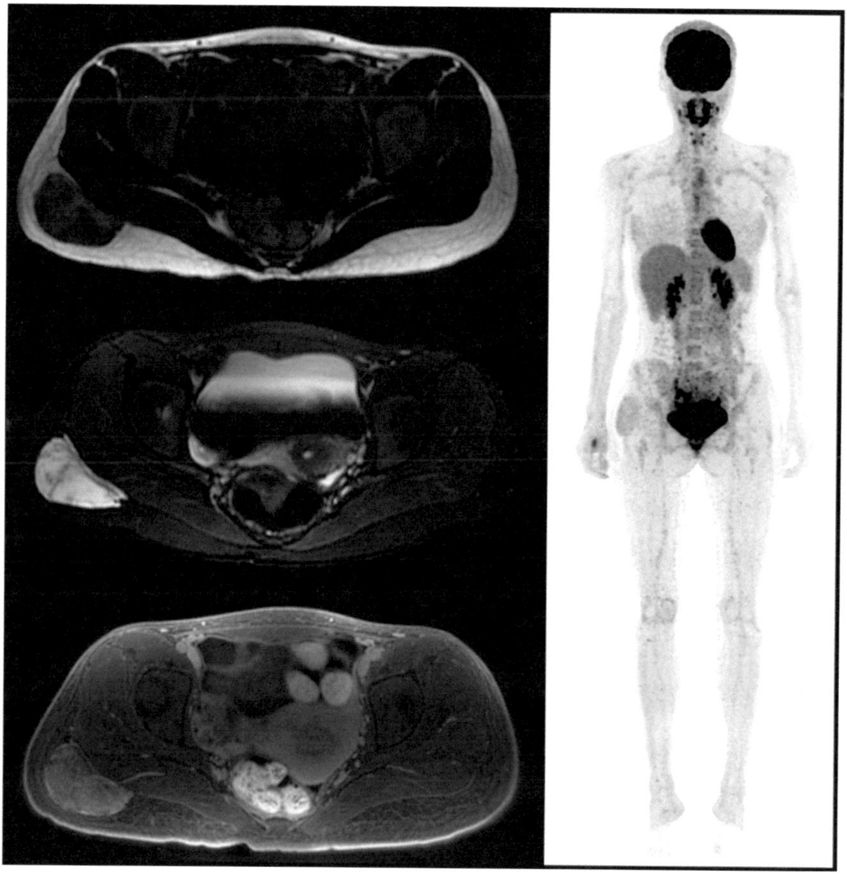

What is the most likely diagnosis:

a) Morel-Lavallée lesion
b) Myxoid Liposarcoma
c) Vascular Malformation
d) Gossypiboma

Case 99: Myxoid Liposarcoma

a) A Morel-Lavallée lesion is a post-traumatic fluid collection in the subcutaneous tissues composed of blood products, lymphatic fluid, and fat. It would not show contrast enhancement on contrast enhanced scans.

b) **Myxoid Liposarcoma: Correct! The axial fat-only MRI demonstrates a well-defined hypointense lesion in the subcutaneous fat above the right gluteus musculature, which contains macroscopic fat. The axial T2-weighted MRI demonstrate very high signal of the lesion and the axial contrast-enhanced T1-weighted MRI demonstrates marked contrast enhancement. The lesion shows minor 18F-FDG uptake on the positron emission tomography (PET) scan, consistent with a low-grade lesion. Taken together, the findings are consistent with a myxoid liposarcoma, as confirmed by histology**.

c) A vascular malformation of the subcutaneous soft tissue would typically demonstrate a lobulated shape with visible vascular structures and/or phleboliths on T1- and T2-weighted MRI scans. It would not contain macroscopic fat.

d) A gossypiboma refers to a retained sponge. Then term is derived from the Latin word "gossipium", which means "cotton" and the Swahili word "boma" which means "place of concealment". There is no history of surgery in this case. A retained sponge typically presents on MRI scans as a soft-tissue mass with a non-enhancing center and a well-defined thick rim of contrast-enhancing granulation tissue. The central sponge can demonstrate T2-hyper- or hypointense signal based on its fluid and cotton/foreign tissue composition.

Patient 100: 14-year-old male with right ankle pain

Author: Heike E. Daldrup-Link, M.D.

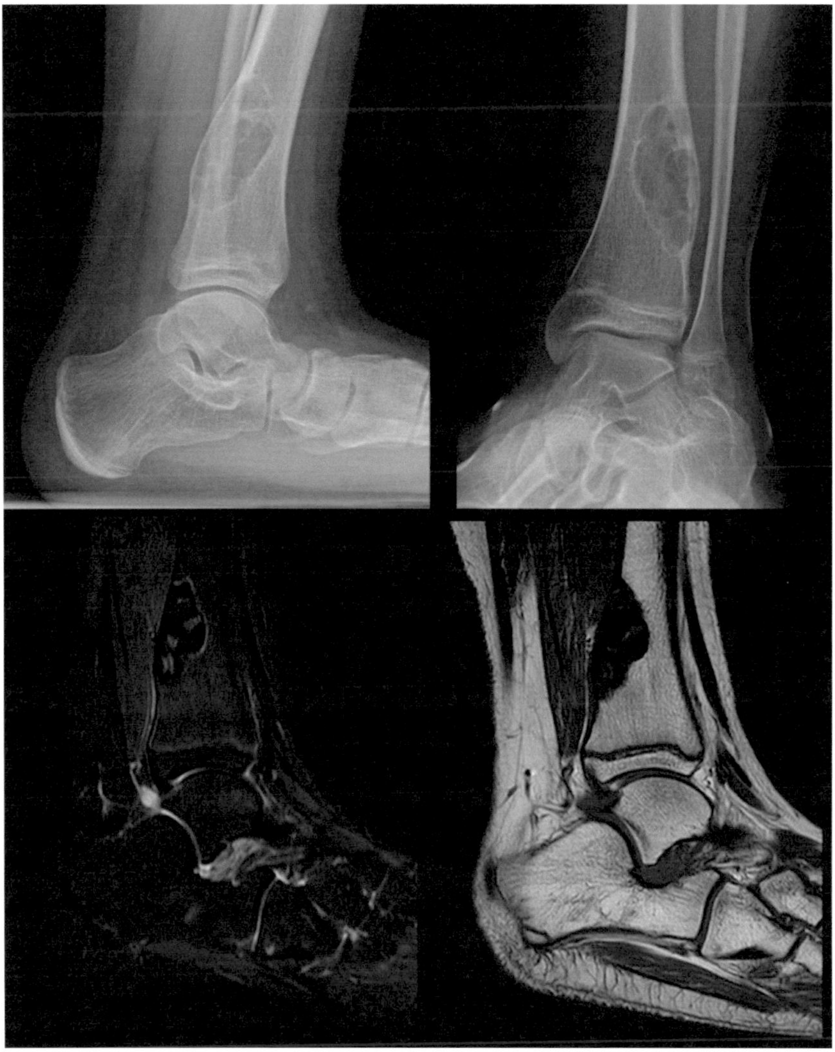

What is the most likely diagnosis:

a) Osteofibrous Dysplasia
b) Giant Cell Tumor
c) Non-Ossifying Fibroma
d) Aneurysmal Bone Cyst

Case 100: Non-Ossifying Fibroma (NOF)

a) An osteofibrous dysplasia presents as a lytic lesion which is centered in the cortex of the tibia. The proximal and distal ends of the lesion are centered in the cortex. The lesion demonstrates interspersed sclerosis and can demonstrate benign periosteal reactions.

b) A giant cell tumor (GCT) typically presents in patients with closed growth plates as a well-defined, radiolucent lesion in the epiphysis of long bones. GCT have a well-defined, non-sclerotic margin. Benign periosteal reactions may be noted.

c) Non-ossifying fibroma (NOF): Correct! The radiograph demonstrates a well-defined, lobulated eccentric lucent lesion in the distal tibial metaphysis. The lesion demonstrates a thin sclerotic rim. There is no periosteal reaction. The MRI demonstrates low signal of the lesion on T1-weighted and T2-weighted scans, consistent with a fibrous matrix and ossification. Note that NOF initially demonstrate high or intermediate T2 signal, with a thin hypointense rim. As the lesion matures and begins to ossify, the signal becomes low on all sequences as seen here. NOF are considered "do not touch" lesions. Most lesions do not require biopsy or follow up, because they have a characteristic imaging appearance, and they heal spontaneously. If a large NOF affects more than 50% of the underlying bone, then clinical follow up and/or orthopedic interventions may rarely be necessary.

d) An aneurysmal bone cyst (ABC) typically presents as a single expansile, well-defined lucent bone lesion with thin sclerotic margin. On MRI, an ABC would demonstrate hyperintense signal on T2-weighted MR images, with or without fluid-fluid levels.

Musculoskeletal, Spine, CNS

7) Trauma

Patient 101: 15-year-old teenager, inversion injury

Author: Heike E. Daldrup-Link, M.D.

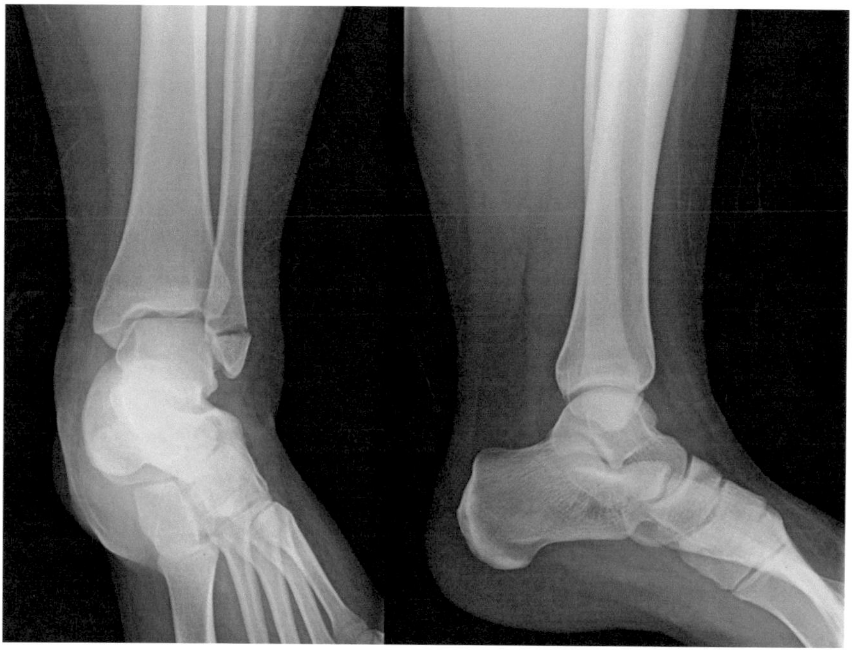

What is the most likely diagnosis:

a) Weber A Fracture
b) Weber B Fracture
c) Weber C Fracture
d) Tilleaux Fracture

Case 101: Weber A Fracture

a) Weber A Fracture (or Danis-Weber A fracture). Correct! The radiograph shows a non-displaced transverse fracture of the distal fibula below the level of the tibiofibular syndesmosis. The tibiofibular syndesmosis and the deltoid ligament are usually intact.

b) A Weber B fracture (or Danis-Weber B fracture) is defined as a fracture through the distal fibula at the level of the tibiofibular syndesmosis. This is often a spiral fracture. This fracture can be associated with injury of tibiofibular syndesmosis and deltoid ligament. It is important to check for widening of the tibiofibular joint and widening of the space between the medial malleolus and talus.

c) A Weber C fracture (or Danis-Weber C fracture) is defined as a fracture through the distal fibula above the level of the tibiofibular syndesmosis. This fracture can be associated with injury of tibiofibular syndesmosis and deltoid ligament.

d) A Tilleaux fracture refers to a fracture of the distal tibia in teenagers with partially closed growth plate, where the medial aspect of the growth plate is closed, and the lateral aspect of the growth plate is still open. The fracture line extends through the anterolateral aspect of the open physis and extends vertically into the epiphysis when it hits the closed part of the growth plate. Weber fractures can be associated with tibia fractures, most commonly fractures of the medial malleolus.

Patient 102: 5-month-old female, fall from couch at home

Author: Heike E. Daldrup-Link, M.D.

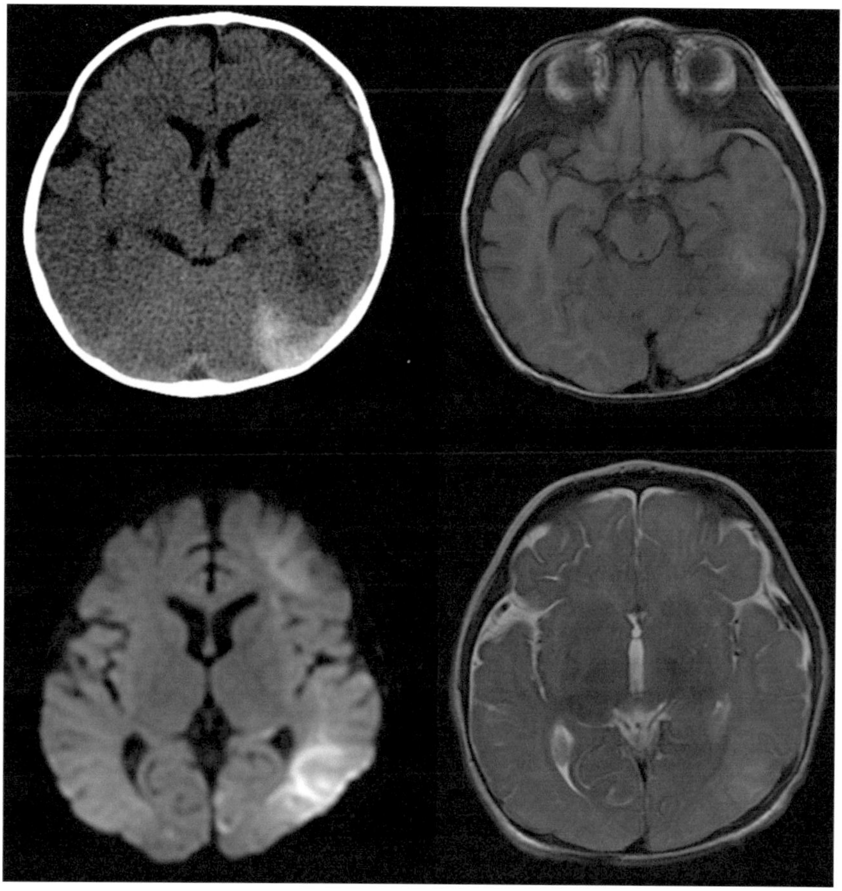

What is the most likely diagnosis:

a) Epidural hematoma
b) Nonaccidental Trauma
c) Bacterial Meningitis
d) MoyaMoya Disease

Case 102: Nonaccidental Trauma

a) An epidural hematoma presents as a biconvex extraaxial blood collection between the skull and dura, which grows over time. CT and MRI scans often show an associated skull fracture. High resolution MRI may show the displaced dura. The underlying injury is usually an arterial bleed, classically due to injury of the middle meningeal artery, which can cause significant mass effect on the brain and require urgent neurosurgical intervention.

b) Nonaccidental trauma: Correct! The axial CT scan shows a crescent shaped hyperdense hematoma over the entire left cerebral convexity and – to a lesser extent - the posterior right cerebral convexity. The hematoma also extends along the left tentorium. The axial T1- and T2-weighted MRI confirms a left sided subdural hematoma over the left frontal, temporal and occipital convexities. The subdural hematoma demonstrates T1-shortening and areas of T2-shortening, consistent with a subacute hemorrhage (2-7 days old). The diffusion weighted MRI demonstrates extensive restricted diffusion involving the subcortical white matter of the left cerebral hemisphere and more subtle signal changes in the posterior right cerebral hemisphere, suggestive of hypoxic ischemic injury. The described trauma does not match the extensive findings noted on the imaging studies. The patient also had subretinal hemorrhages on the ophthalmoscopic exam. Taken together, these findings are consistent with nonaccidental trauma.

c) Bacterial meningitis presents with sulcal effacement on CT and MRI studies, sulcal restricted diffusion on diffusion-weighted MRI and marked contrast-enhancement of the meninges.

d) Moyamoya disease is a vasculopathy which is best diagnosed on conventional, or MRI angiography based on different degree of stenosis and occlusions of large arteries of the anterior part of the Willis circle, and development of collateral vessels that produces a typical 'cloud of smoke' or 'puff of cigarette smoke' appearance.

Patient 103: Teenage male, football injury

Author: Heike E. Daldrup-Link, M.D.

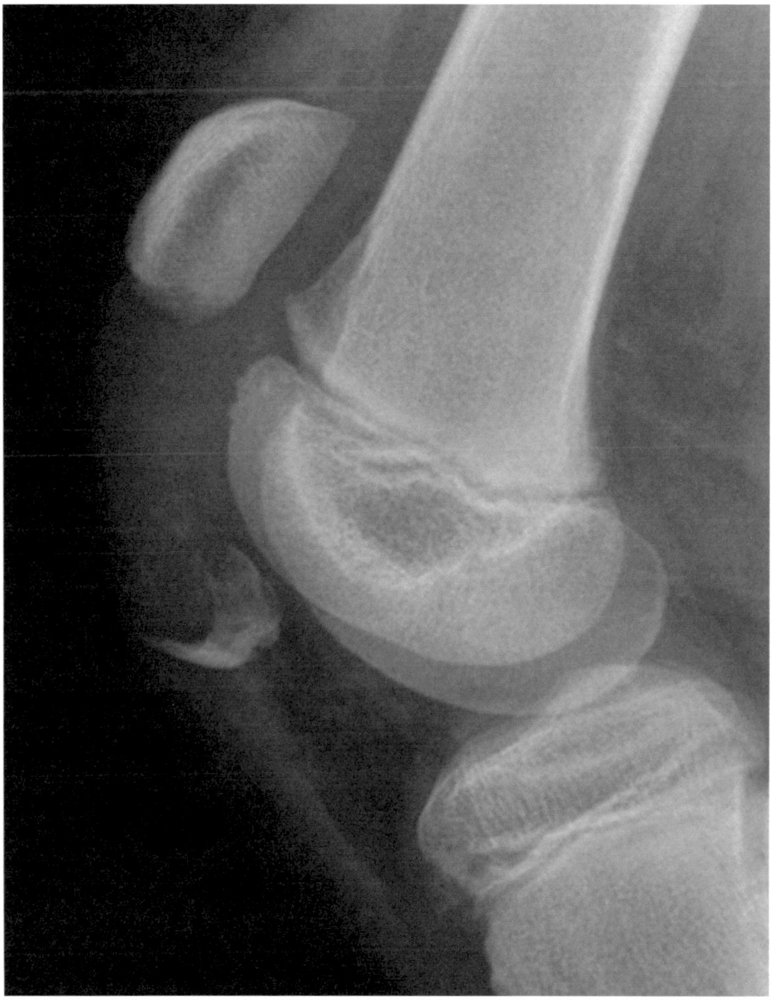

What is the most likely diagnosis:

a) Osgood-Schlatter Disease
b) Sinding Larsen Disease
c) Patella Sleeve Fracture
d) Quadriceps Tendon Rapture

Case 103: Patella Sleeve Fracture

a) Osgood Schlatter Disease is a lesion at the distal end of the patella tendon. Radiographs typically show fragmentation and soft tissue swelling at the proximal apophysis of the tibia.

b) Sinding Larsen Johannsson disease is characterized by thickening of the proximal patella tendon as a result of a chronic traction injury. Mild beaking and/or calcifications of the inferior patella might be seen.

c) Patella Sleeve Fracture: Correct! The radiograph shows a soft tissue swelling at the inferior pole of the patella and a curvilinear bone fragment in front of the distal femoral epiphysis, consistent with an acute osteochondral avulsion injury of the inferior pole of the patella.

d) A quadriceps tendon rapture is more commonly seen in adults and characterized by a soft tissue swelling above the patella and downward angulation of the patella.

Patient 104: 11-year-old teenager, fall on outstretched hand
Author: Heike E. Daldrup-Link, M.D.

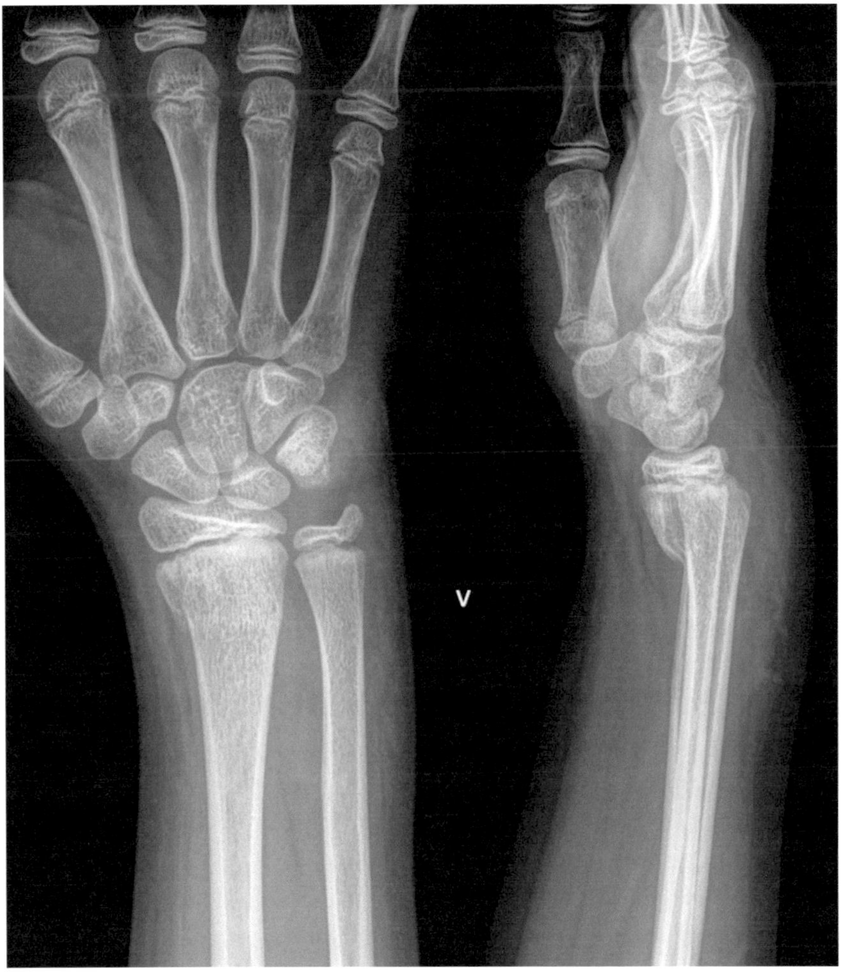

What is the most likely diagnosis:

a) Salter-Harris Type 1 Fracture
b) Salter-Harris Type 2 Fracture
c) Salter-Harris Type 3 Fracture
d) Salter-Harris Type 4 Fracture

Case 104: Salter-Harris Type 2 Fracture

a) A Salter-Harris type 1 fracture describes a fracture through the growth plate, not extending into the epiphysis or metaphysis.

b) Salter-Harris type 1 fracture. Correct! The radiograph shows a fracture through the growth plate of the distal radius, which extends into the metaphysis. Salter-Harris type II fractures are the most common physeal fractures that occur in children.

c) A Salter-Harris type 3 fracture is defined as a fracture through the growth plate, which extends into the epiphysis. This is an intra-articular fracture.

d) A Salter-Harris type 4 fracture is defined as a fracture through the metaphysis, growth plate and epiphysis. This is an intra-articular fracture.

All Salter-Harris fractures either involve or extend through the growth plates. Therefore, by definition, they only occur in children with open growth plates. There are five common types of Salter-Harris fractures. Type 1-4 are mentioned above. A Salter-Harris type 5 fracture is defined as a crush injury of the growth plate.
Various authors have described additional types of epiphyseal injuries: Rang et al. described a sixth type of an open injury that led to damage of the perichondral ring. Ogden et al. described nine types of injuries, adding four new types of epiphyseal injuries. However, these new types have received limited acceptance in most clinical practices.

Patient 105: Teenage soccer player
Author: Heike E. Daldrup-Link, M.D.

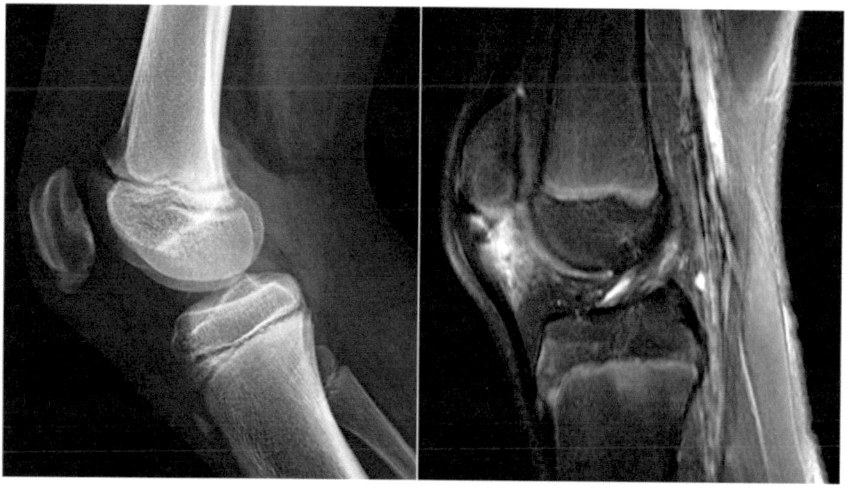

What is the most likely diagnosis:

a) Osgood-Schlatter Disease
b) Sinding Larsen Disease
c) Patella Sleeve Fracture
d) Quadriceps Tendon Rapture

Case 105: Sinding Larsen Johannsson Disease

a) Osgood Schlatter Disease is a lesion at the distal end of the patella tendon. Radiographs typically show fragmentation and soft tissue swelling at the proximal apophysis of the tibia.

b) Sinding Larsen Johannsson disease: Correct! The radiograph shows thickening of the proximal patella tendon as a result of a chronic traction injury. Mild beaking of the inferior patella is also seen. The T2-weighted MRI demonstrates marked edema of the proximal patella tendon.

c) A patella sleeve fracture presents with soft tissue swelling at the inferior pole of the patella and a curvilinear bone fragment in front of the distal femoral epiphysis as a result of an acute osteochondral avulsion injury of the inferior pole of the patella.

d) A quadriceps tendon rapture is more commonly seen in adults and characterized by a soft tissue swelling above the patella and downward angulation of the patella.

Patient 106: Twelve-year-old female with soccer injury

Author: Lisa Adams, M.D.

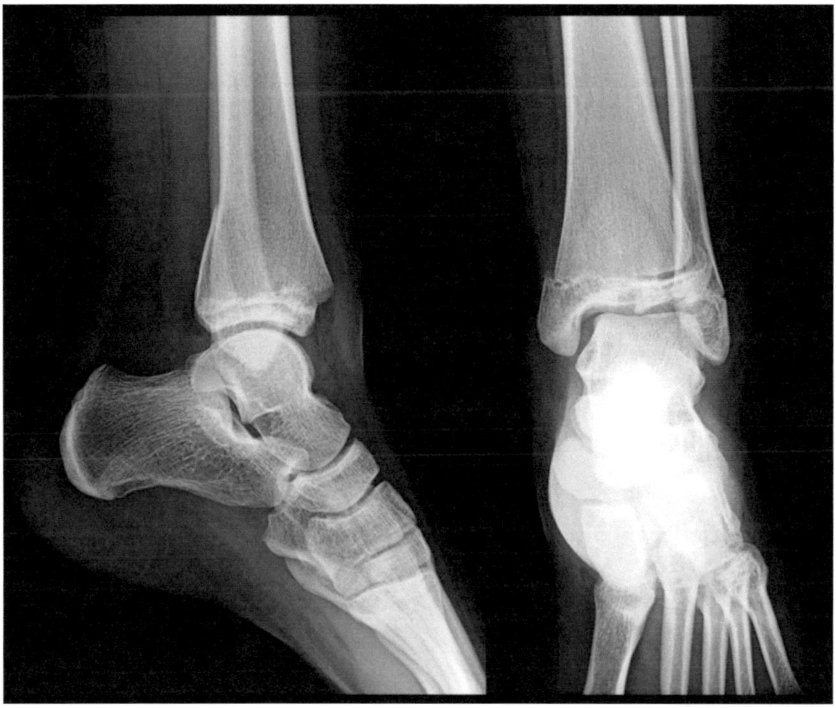

What is the most likely diagnosis:

a) Tillaux fracture
b) Salter Harris type II fracture
c) Triplane fracture
d) Calcaneal fracture

Case 106: Triplane fracture of the distal tibia

a) A Tillaux fracture is a two-part intraarticular fracture with involvement of the physis and the epiphysis (corresponding to a Salter-Harris type III fracture of the lateral part of the physis). The metaphysis is not involved.

b) A Salter Harris type II fracture is the most common pediatric physeal fracture. It involves a fracture through the growth plate and metaphysis. The epiphysis remains intact.

c) Triplane fracture of the distal tibia: Correct! The radiographs demonstrate an acute Salter-Harris type IV (triplane) fracture involving the distal tibia. There is a vertically oriented fracture of the tibial plafond with lateral distraction. The fracture line extends through the anterolateral aspect of the tibial physis resulting in physeal widening. On the oblique view, an obliquely oriented fracture of the distal tibia metaphysis is noted.

d) The radiographs show a normal calcaneus.

Patient 107: 16-year-old female, chronic ulnar sided wrist pain. History of fall on outstretched hand several years ago

Authors: Praveen Jayapal, M.D., Ali Rashidi, M.D.

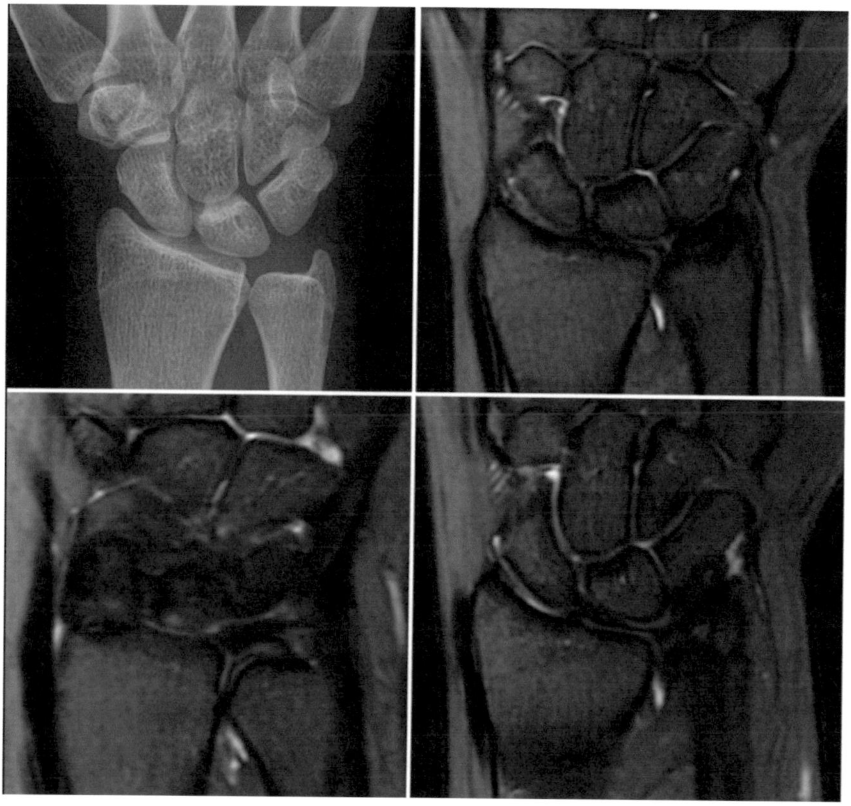

What is the most likely diagnosis:

a) Ulnocarpal abutment
b) Negative ulnar variance
c) Isolated effusion at the distal radioulnar joint (DRUJ)
d) Triangular fibrocartilage complex (TFCC) tear

Case 107: Triangular Fibrocartilage Complex (TFCC) Tear

a) Ulnocarpal abutment is incorrect since the ulnar variance is normal and there are no degenerative or cystic changes in the ulnar epiphysis, lunate or triquetrum.

b) Negative ulnar variance is incorrect. The relationship between distal radius and ulna is normal.

c) While there is a small effusion at the Distal Radioulnar Joint (DRUJ), this finding is secondary to a TFCC tear. The effusion alone does not directly explain the cause of the patient's pain.

d) Triangular fibrocartilage complex (TFCC) Tear: Correct! The patient has characteristic history and imaging findings of TFCC tear. The radiograph is normal. The coronal T2 weighted Fat saturated image demonstrates a focal 2 mm perforation in the triangular fibrocartilage disc proper. The MR images in the lower row demonstrate a normal dorsal and volar radioulnar ligament. There is a small effusion at the DRUJ (Distal Radioulnar Joint) which is a secondary finding.

The TFCC complex is composed of:

1. **Dorsal radioulnar ligament**
2. **Volar radioulnar ligament**
3. **Triangular fibrocartilage disc proper**
4. **Meniscal homologue**
5. **Extensor carpi ulnaris tendon sheath**
6. **Ulnocapitate, ulnolunate, ulnotriquetral and ulnocarpal collateral ligaments**

The triangular fibrocartilage disc proper is a triangular sheet-like structure interposed between the dorsal and volar radioulnar ligaments. Isolated tears involving this TFCC component are a common cause for ulnar sided wrist pain.

Patient 108: 9-year-old female, shoulder pain after bike injury
Author: Heike E. Daldrup-Link, M.D.

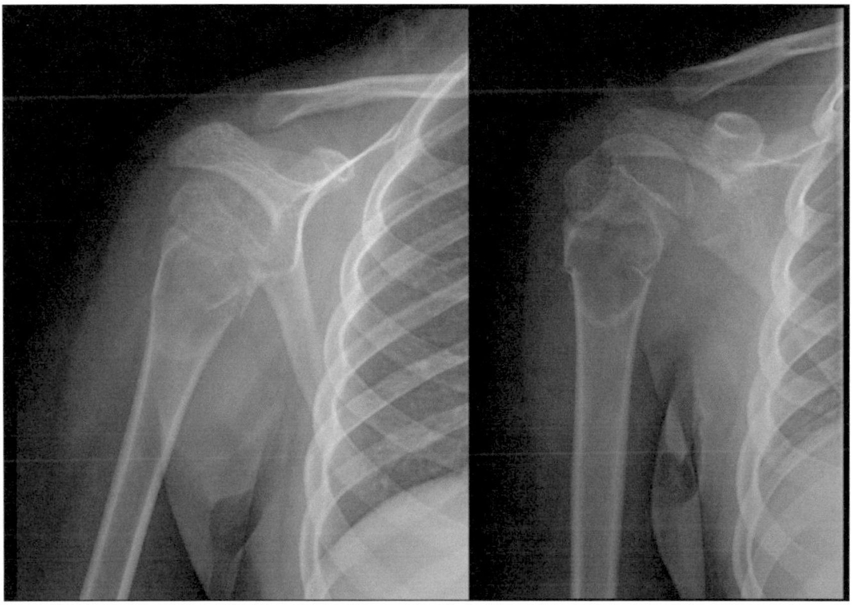

Which radiographic sign is seen here?

a) Lightbulb sign
b) Fallen fragment sign
c) Grey cortex sign
d) Rind sign

Case 108: Fallen Fragment Sign

a) The *lightbulb sign* describes a specific shape of the humeral head after a posterior shoulder dislocation. The humeral head rotates internally, which leads to a "light bulb" like appearance.

b) Fallen fragment sign: Correct! The radiograph shows a bone fracture fragment in the dependent portion of a well defined, expansile, lucent lesion in the proximal humeral metaphysis and diaphysis. There is a bilateral cortical break, consistent with an acute pathological fracture. The *fallen fragment sign* is pathognomonic of a fracture through a unicameral bone cyst. The bone fragment can descent through the cystic content of a bone cyst. It would not be able to descent through solid lesions, such as a fibrous dysplasia or an eosinophilic granuloma, which could be otherwise considered in the differential diagnosis of well-demarcated lucent bone lesions.

c) The *grey cortex sign* describes a subtle, ill-defined lucency at the site of a stress fracture.

d) The *rind sign* refers to a dense layer of sclerosis around a lucent bone lesion. In the pediatric population, it is suggestive of fibrous dysplasia.

Patient 109: Ten-year-old child with left elbow injury

Authors: Marcello Chang, Jayne Seekins, D.O.

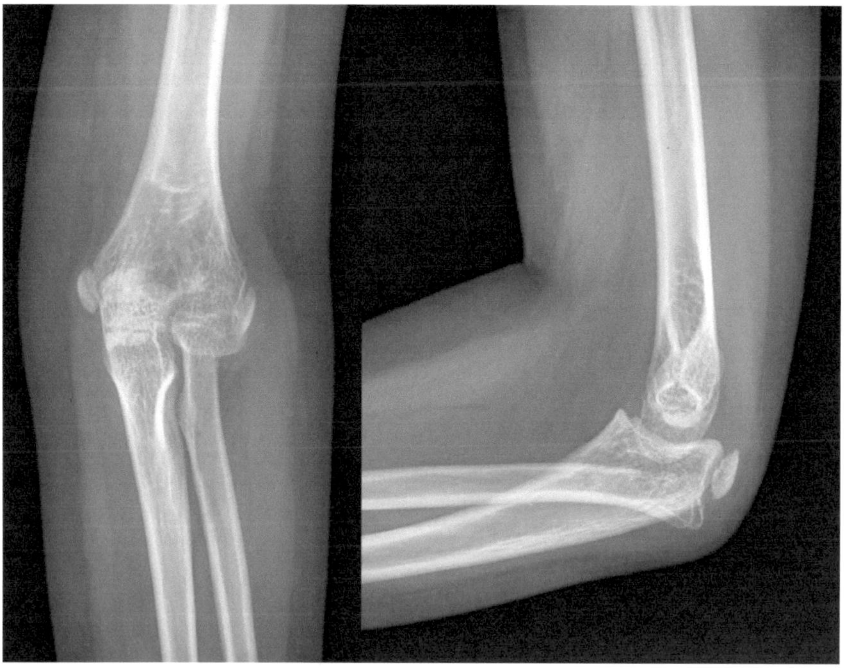

What is the most likely diagnosis:

a) Radial Head Subluxation
b) Bowing Deformity
c) Radial Head Dislocation
d) Incomplete Fracture

Case 109: Radial Head Dislocation

a) Radial head subluxation is a common elbow injury in young children where the radial head slips under the annular ligament without any osseous displacement or fracture. The patient is unable to supinate the forearm. Radiography usually is not required. But if an x-ray is obtained, it typically demonstrates minimal malalignment of the proximal radius without frank dislocation or fracture.

b) A bowing deformity of the radius or ulna present with a bending deformity of the bone on a radiograph. There is often no detectable fracture line or cortical defect of the bone. Note that the paired bone (e.g., ulna or radius) besides the bone with the bowing deformity can have an associated non-bowing fracture.

c) Dislocation of the radial head: Correct! The frontal and lateral radiograph of the elbow shows a posterior dislocation of the left radial head away from the capitellum. Instead, the radial head is now abutting the left olecranon apophysis. A line drawn along the shaft of the radial neck does not intersect with the capitellum, consistent with a malalignment of the radiocapitellar line. Dislocation of the radial head typically requires open reduction.

d) Incomplete fractures can present on conventional radiographs with a focal deformity of the bone cortex, usually without displacement or discrete fracture line, classically at the distal radial metaphysis.

Patient 110: Adolescent female with soccer injury

Author: Heike E. Daldrup-Link, M.D.

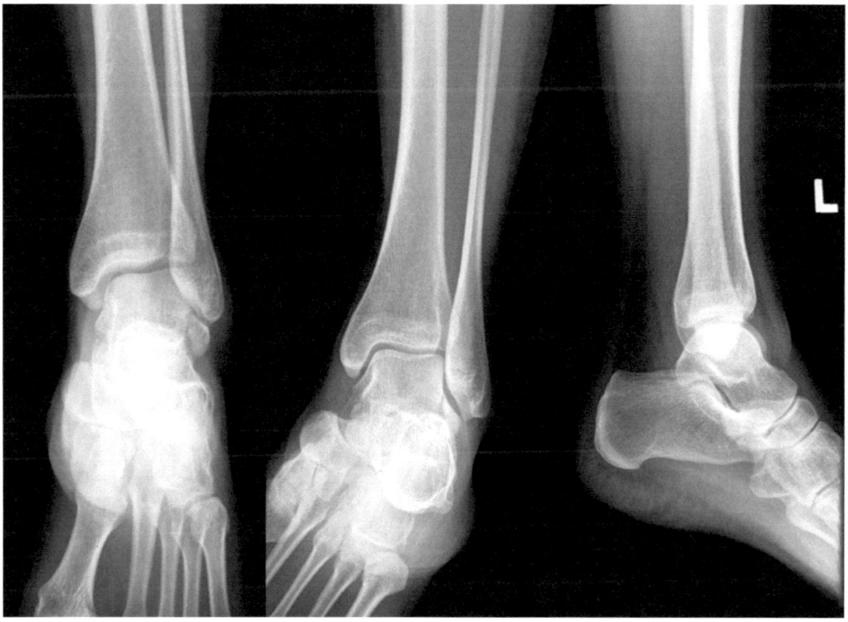

What is the most likely diagnosis:

a) Tilleaux Fracture
b) Talus Fracture
c) Calcaneus Fracture
d) Os Trigonum

Case 110: Lateral Talus Fracture

a) A Tilleaux fracture of the distal tibia occurs in teenagers with partially closed growth plate, where the medial aspect of the growth plate is closed, and the lateral aspect of the growth plate is still open. The fracture line extends through the open anterolateral physis. When it hits the closed part of the growth plate, it extends downwards into the epiphysis

b) Talus Fracture: Correct! The frontal and lateral radiograph of the left ankle shows a fracture through the lateral talus with an associated joint effusion.

c) There is no fracture of the calcaneus noted on this radiograph.

d) An os trigonum represents an accessory ossicle posterior to the talus.

Patient 111: Two-year-old male, leg pain

Author: Heike E. Daldrup-Link, M.D.

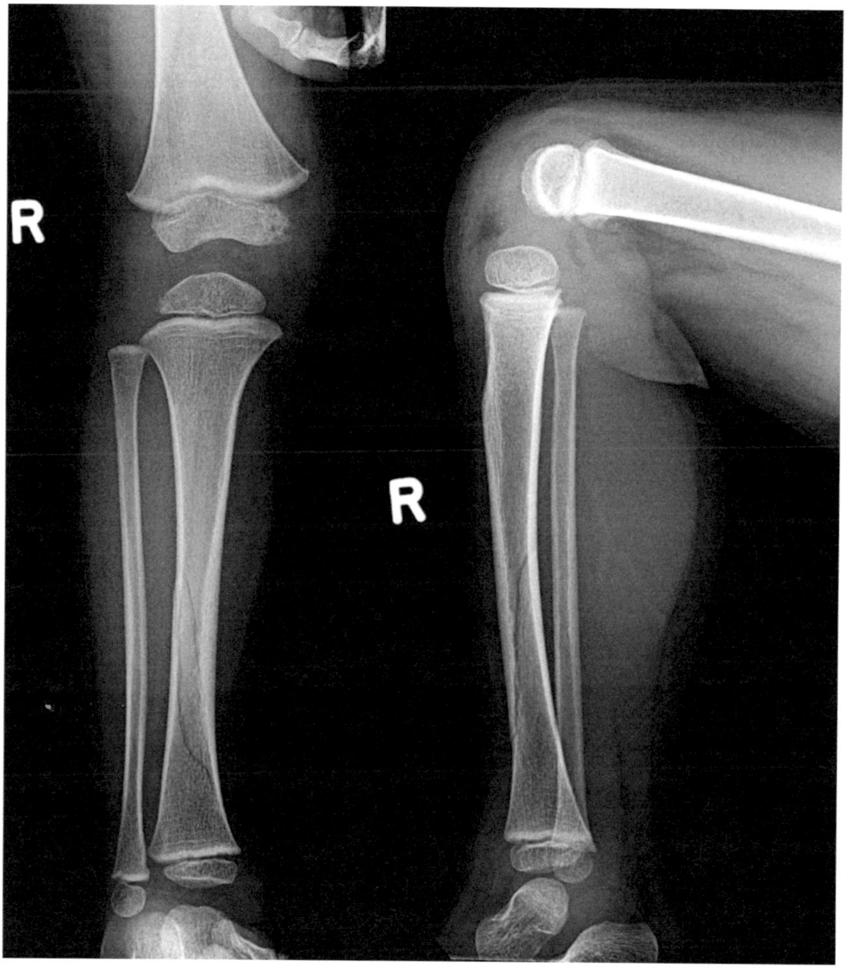

What is the most likely diagnosis:

a) Tilleaux Fracture
b) Toddler's Fracture
c) Weber Fracture
d) Maisoneuve fracture

Case 111: Lateral Talus Fracture

a) A Tilleaux fracture of the distal tibia occurs in teenagers with partially closed growth plate, where the medial aspect of the growth plate is closed, and the lateral aspect of the growth plate is still open. The fracture line extends through the open anterolateral physis. When it hits the closed part of the growth plate, it extends downwards into the epiphysis

b) Toddlers Fracture: Correct! The frontal and lateral radiograph of the left leg shows a non-displaced spiral fracture through the shaft of the right tibia. The fracture typically occurs in young children (age 1-3 years) when the foot is trapped somewhere and the leg twists around its long axis while the child is tripping/falling.

c) A Weber fracture refers to a fracture of the fibula below the level of the tibiofibular syndesmosis (Weber A), at the level of the syndesmosis (Weber B) or above the level of the syndesmosis (Weber C).

d) A Maisoneuve fracture refers to a fracture of the proximal fibula plus an injury of the tibiofibular syndesmosis with widening of the medial ankle joint space. The condition can be also associated with a fracture of the medial malleolus.

Patient 112: 16-year-old male with hip pain

Author: Heike E. Daldrup-Link, M.D.

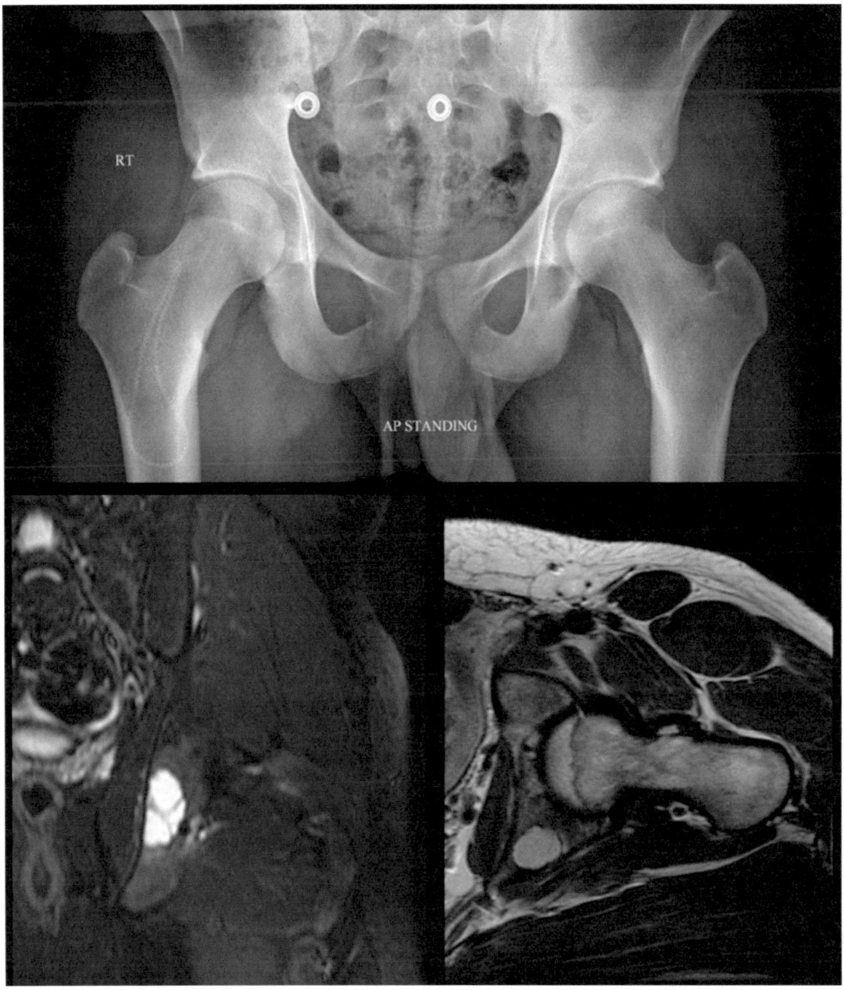

What is the most likely diagnosis:

a) Unicameral Bone Cyst
b) Giant Cell tumor
c) Chondroblastoma
d) Langerhans Cell Histiocytosis

Case 112: Unicameral Bone Cyst

a) Unicameral bone cyst (UBC): Correct! The radiograph shows a well-circumscribed lytic bone lesion in the left ischium with a narrow zone of transition and thin sclerotic margin. On the MRI, the lesion shows fluid-equivalent signal. UBCs can contain fibrous septations, as seen here. UBCs are most found in the proximal long bones. A location in the pelvis is unusual.

b) A giant cell tumor would be more common older patients with closed growth plates. Giant cell tumors do not usually have a sclerotic rim (although few cases with sclerotic rim have been described).

c) A chondroblastoma presents as a lytic lesion with thin sclerotic margin and a narrow zone of transition. Chondroblastomas are most located in the epiphyses of long bones. They do not show an associated periosteal reaction. The MRI scan shows a well-defined T2-hyperintense, heterogenous lesion with characteristic extensive bone marrow edema.

d) Langerhans cell histiocytosis. While this would be a potential differential diagnosis, the sclerotic rim and fluid-equivalent MRI signal would be unusual.

Patient 113: Four-year old female, bike accident

Author: Heike E. Daldrup-Link, M.D.

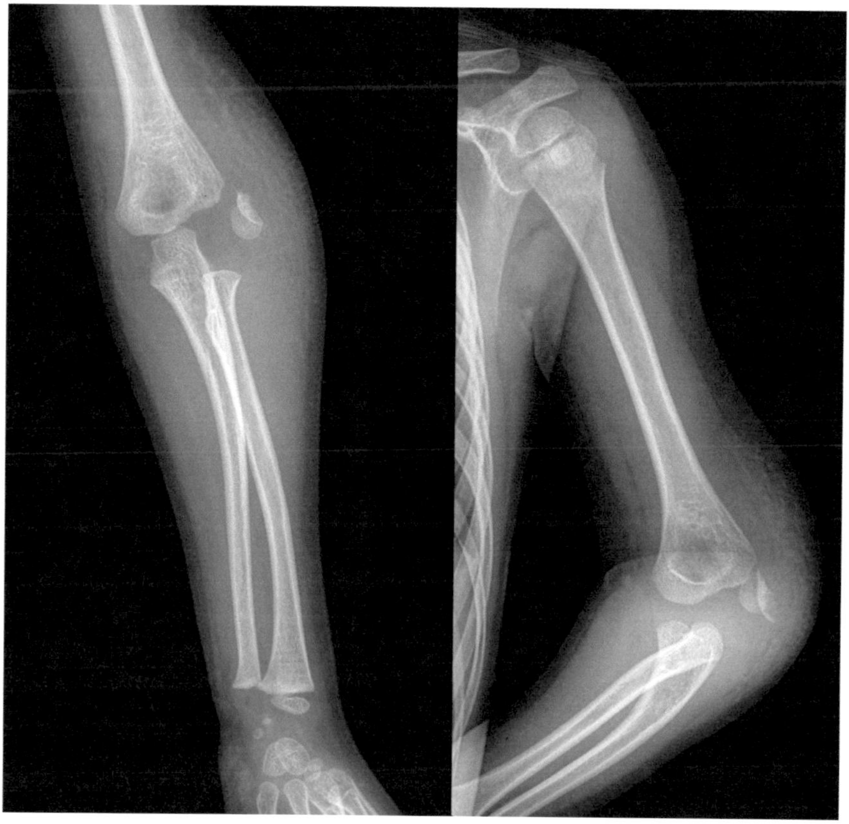

What is the most likely diagnosis:

a) Medial epicondyle avulsion fracture
b) Radial head fracture
c) Lateral epicondyle avulsion fracture
d) Olecranon fracture

Case 113: Lateral Epicondyle Avulsion Fracture

a) The medial epicondyle is normal.

b) The ossification center of the radial head is not yet ossified. Remember the mnemonic CRITOE for the ossification centers of the elbow: C – capitellum, R – radial head, I – internal epicondyle, T - trochlea, O – olecranon, E – external epicondyle. In this patient, only the ossification center of the capitellum is ossified.

c) Lateral epicondyle fracture: Correct! The radiograph shows an avulsion fracture of the lateral epicondyle and lateral displacement of the ossification center of the capitellum. The fracture line likely extends through the cartilaginous epiphysis.

d) The olecranon is normal.

Patient 114: 13-year-old female, foot pain

Author: Heike E. Daldrup-Link, M.D.

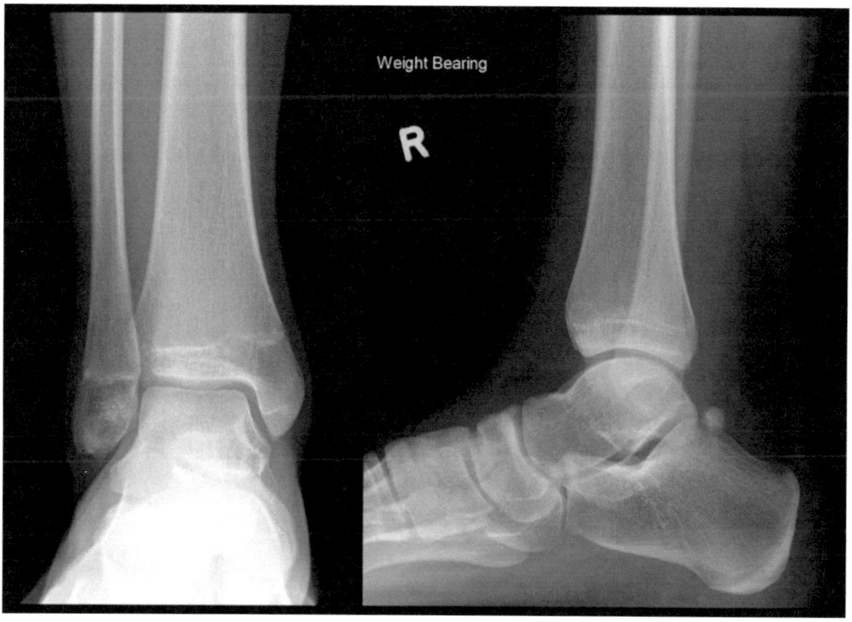

What is the most likely diagnosis:

a) Talus fracture
b) Os subtibiale
c) Calcaneus fracture
d) Os trigonum

Case 114: Os Trigonum

a) The talus is normal.

b) An os subtibiale is an accessory ossicle that is located below the medial malleolus of the tibia.

c) The calcaneus is normal.

d) Os trigonum: Correct! The radiograph shows a well corticated accessory ossicle posterior to the talus, an os trigonum. It can be associated with posterior ankle impingement syndrome.

Patient 115: 7-year-old female, bike accident
Author: Heike E. Daldrup-Link, M.D.

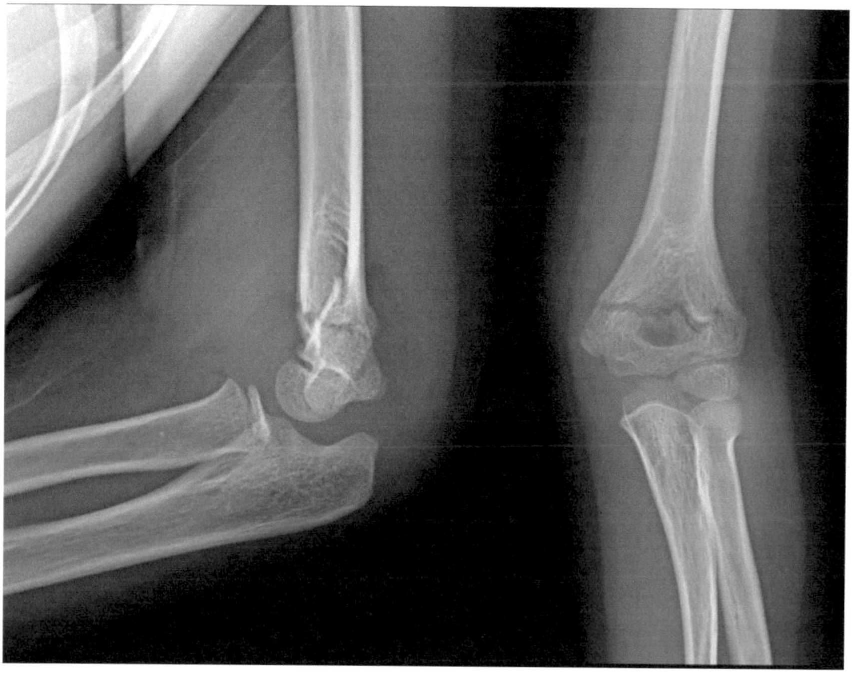

What is the most likely diagnosis:

a) Medial epicondyle fracture
b) Radial neck fracture
c) Lateral epicondyle fracture
d) Supracondylar humerus fracture

Case 115: Supracondylar Humerus Fracture

a) The medial epicondyle is normal.

b) The proximal radius is normal. There is no kinking/irregularity of the radial neck. The ossification center of the proximal radius is well centered towards the capitellum.

c) The lateral epicondyle is normal.

d) Supracondylar humerus fracture: Correct! The lateral radiograph shows a fracture line through the distal humerus with posterior angulation of the distal humerus/capitellum compared to the more proximal shaft of the humerus. The anterior humeral line passes through the anterior third rather than the middle third of the capitellum. In addition, there is an elevated anterior fat pad and an elevated posterior fat pad, consistent with an accompanying elbow joint effusion. Note that lateral radiographs of the elbow in young children are often taken by elevating the arm above the head (with flexed elbow). This was not possible in this patient due to pain. The frontal radiograph demonstrates a transverse fracture line through the distal humerus.

Remember the mnemonic CRITOE for the ossification centers of the elbow: C – capitellum, R – radial head, I – internal epicondyle, T - trochlea, O – olecranon, E – external epicondyle.

Musculoskeletal, Spine, CNS

8) Metabolic, endocrine, and toxic

Patient 116: Young woman, treated lymphoma, now hip pain
Author: Heike E. Daldrup-Link, M.D.

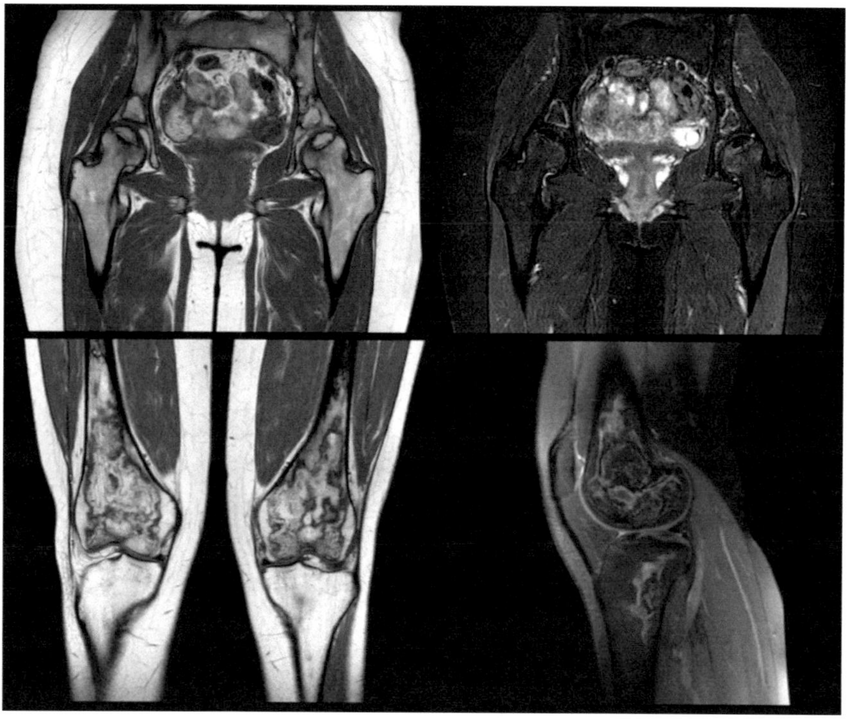

What is the most likely diagnosis?

a) Leg Calve Perthes disease
b) Bone marrow metastases
c) Osteonecrosis
d) Chronic recurrent multifocal osteomyelitis (CRMO)

Case 116: Osteonecrosis

a) Perthes disease could lead to avascular necrosis of the hip joint. It would typically present with flattening of the femoral epiphysis in a younger child, before closure of the growth plates. Perthes disease would not cause any changes of the lower femur.

b) Metastases would more commonly present as focal lesions in the bone marrow with T1-hypointense and T2-hyperintense signal (or T1- and T2-hypointense sclerotic lesions), rather than serpiginous lines with a fatty center seen here.

c) Osteonecrosis: Correct! The The T1-weighted (left) and T2-weighted (right) MRI of the hip joints shows lesions in the proximal epiphyses of the bilateral femur with a central area of fatty marrow conversion and a characteristic "double line sign": an inner brighter line representing reparative granulation tissue and an outer dark line representing adjacent sclerotic bone. There are also similar lesions noted in the lower ilium and ischium bilaterally. The T1-weighted (left) and T2-weighted (right) MRI of the lower femur and proximal tibia demonstrates additional bone infarcts in the bilateral the lower femur and proximal tibia. This patient had been treated with high dose corticosteroids. Note that osteonecrosis is the umbrella term for avascular necrosis (which affects the epiphyses and specifically the hip joints) and bone infarcts (affecting other bone areas).

d) Chronic recurrent multifocal osteomyelitis (CRMO) presents with bone marrow edema, periostitis and bone sclerosis. It does not typically present with bone infarcts.

Patient 117: Hospitalized infant, painful swelling of the hand and forearm

Author: Heike E. Daldrup-Link, M.D.

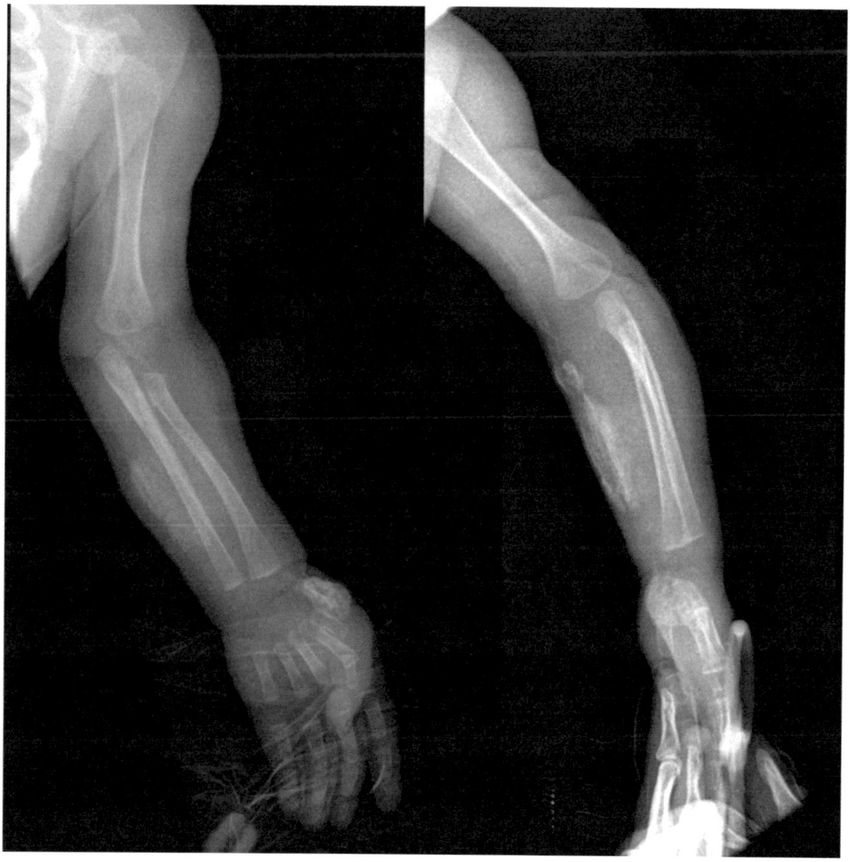

What is the most likely diagnosis:

a) Non-accidental trauma
b) Calcium Gluconate Extravasation
c) Teratoma
d) Scleroderma

Case 117: Calcium Gluconate Extravasation

a) Non-accidental trauma can present with fractures of different ages. Soft tissue bruises and hematomas can also occur. However, the calcifications shown here follow the distribution of the brachial vein.

b) Calcium gluconate extravasation: Correct! The radiograph of the left arm demonstrates calcifications in the subcutaneous soft tissues of the left hand and left forearm, with linear calcifications extending superiorly along the brachial vein. Calcium gluconate is administered on neonatal wards and intensive care units to correct hypocalcemia. Extravasation is a medical emergency, which can lead to severe tissue necrosis. Soft tissue calcifications develop in the affected areas over several days or weeks and can gradually resolve over time.

c) Teratomas are most found in the ovaries, testes, mediastinum and sacrococcygeal region. In principle, they can occur anywhere in the body, but a location in the hand and forearm would be exceedingly rare. Non-seminomatous germ cell tumors (NSGCT) can metastasize everywhere in the body and metastases into the extremities have been described, causing growing calcified masses. The absence of a cancer history and presence of linear calcifications along the brachial vein make this diagnosis unlikely.

d) Scleroderma typically manifests in adolescents or young adults. Juvenile systemic scleroderma can affect children, but it is extremely rare in early childhood. Radiographic manifestations can include irregularly shaped calcific densities in the subcutaneous soft tissues, often around articular joints. However, the calcifications shown here follow the distribution of the brachial vein.

Patient 118: Two-week old child

Author: Heike E. Daldrup-Link, M.D.

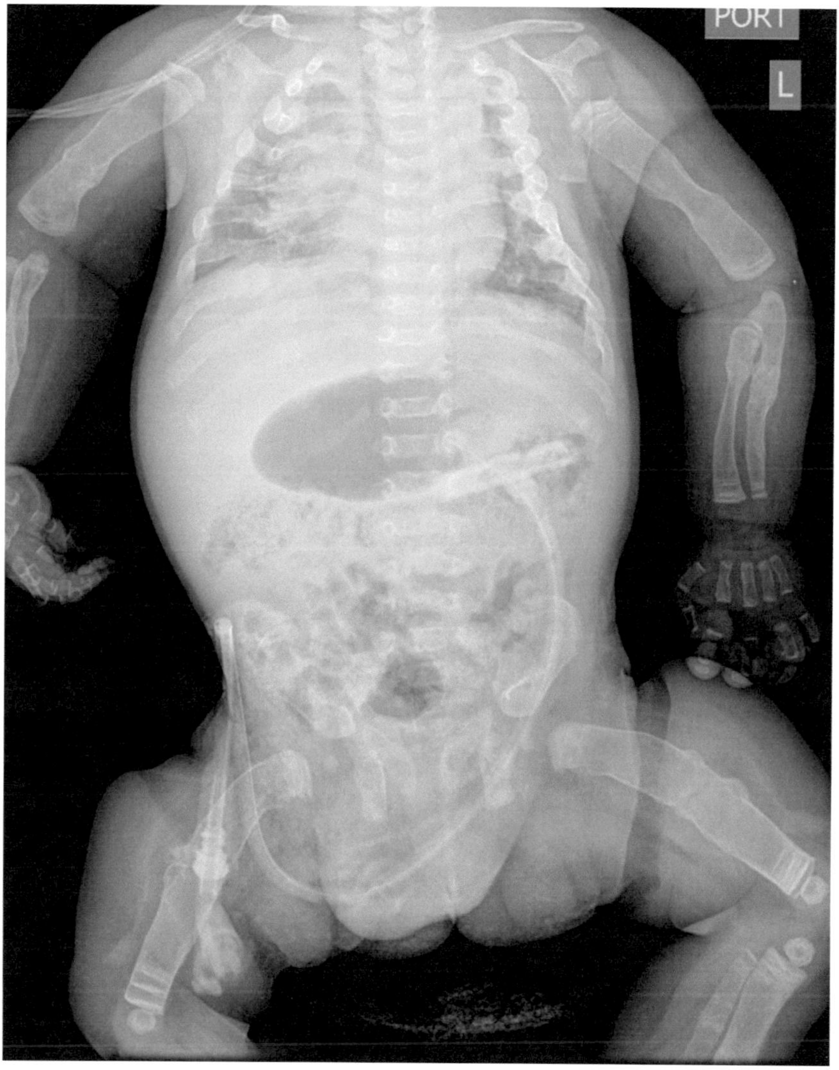

What is the most likely diagnosis:

a) Non-accidental trauma
b) Rickets
c) Osteogenesis Imperfecta
d) Menkes syndrome

Case 118: Osteogenesis Imperfecta

a) Non-accidental trauma can present with fractures of different ages. However, the radiograph shown here demonstrates an additional, markedly decreased bone density.

b) Rickets usually presents in older children, although neonatal forms have been described. While radiographs can also show a generally decreased bone density, there are additional findings such as irregular fraying of the provisional zone of calcification of the distal metaphyses of long bones, which are not seen here.

c) Osteogenesis Imperfecta. Correct! The radiograph shows a markedly decreased bone density and multiple fractures of the ribs and long bones. The fractures of the humerus and femur have led to bone deformities. The fractures demonstrate different degrees of callus formation, indicative of different ages.

d) Menkes syndrome is an x-linked recessive disorder which is associated with metaphyseal and diaphyseal bone fractures. The patients typically have associated neurological symptoms.

Patient 119: Two-month-old female

Author: Heike E. Daldrup-Link, M.D.

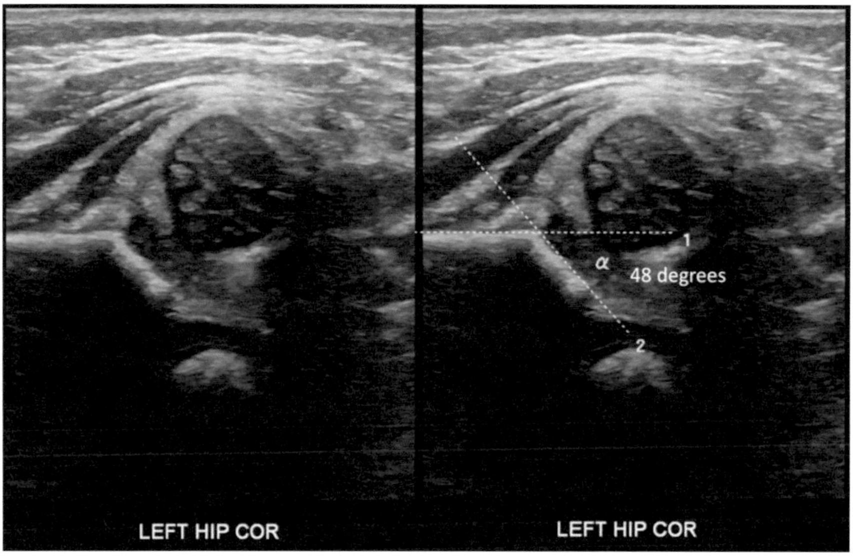

What is the most likely diagnosis:

a) Hip Effusion
b) Normal Hip Ultrasound
c) Developmental Dysplasia
d) Immature Hip

Case 119: Developmental Dysplasia of the Hip

a) A hip joint effusion would present with hypoechogenic fluid in the joint space. An US examination along the long axis of the femoral head would show the anterior joint capsule as a hyperechogenic band between the anterior surface of the femoral neck and the fascial layer of the iliopsoas muscle. A joint effusion would be best noted in the the anterior recess of the joint capsule.

b) The images shown here are not normal.

c) **Developmental Dysplasia of the Hip (DDH): Correct! The ultrasound shows a shallow acetabulum with decreased acetabular angle, less than 50% coverage of the cartilaginous femoral head and lateral luxation of the femoral head.**

d) An immature hip is defined as a hip joint with an alpha angle of 50-59 degrees in an infant less than 3 months of age (physiological immature hip) or more than 3 months of age (pathological immature hip, requires treatment).

Sonographic classification of DDH according to Graf:

Type	alpha angle	beta angle	Description
I	≥ 60°	< 50°	Normal Hip
IIa	50-59°	55-77°	< 3 months of age, physiological immature hip, appropriate for age
IIb	50-59°	55-77°	> 3 months of age, pathological immature hip, requires treatment
IIc	43-49°	< 77°	Centered hip, dysplastic, unstable
IId	43-49°	≥ 77°	Decentered hip
III	< 43°	≥ 77°	Dislocated femoral head
IV	< 43°	≥ 77°	Dislocated femoral head, inverted labrum (labrum pressed downwards)

Patient 120: Child with Hip Pain

Author: Heike E. Daldrup-Link, M.D.

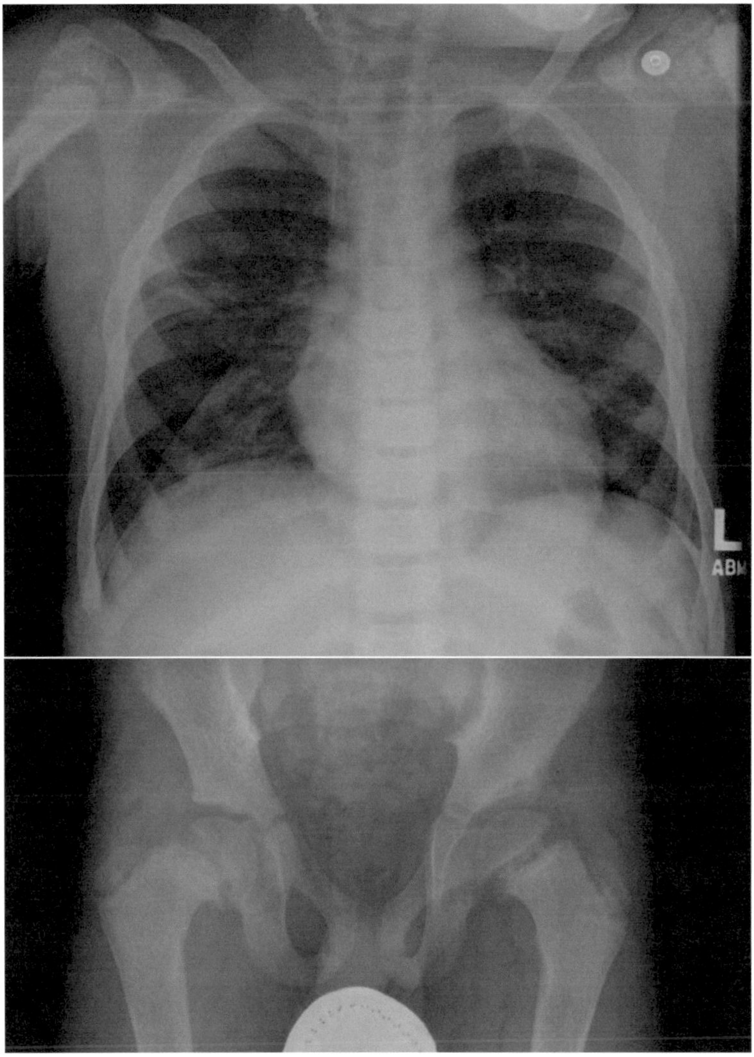

What is the most likely diagnosis:

a) Rickets
b) Osteogenesis Imperfecta
c) Secondary Hyperparathyroidism
d) Osteopetrosis

Case 120: Secondary Hyperparathyroidism

a) Rickets usually presents with diffusely decreased bone density, broadening and irregular fraying of the provisional zone of calcification of the metaphyses of the long bones. Fraying is usually more prominent in the distal compared to the proximal metaphyses. Chest x-rays may demonstrate broadening of the anterior ends of the ribs, the so-called "rachitic rosary".

b) Osteogenesis imperfecta would present with diffuse osteopenia and pathological fractures. The radiographs here demonstrate coarse, dense bones.

c) Secondary Hyperparathyroidism due to renal osteodystrophy. Correct! The radiographs here demonstrate coarse, dense bones with bilateral symmetrical resorption of the humeral epiphyses and femoral epiphyses, consistent with bone resorption due to secondary hyperparathyroidism. The patient had a history of renal insufficiency and dialysis. The radiograph of the pelvis demonstrates bilateral symmetrical resorption of the femoral epiphyses and slippage of the right epiphysis. Patients with renal osteodystrophy are at risk for developing slipped capital femoral epiphyses. Stabilization of one side can provoke slippage of the other side. Therefore, this patient here was treated with bilateral cannulated screws.

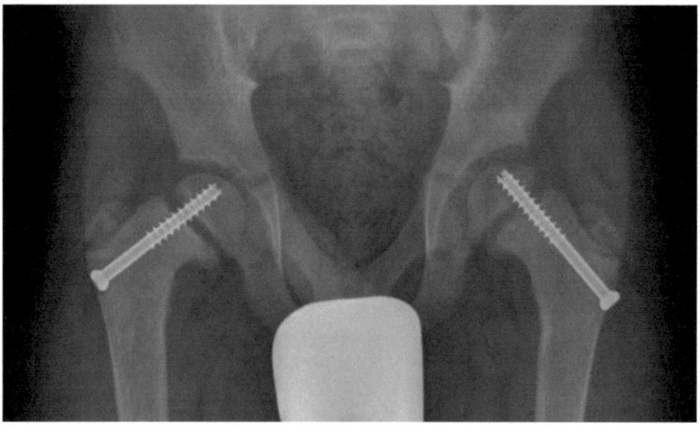

d) Patients with osteopetrosis present with diffusely increased bone density and dense bands along the distal metaphyses.

Patient 121: 17-year-old male, chest pain after e-cigarette smoking
Author: Heike E. Daldrup-Link, M.D.

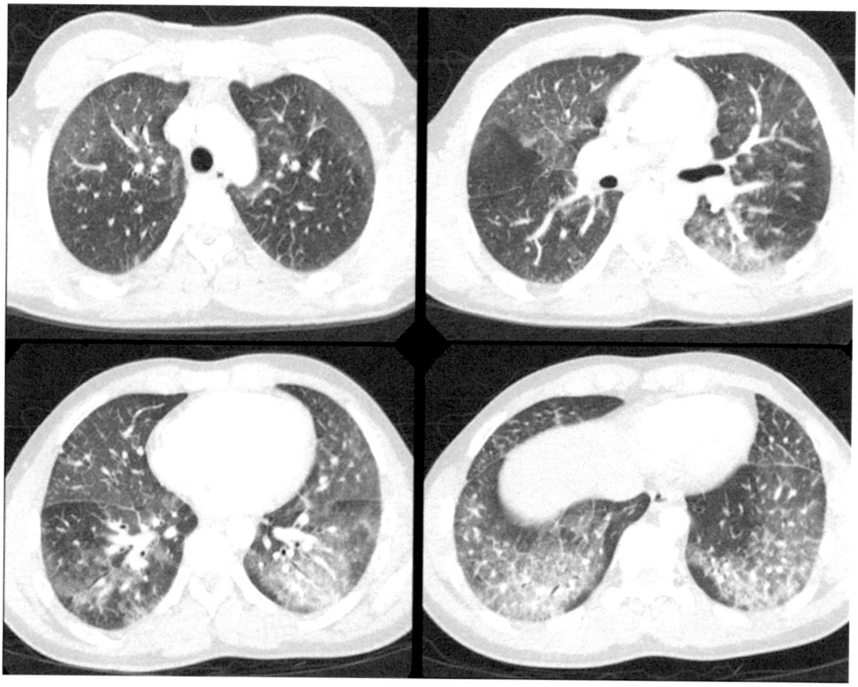

What is the most likely diagnosis:

a) Pneumocystis jiroveci pneumonia
b) Cardiogenic pulmonary edema
c) Asthma
d) EVALI

Case 121: EVALI (e-cigarette or vaping use-associated lung injury)

a) Pneumocystic jiroveci pneumonia (aka pneumocystis carinii pneumonia) presents in immunocompromised patients with predominantly perihilar ground glass opacities and pneumatoceles of varying size and shapes. Interlobular septal thickening with a crazy paving pattern can also be seen. However, the patient here is not immunocompromised.

b) Cardiogenic pulmonary edema is most associated with perihilar airspace opacities. Associated clinical findings would include left heart failure, myocarditis or other cardiac pathologies that lead to pulmonary congestion. Associated pleural effusions are often noted as well.

c) Asthma could present with bronchial wall swelling, inspiratory ground glass opacities and expiratory peripheral air trapping. Uncomplicated asthma often shows few if any abnormalities on a standard CT scan.

d) EVALI (e-cigarette or vaping use-associated lung injury): Correct! The CT scan shows basilar predominant centrilobular ground glass opacities and thickened interlobular septae with a crazy paving pattern, consistent with diffuse alveolar damage and interstitial lung disease. The subpleural areas are spared.

Patient 122: 2-month-old infant, tetralogy of Fallot
Author: Heike E. Daldrup-Link, M.D.

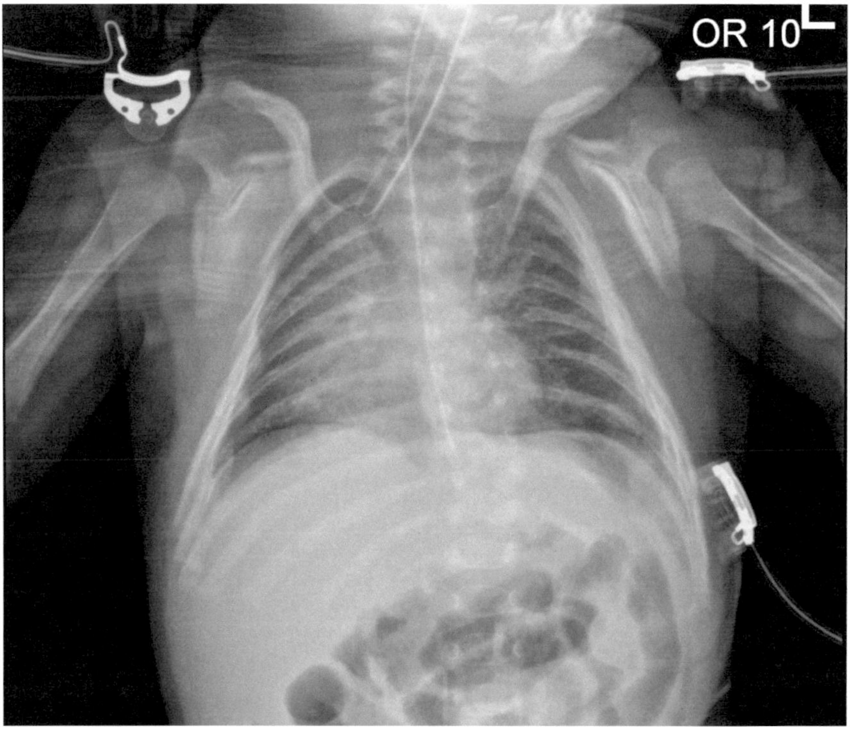

What is the most likely diagnosis:

a) Non-Accidental Trauma
b) Caffey Disease
c) Osteogenesis Imperfecta
d) Prostaglandin-Induced Hyperostosis

Case 122: Prostaglandin-Induced Hyperostosis

a) Non-accidental trauma can present with fractures of different ages. The radiograph shown here does not show any fractures. Periosteal reactions noted here involve the long bones, clavicles, scapulae, and ribs in a symmetric fashion.

b) Caffey disease (infantile cortical hyperostosis) is an inflammatory periostitis which typically presents in infants between 6 weeks and 6 months of age with fever, irritability and soft tissue swelling over the affected bones. Typical radiographic findings include abundant lamellated subperiosteal new bone formation along the diaphysis of affected bones which progress to a markedly thickened cortex and markedly increased diameter of the bone. The most commonly involved bones are the mandible, ulna, ribs, and clavicle.

c) Osteogenesis Imperfecta would present with generalized osteopenia, fractures of multiple bones with different degrees of callus formation, indicative of different ages.

d) Prostaglandin-Induced Hyperostosis. Correct! Newborns with Tetralogy of Fallot and pulmonary atresia rely on the ductus arteriosus as an important source of pulmonary blood flow. Therapy with prostaglandin maintains patency of the ductus. A well-known side-effect of this therapy is direct activation of osteoblasts. The radiograph here shows marked periosteal reactions along the bilateral humeri, clavicles, scapulae, and ribs in a symmetric fashion. There is a typical periosteal elevation along the diaphysis of the long bones with relative sparing of the metaphyses. Also note that the partially visualized mandible is not affected.

Musculoskeletal, Spine, CNS

9) Other, systemic and osteochondroses

Patient 123: 17-year-old female, knee pain
Author: Heike E. Daldrup-Link, M.D.

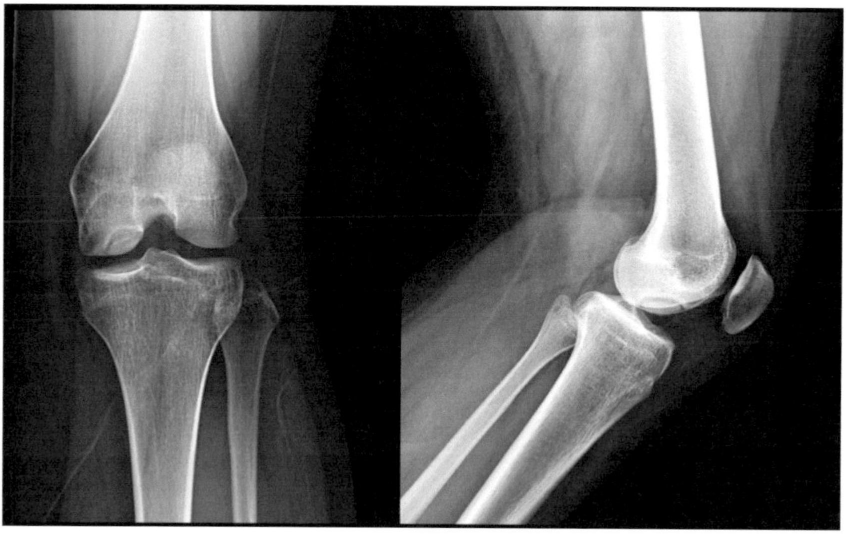

What is the most likely diagnosis:

a) Brodie abscess
b) Osteochondritis dissecans
c) Chondroblastoma
d) Acute fracture of the medial femoral condyle

Case 123: Osteochondritis dissecans (OCD)

a) Brodie's abscess describes an intra-osseous abscess due to a subacute or chronic osteomyelitis. It is most commonly found in the metaphysis of long bones. A Brodie's abscess in the epiphysis is more commonly seen in children with unfused epiphyseal plates. It typically presents as a lytic lesion with sclerotic rim.

b) Osteochondritis dissecans (OCD): Correct! The radiograph shows a classic, well defined, crescent-shaped lesion in the medial femoral condyle with lucent rim and a sclerotic base. OCD classically involves the lateral (intercondylar) of the medial condyle of the distal femur. OCD lesions are graded as follows:

- **Grade I: Compression injury, no visible fragmentation.**
- **Grade II: Localized fragment, no detachment.**
- **Grade III: Complete detachment without displacement.**
- **Grade IV: Complete detachment with intra-articular loose body.**

c) Chondroblastoma typically presents as an epiphyseal lucent lesion.

d) Acute fracture of the medial femoral condyle: The lesion shown here has a sclerotic base, which implies a long-standing pathology.

Patient 124: Teenage female

Author: Heike E. Daldrup-Link, M.D.

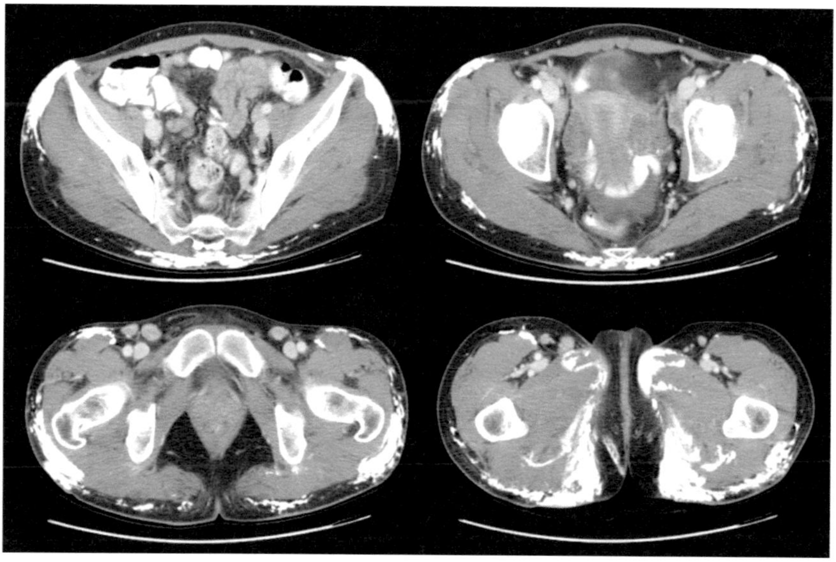

What is the most likely diagnosis:

a) Vascular Malformation
b) Scleroderma
c) Juvenile dermatomyositis
d) Myositis ossificans progressiva

Case 124: Juvenile Dermatomyositis

a) A vascular malformation could demonstrate a similar distribution and contain phleboliths, but it would not be calcified like the lesion here.

b) Scleroderma (Systemic Sclerosis): Imaging findings in patients with scleroderma include (but are not limited to) sclerosis along the skin, acroosteolysis of the distal phalanges of the hands, pulmonary fibrosis, right ventricular hypertrophy, and a range of gastrointestinal abnormalities.

c) Juvenile dermatomyositis: Correct! The CT shows coarse dystrophic calcifications in the subcutaneous soft tissues of the pelvis and upper thighs. There are also calcifications along the muscle fascias and in the muscles of the posteromedial thigh. These findings are most consistent with the diagnosis of juvenile dermatomyositis.

d) Myositis ossificans progressiva describes an inherited debilitating systemic fibrosis and ossification of muscles and tendons across joints, which leads to progressive immobility. Fibrosis and ossification along the posterior elements of the cervical spine and fusion of the facet joints between C2 and C7 lead to early ankylosis. Ankylosis of the jaw leads to weight loss and ankylosis of the costovertebral joints and ossification of intercostal muscles leads to thoracic insufficiency. The disease is ultimately fatal.

Patient 125: 7-year-old child, bilateral hip pain

Author: Heike E. Daldrup-Link, M.D.

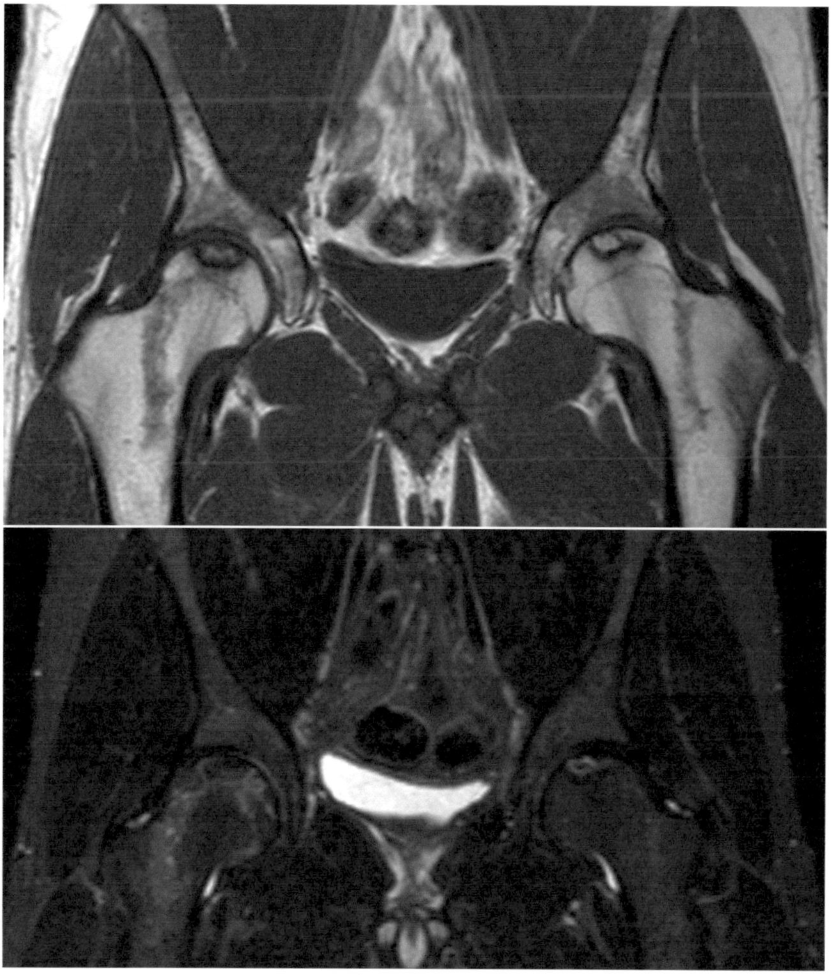

What is the most likely diagnosis:

a) Slipped capital femoral epiphysis
b) Legg-Calvé Perthes disease
c) Bilateral femur fracture
d) Meyer dysplasia

Case 125: Legg-Calvé Perthes disease

a) Slipped capital femoral epiphysis: The femoral epiphysis is not posteromedially displaced.

b) Legg-Calvé Perthes disease: Correct! The MRI demonstrates focal lesions of the bilateral femoral epiphysis, consistent with an idiopathic osteonecrosis of the right and left femoral head. The necrotic bone in the center of the lesion undergoes fatty conversion, which leads to fat-equivalent signal on both T1- and T2-weighted MR images. The central osteonecrosis is surrounded by a rim of granulation tissue and sclerosis, which leads to a characteristic "double line sign". The "double line sign" presents with intermediate-hypointense granulation tissue and hypointense sclerotic on the coronal T1-weighted image and hyperintense granulation tissue and hypointense sclerotic rim on the coronal STIR image.

c) There is no fracture noted here. The epiphyseal lesions demonstrate characteristic imaging patents of bilateral osteonecrosis. Osteonecrosis can be associated with a subchondral fracture or collapse of the epiphysis. However, this is not seen in this patient. The vertical linear T1-hypointense signal in the femoral neck bilaterally represents hematopoietic bone marrow.

d) Meyer dysplasia refers to a developmental variation which leads to fragmentation and delayed ossification of the femoral capital epiphyses. This condition is not associated with focal epiphyseal lesions as seen here.

Patient 126: 9-year-old female, pain in the right wrist

Author: Heike E. Daldrup-Link, M.D.

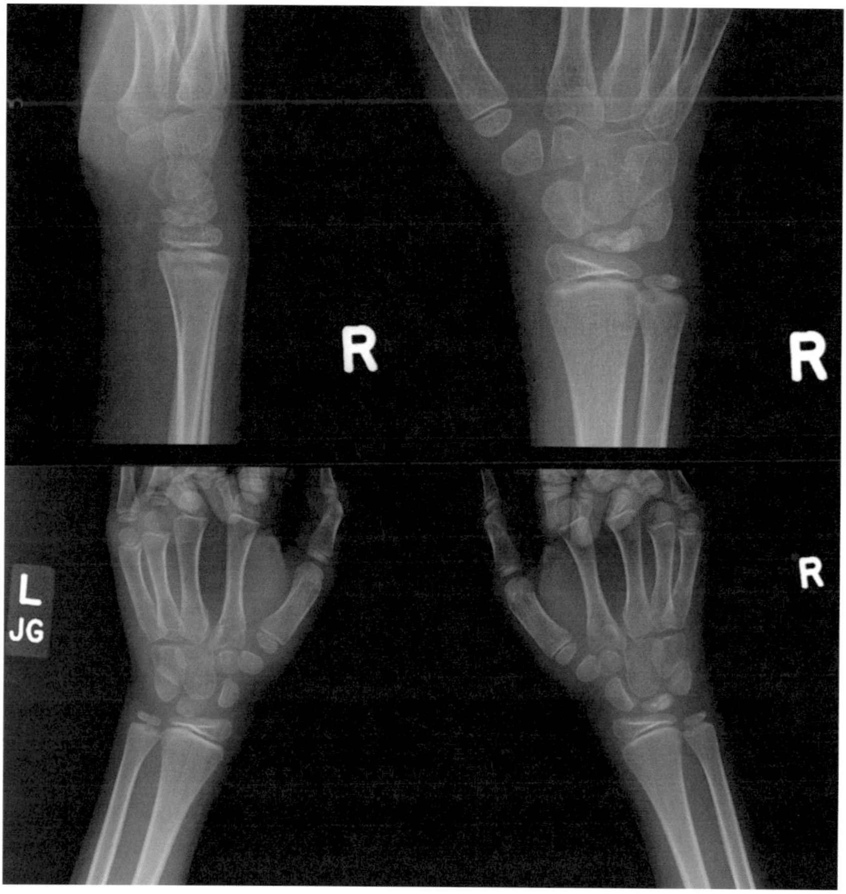

What is the most likely diagnosis:

a) Freiberg disease
b) Panner disease
c) Ulnar impaction syndrome
d) Kienböck disease

Case 126: Kienböck Osteonecrosis

a) Freiberg disease refers to an avascular necrosis of the metatarsal heads, most commonly the second metatarsal head.

b) Panner disease refers to an avascular necrosis of the capitellum of the humerus.

c) Ulnar impaction syndrome presents with sclerosis of the radial aspect of the lunate bone, most commonly in patients with positive ulnar variance or Madelung deformity.

d) Kienböck disease: Correct! The radiograph shows flattening, sclerosis, and fragmentation of the right lunate bone, consistent with an avascular necrosis of the lunate bone, also termed Kienböck osteonecrosis.

Patient 127: 7-year-old female, neurofibromatosis 1

Author: Heike E. Daldrup-Link, M.D.

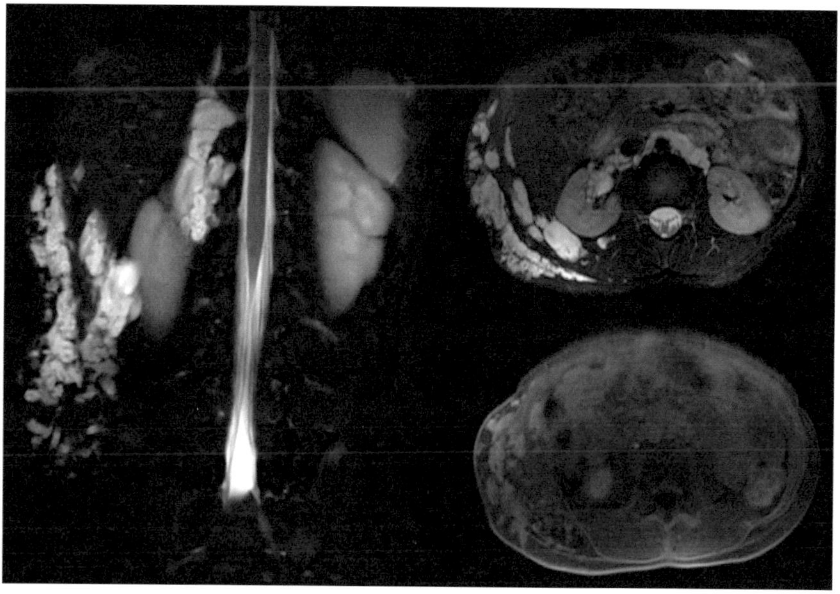

What is the most likely diagnosis:

a) Angiofibroma
b) Plexiform neurofibroma
c) Malignant peripheral nerve sheath tumor
d) Vascular malformation

Case 127: Plexiform Neurofibroma

a) Facial angiofibromas (adenoma sebaceum) are typically found in patients with Tuberous Sclerosis.

b) Plexiform neurofibroma: Correct! The MRI demonstrates serpiginous lesions in the right paraspinal area, anterior to the spine, around the right kidney, in the right retroperitoneal space and in the subcutaneous tissues of the right postero-lateral chest wall. The lesions are following the distribution of the nerve roots and demonstrate a typical "target sign" on T2-weighted scans, consisting of a central area of low intensity and a T2-hyperintense rim. The lesions demonstrate enhancement on contrast-enhanced T1-weighted MRI scans. The finding is characteristic of a plexiform neurofibroma, a benign tumor of peripheral nerves.

c) Malignant peripheral nerve sheath tumor (MPNST). Patients with NF1have a risk of developing MPNST. MPNST can develop within plexiform neurofibromas. Therefore, it is important to carefully evaluate plexiform neurofibromas for any interval changes on follow up scans. Imaging findings that can suggest malignant transformation include a soft tissue nodule with rapid interval growth, loss of the target sign, inhomogeneous contrast enhancement, more than 20% internal necrosis, restricted diffusion on diffusion weighted MRI (less than 1000 mm^2/s), increased metabolism on 18F-FDG PET and increasing 18F-FDG tumor accumulation between an initial PET scan (e.g., 1 hour after radiotracer injection) and delayed PET scan (e.g., 4 hours after radiotracer injection). None of these criteria have 100% sensitivity and specificity. The diagnosis is usually made by a combination of these findings.

d) Vascular malformation: The location of the lesion in the neuroforamina, distribution along the peripheral nerve roots, the target sign and the history of NF-1 suggests a different diagnosis.

Patient 128: 14-year-old male, migratory joint pain
Author: Heike E. Daldrup-Link, M.D.

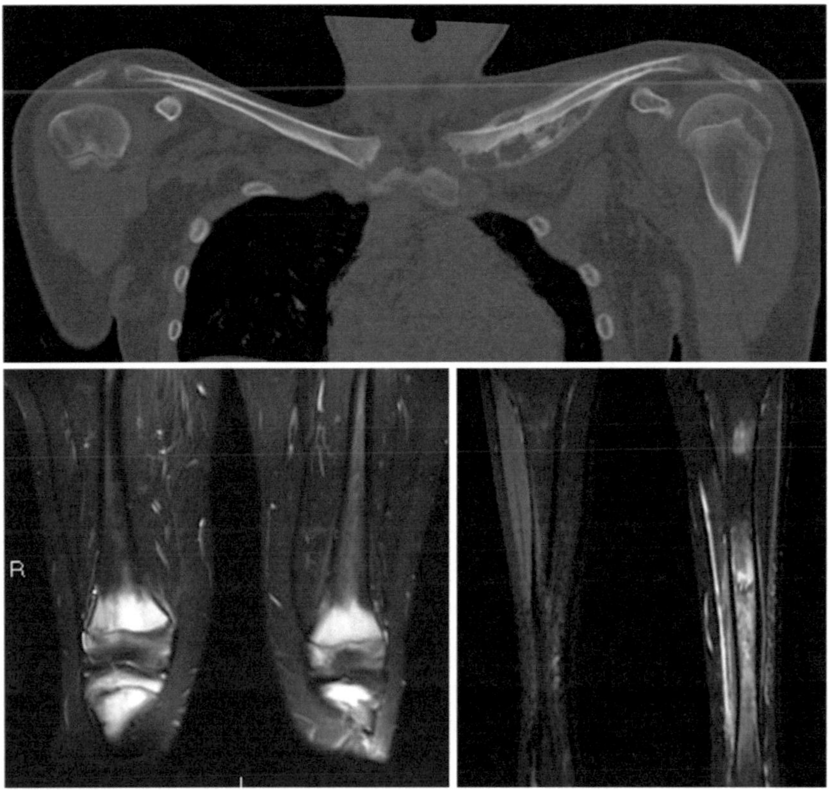

What is the most likely diagnosis:

a) Ewing Sarcoma
b) Langerhans Cell Histiocytosis
c) Chronic Recurrent Multifocal Osteomyelitis (CRMO)
d) SAPHO Syndrome

Case 128: Chronic Recurrent Multifocal Osteomyelitis

a) Ewing sarcoma would present with a more aggressive periosteal reaction and an associated soft tissue mass, which is not noted here. A location in the clavicle is not impossible but would be unusual.

b) Langerhans cell histiocytosis. While this would be a potential differential diagnosis, the sclerotic rim of the clavicle lesion and extensive multi-focal bone marrow edema would be unusual. The lesions in the distal femur and proximal tibia present as ill-defined diffuse marrow disease rather than focal lesions.

c) Chronic Recurrent Multifocal Osteomyelitis (CRMO). Correct! CRMO or chronic nonbacterial osteomyelitis (CNO) is a non-bacterial bone inflammation that causes bone pain. The T scan shows a classic expansile lytic lesion with sclerotic rim and solid periosteal reaction in the left clavicle. Erosions of the bilateral sternoclavicular joint are also noted. The T2-weighted fat saturated MRIs demonstrate T2-hyperintense lesions in the bone marrow of the bilateral distal femoral metaphyses and epiphyses, the bilateral proximal tibial metaphyses and epiphyses, and the diaphysis of the left tibia. Note the extension of the inflammatory disorder across the physis.

d) SAPHO syndrome represents the adult equivalent of CRMO. It could present with the same bone lesions shown here. However, patients typically have an associated skin condition, often acne. SAPHO is an acronym for synovitis, acne, pustulosis, hyperostosis and osteitis.

Patient 129: 7-year-old male, heel pain
Author: Heike E. Daldrup-Link, M.D.

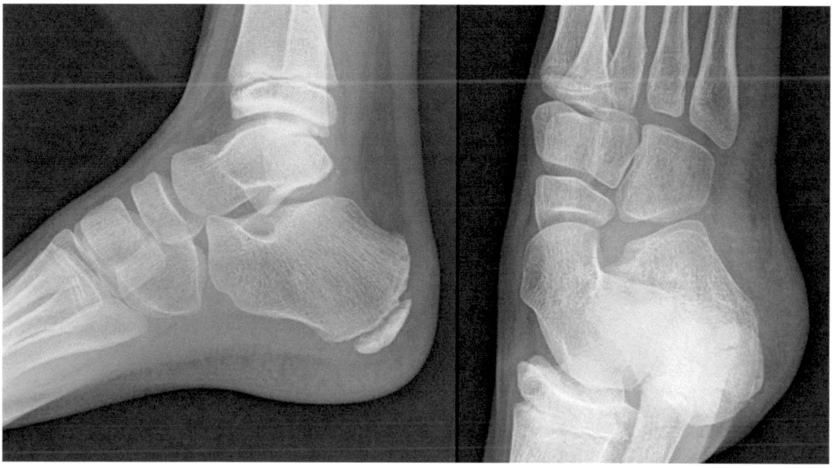

What is the most likely diagnosis:

a) Freiberg disease
b) Sever disease
c) Achilles tendinosis
d) Hegemann disease

Case 129: Sever Disease

a) Freiberg disease refers to an avascular necrosis of the metatarsal heads, most commonly the second metatarsal head.

b) Sever disease: Correct! The radiograph shows sclerosis and superior fragmentation of the apophysis of the calcaneus. There is loss of the fat/soft tissue plane in the region of the calcaneal bursa. Findings are consistent with calcaneal apophysitis, also termed Sever disease, the most common source of heel pain in physically active children.

c) Achilles tendinosis presents with thickening of the achilles tendon several centimeters above the calcaneus. The Achilles tendon in this case is normal.

d) Hegemann disease refers to an avascular necrosis of the humeral trochlea.

Patient 130: Young adult female, tuberous sclerosis complex

Author: Heike E. Daldrup-Link, M.D.

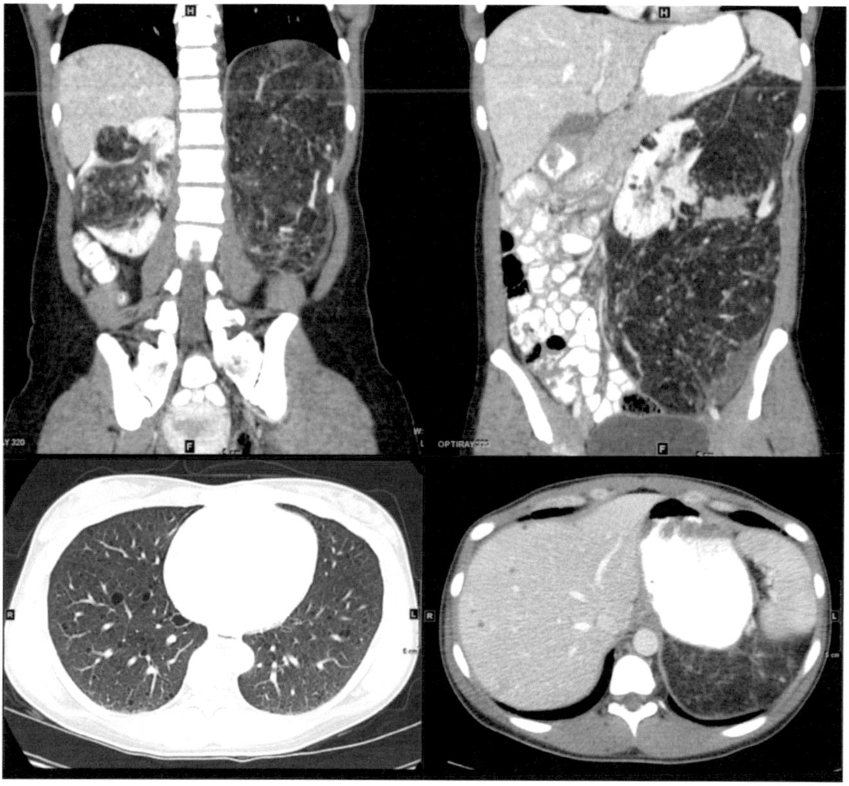

What is the most likely diagnosis:

a) Ewing Sarcoma
b) Langerhans Cell Histiocytosis
c) Lymphangioleiomyomatosis
d) Multilocular Cystic Nephroma

Case 130: Lymphangioleiomyomatosis

a) Ewing sarcoma would present as a predominantly solid, aggressive soft tissue mass, which is not noted here. Ewing sarcomas are not associated with tuberous sclerosis.

b) Langerhans cell histiocytosis (LCH). While LCH can present with lesions in all the shown organ systems, it would usually present as soft tissue masses, not cystic lesions. The most affected organ system in LCH is the bone/bone marrow.

c) Lymphangioleiomyomatosis (LAM). Correct! LAM presents in patients with tuberous sclerosis complex with a typical triad of renal angiomyolipoma (AML), cystic lymphangio-leiomyoma and small cysts in the lungs. The disease may be accompanied by a chylothorax or chyloperitoneum, which is not seen in this case. The CT scan demonstrates large lungs with multiple scattered thin-walled cysts, scattered small cystic lesions in the liver, bilateral low density focal lesions in the kidneys, consistent with angiomyolipomas, as well as a multi-cystic mass in the right kidney and a large multi-cystic mass in the left retroperitoneum, consistent with a lymphangioleiomyoma.

d) A multilocular cystic nephroma presents as a predominantly cystic mass in the kidney in young children. The additionally seen lesions in and around the left kidney, in the liver and lung would not be explained by this diagnosis.

Patient 131: 12-year-old female with knee pain

Authors: Marcello Chang, Jayne Seekins, D.O.

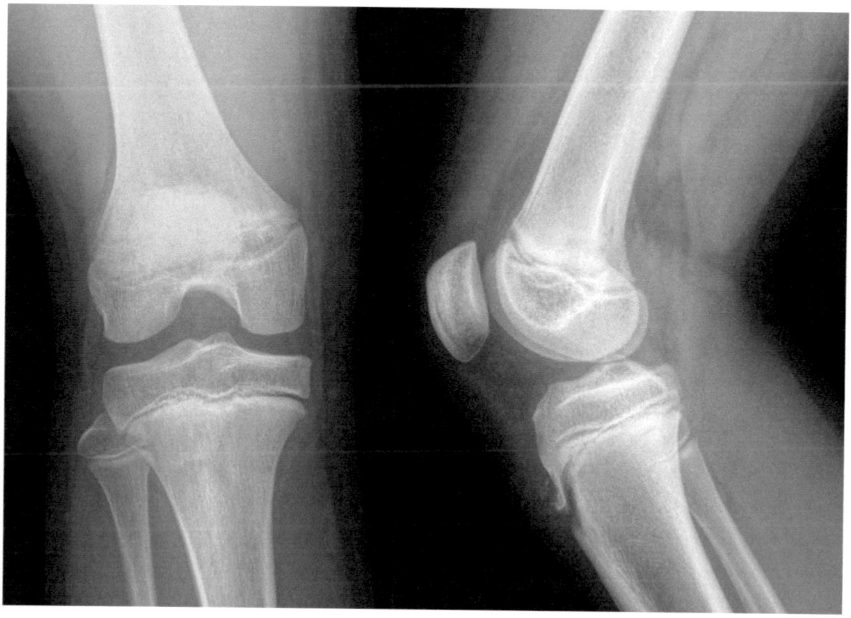

What is the most likely diagnosis:

a) Apophysitis of the tibial tubercle
b) Patellar Fracture
c) Sinding Larsen Johannsen disease
d) Prepatellar bursitis

Case 131: Apophysitis of the Tibial Tubercle (Osgood Schlatter)

a) Apophysitis of the tibial tubercle (Osgood-Schlatter disease): Correct! The lateral knee radiograph shows fragmentation and prominence of the anterior tibial tubercle/apophysis with associated soft tissue swelling and haziness of the inferior part of Hoffa's fat pad, consistent with an apophysitis and Osgood-Schlatter's disease.
Apophysitis of the tibial tubercle occurs due to overuse at the patellar insertion site on the tibia usually affecting growing adolescents, specifically males around 10-14 years of age and females around 8-12 years of age. The apophysitis leads to pain and swelling over the tibial tuberosity which worsens with exercise. Usually, conservative treatment is sufficient, and the condition spontaneously resolves.

b) A patellar fracture would show a fracture of the patella, typically associated with a joint effusion and/or hemarthrosis.

c) An inferior patellar apophysitis (Sinding Larsen Johannsen) may show thickening of the proximal patellar tendon near the inferior pole of the patella. Early stages if the disease may not have significant radiographic findings. At advanced stages, the radiograph may show stranding of Hoffa's fat pad or dystrophic calcifications below the patella. Both Sinding Larsen Johannsen disease and Osgood Schlatter disease occur due to a chronic traction injury of the patella tendon. The major difference is the location: At/above the tibial tuberosity in Osgood-Schlatter versus at/below the inferior pole of the patella in Sinding Larsen Johannsen disease.

d) A prepatellar bursitis would also present with knee pain but would show soft tissue swelling anterior to the patella. If the inflammation is chronic, the prepatellar tissue may demonstrate calcifications.

Patient 132: 13-year-old female, tennis player, knee pain
Author: Heike E. Daldrup-Link, M.D.

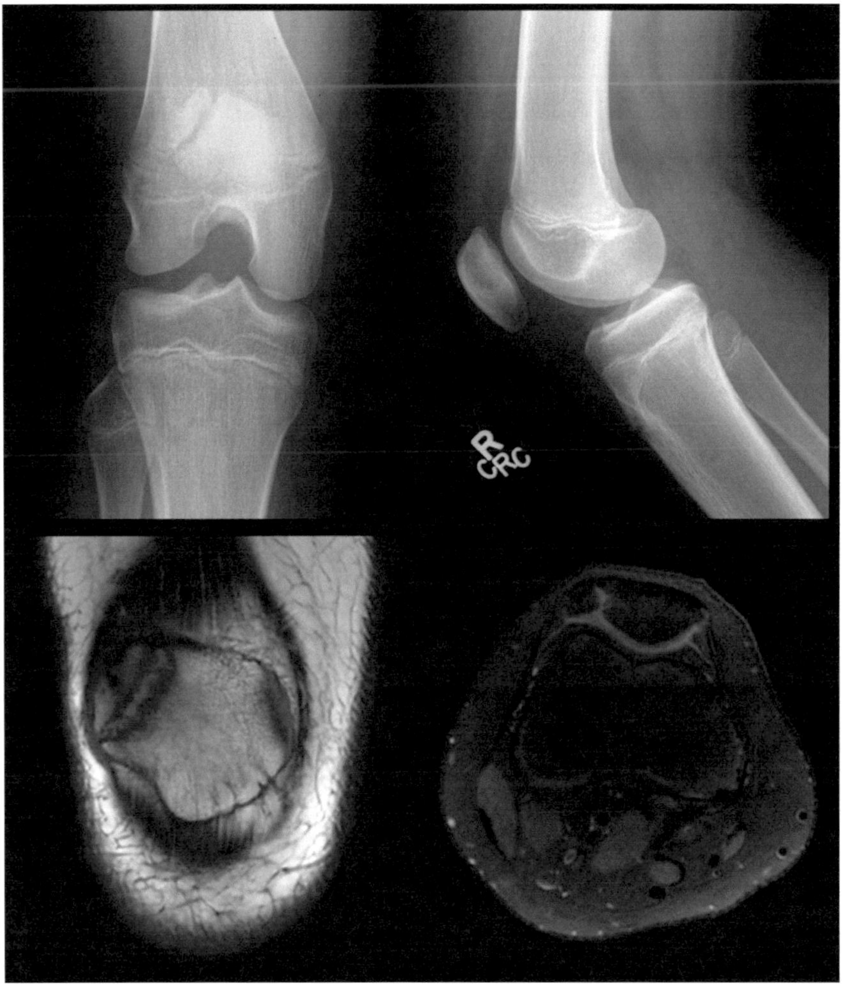

What is the most likely diagnosis:

a) Osgood-Schlatter Disease
b) Bipartite Patella
c) Patella Sleeve Fracture
d) Sinding Larsen Johannsen Disease

Case 132: Bipartite Patella

a) Osgood Schlatter Disease is a traction osteochondritis at the caudal insertion site of the patella tendon. Imaging studies show fragmentation of the tibial tuberosity and overlying soft tissue swelling.

b) Bipartite Patella: Correct! The radiograph shows a radiolucent line across the superolateral aspect of the patella with a well corticated ossicle antero-lateral to the main patella, consistent with an unfused accessory ossification center. The coronal T1-weighted and axial T2-weighted MRI demonstrates division of the patella in two parts, with extension of cartilage into the synchondrosis between the patella and the accessory bone. There is no bone marrow edema and no joint effusion. A bipartite patella is usually asymptomatic and noted as an incidental finding. There are three types based on the location of the accessory bone at the inferior pole (type I), lateral patellar border (type II) and superolateral margin (type III, most common).

c) A patella sleeve fracture is an avulsion injury of the inferior pole of the patella.

d) Sinding Larsen Johannsen disease is a traction injury of the patella tendon at the inferior pole of the patella due to repetitive trauma or sports activities that involve jumping, running, squatting, etc. Imaging studies show fragmentation of the lower pole of patella, marrow edema within the fragments, thickening and edema of the patellar tendon at its insertion at the lower pole of the patella and edema of Hoffa's fat pad.

Patient 133: 10-year-old female, supracondylar humerus fracture a few months ago, now new elbow pain
Author: Heike E. Daldrup-Link, M.D.

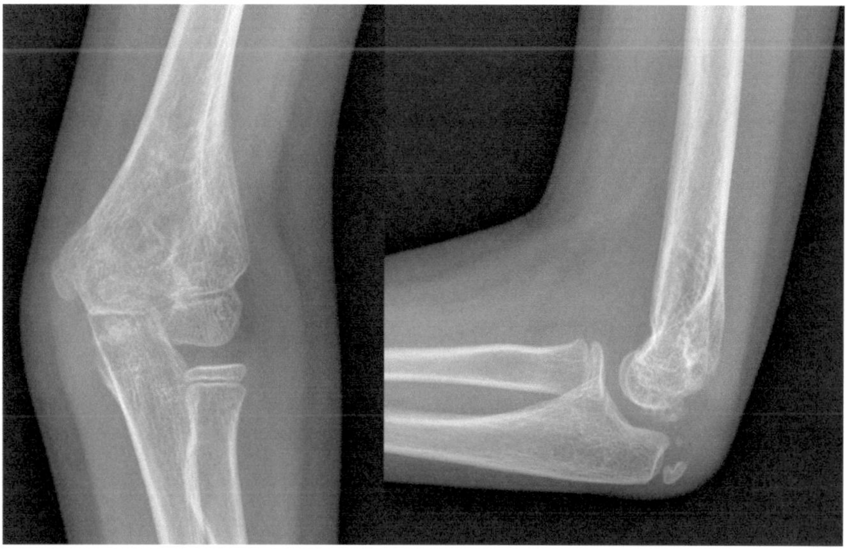

What is the most likely diagnosis:

a) Freiberg disease
b) Panner disease
c) Ulnar impaction syndrome
d) Hegemann disease

Case 133: Hegemann Osteonecrosis

a) Freiberg disease refers to an avascular necrosis of the metatarsal heads, most commonly the second metatarsal head.

b) Panner disease refers to an avascular necrosis of the capitellum of the humerus.

c) Ulnar impaction syndrome presents with sclerosis of the radial aspect of the lunate bone, most commonly in patients with positive ulnar variance or Madelung deformity.

d) Hegemann disease: Correct! The radiograph shows a healed distal humers fracture with callus formation along the distal humeral shaft. In addition, there is sclerosis, and fragmentation of the humeral trochlea, consistent with an avascular necrosis, also termed Hegemann osteonecrosis. The trochlea ossifies around 7 years of age and fuses with the humerus around 12 years of age. An injury of the distal humerus can affect the blood supply to the trochlea and cause ischemia and collapse of the trochlear ossification center. While an osteonecrosis of the trochlea is rare, patients between 10-12 years of age are most commonly affected.

Musculoskeletal, Spine, CNS

10) Bone dysplasias

Patient 134: A child with short stature

Author: Wipawee Morakote, M.D.

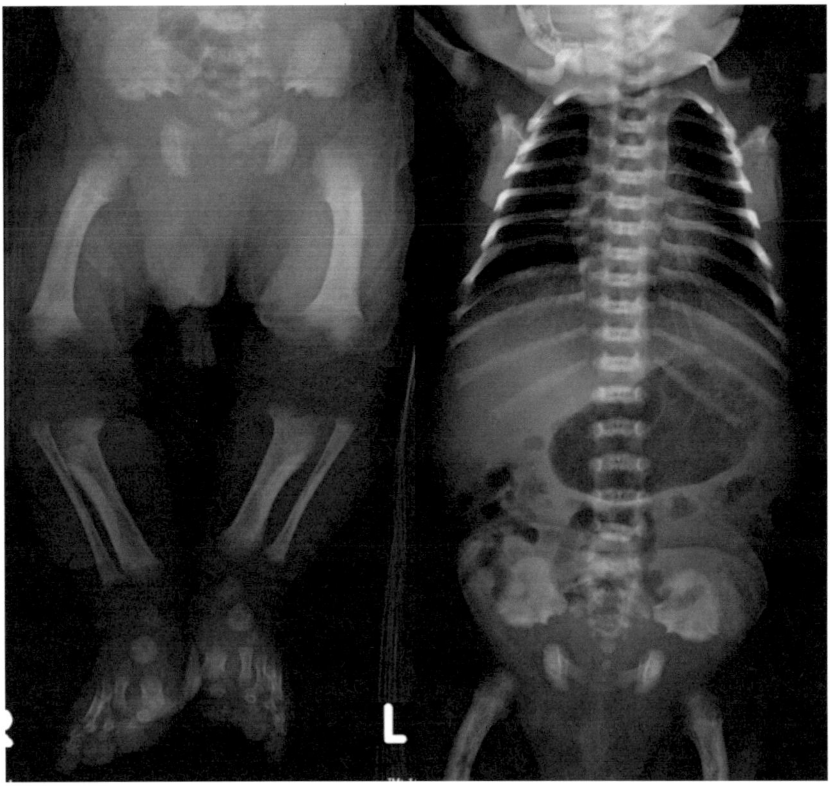

What is the most likely diagnosis:

a) Osteogenesis imperfecta
b) Achondroplasia
c) Morquio syndrome
d) Rickets

Case 134: Achondroplasia

a) An osteogenesis imperfecta typically presents with osteopenia and multiple fractures, which are not noted here.

b) Achondroplasia. Correct! The radiograph of the lower extremities shows short femurs with proximal "fade out" and metaphyseal flaring which is characteristic of achondroplasia. The anteroposterior view of the spine reveals a decreasing interpedicular distance of the lumbar spine. In addition, there is an "elephant ear appearance" of the iliac wings with horizontal acetabular roof, small squared iliac wings, and short sacroiliac notches. The fibula is unusually long. The proximal fibula ends at the level of the of the tibial plateau. Other typical findings include a relatively large cranial vault with frontal bossing and small skull base.

c) Morquio syndrome is one of the mucopolysaccharidoses and presents with short stature, anterior central vertebral beaking, platyspondyly, wide ribs with proximal narrowing. goblet shaped and flared iliac wings, increased acetabular angles, short and wide tubular bones, flattened proximal femoral epiphyses and wide metacarpals with proximal pointing.

d) Rickets presents with an abnormal provisional zone of calcification with irregularity and widening of the metaphysis of the long bones.

Patient 135: A newborn child
Author: Heike E. Daldrup-Link, M.D.

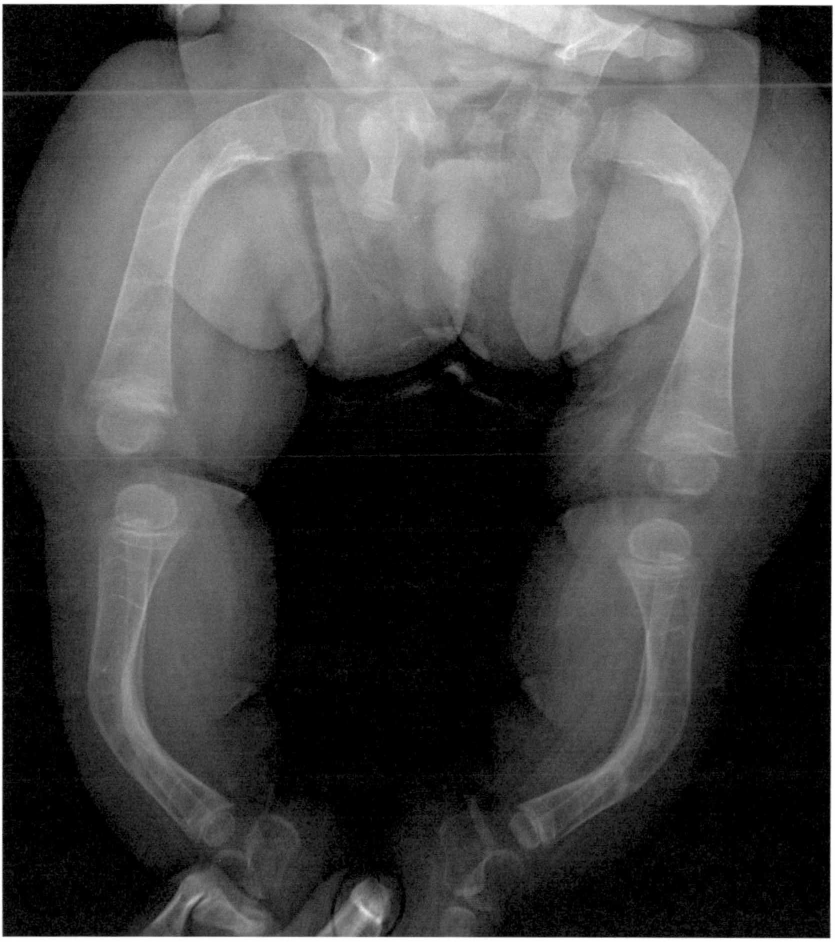

What is the most likely diagnosis:

a) Osteogenesis imperfecta
b) Achondroplasia
c) Morquio syndrome
d) Menkes syndrome

Case 135: Osteogenesis Imperfecta

a) Osteogenesis Imperfecta: Correct! The radiographs demonstrate diffuse osteopenia of all bones with cortical thinning, marked bowing and pathologic fractures of the left proximal femur and left distal tibia. The long bones also demonstrate multiple sclerotic growth arrest lines.

b) Achondroplasia would present with normal bone density, squared iliac wings, horizontal acetabular roofs and flared metaphyses of long bones. Patients with osteogenesis do not have an increased risk of developing bone fractures.

c) Morquio syndrome is one of the mucopolysaccharidoses and presents with goblet shaped and flared iliac wings, steep acetabular angles, short and wide tubular bones and flattened proximal femoral epiphyses.

d) Menkes syndrome is a rare x-linked disorder of copper metabolism. Menkes syndrome can present with osteopenia, an abnormal provisional zone of calcification and symmetrically distributed metaphyseal cupping, fraying and sickle-shaped fractures. The degree of bone deformity seen here would be unusual. Infants with Menkes disease appear healthy at birth and typically start developing clinical symptoms after 2-3 months.

Patient 136: 3-year-old male with short stature

Author: Heike E. Daldrup-Link, M.D.

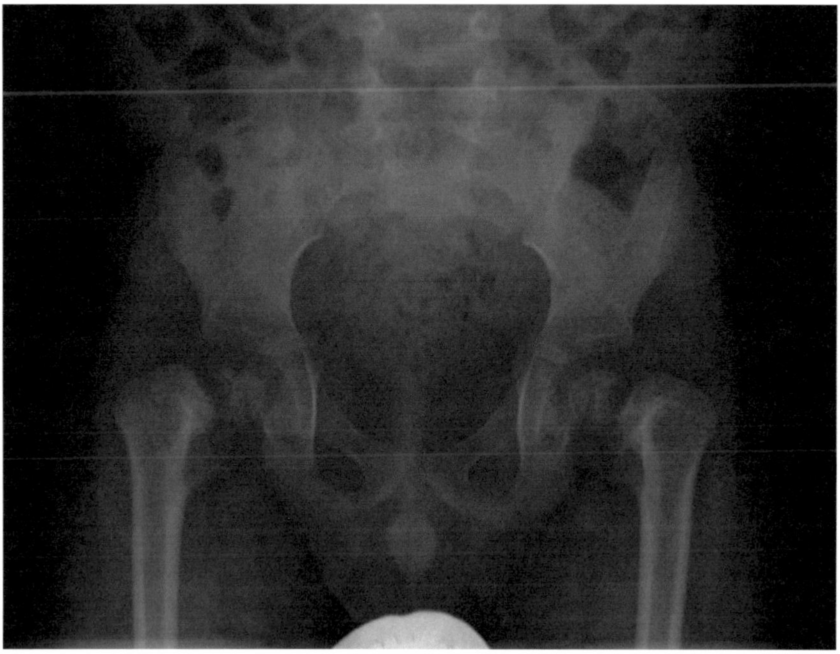

What is the most likely diagnosis:

a) Slipped Capital Femoral Epiphyses (SCFE)
b) Achondroplasia
c) Morquio syndrome
d) Metaphyseal Chondrodysplasia

Case 136: Metaphyseal Chondrodysplasia

a) Slipped Capital Femoral Epiphyses (SCFE) would typically present during puberty, i.e., at age 12 - 16 in boys, and age 10 - 14 in girls. A radiograph of the pelvis would show widening of the proximal epiphyseal plate and slippage of the proximal femoral epiphysis in the posterior medial direction. The femoral ossification centers and metaphyses would not be dysplastic.

b) Achondroplasia would present with squared iliac wings, horizontal acetabular roofs and flared metaphyses of the long bones.

c) Morquio syndrome is one of the mucopolysaccharidoses and presents with goblet shaped and flared iliac wings, steep acetabular angles, short and wide tubular bones and flattened proximal femoral epiphyses.

d) Metaphyseal Chondrodysplasia: Correct! The radiograph of the pelvis demonstrates bilateral coxa vara, with enlarged proximal femur ossification centers, widened growth plates and flared proximal metaphyses. The patient was diagnosed with the Schmid type of metaphyseal chondrodysplasia, which is due to defective type X collagen and characterized by failure of normal mineralization of the zone of provisional calcification.

Patient 137: A newborn child

Author: Heike E. Daldrup-Link, M.D.

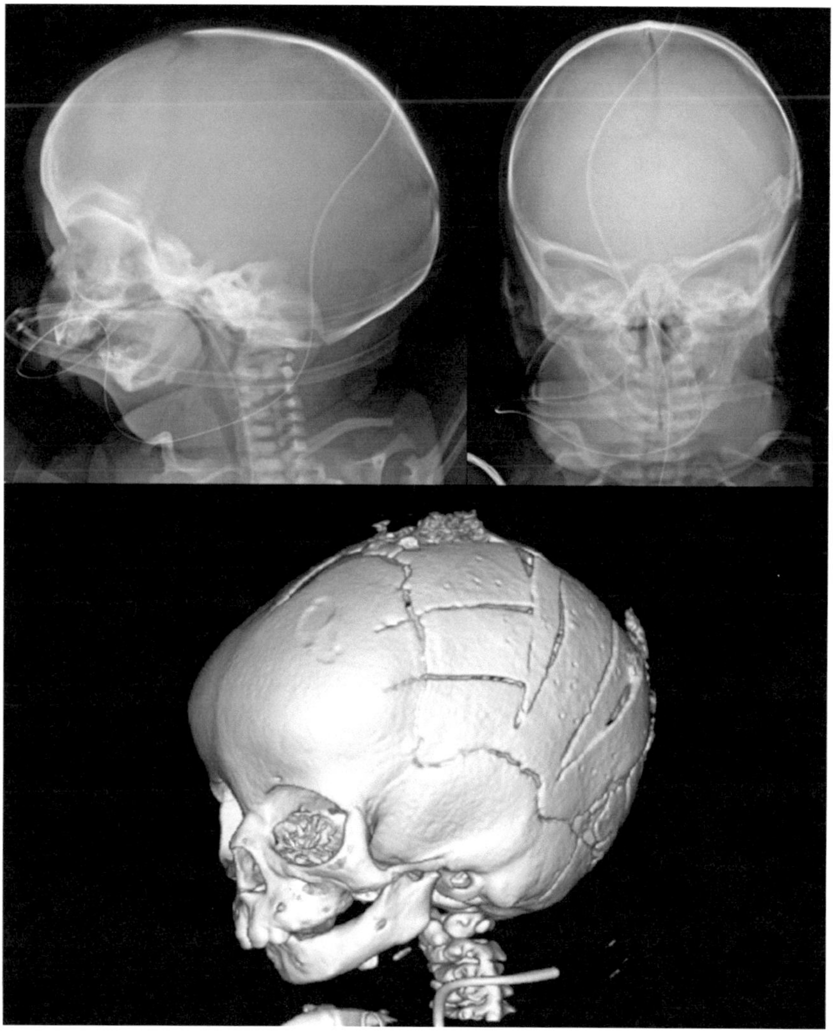

What is the most likely diagnosis:

a) Agnathia
b) Achondroplasia
c) Pierre Robin Sequence
d) Maxillary hypoplasia

Case 137: Pierre Robin Sequence

a) Agnathia describes a congenital absence of the condyloid process, with or without absence of the coronoid process, the mandibular ramus, and parts of the mandibular body. In this case here, the mandibula is present, but hypoplastic.

b) Achondroplasia is associated with frontal bossing, small skull base and narrow foramen magnum. But micrognathia is not a typical characteristic of achondroplasia.

c) Pierre Robin Sequence: Correct! The radiograph of the head and 3D reconstructed CT scan demonstrates hypoplasia of the mandibula (micrognathia) and posteroinferior displacement of the tongue (glossoptosis) which leads to obstruction of the oropharynx. The hard palate is shortened in length. The micrognathia and glossoptosis affect prenatal development of the hard palate, which often leads to an associated cleft palate. The patient underwent glossopexy to advance the tongue.

d) Maxillary hypoplasia presents with underdevelopment of the maxillary bones which leads to midfacial retrusion and apparent protuberance (rather than retropulsion) of the mandibula.

Patient 138: Newborn male

Author: Heike E. Daldrup-Link, M.D.

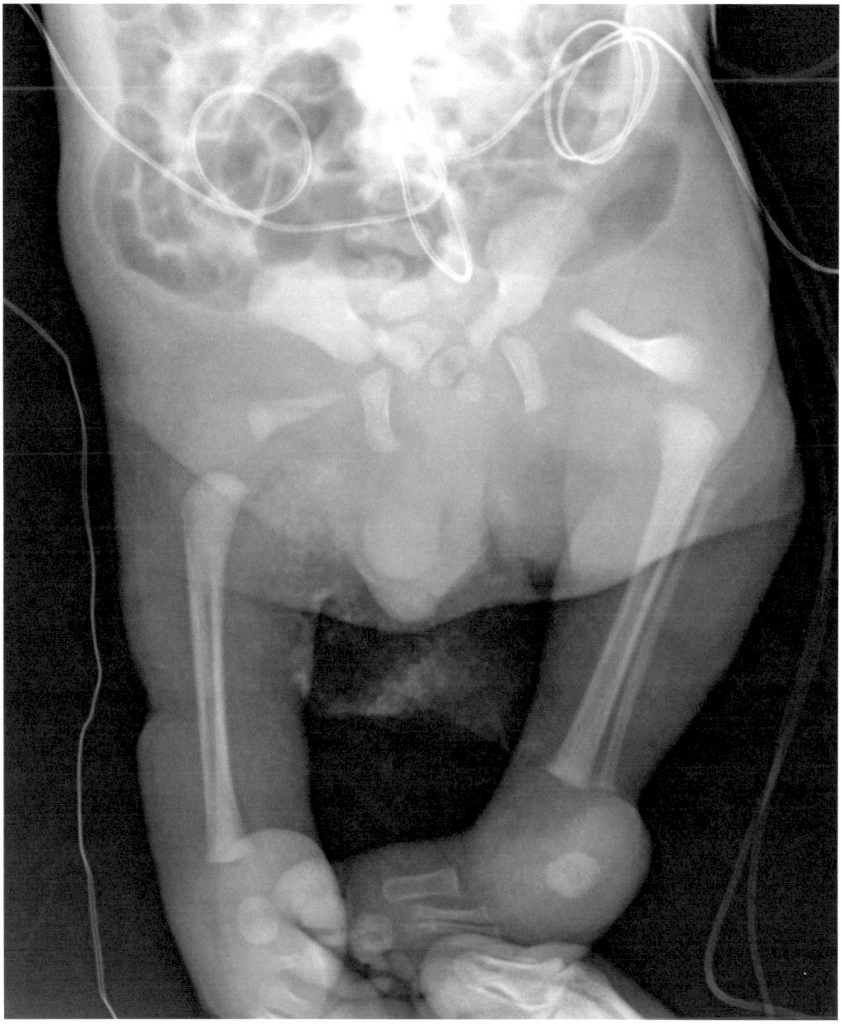

What is the most likely diagnosis:

a) Turner Syndrome
b) Proximal Femoral Focal Deficiency
c) Campomelic Dysplasia
d) Achondroplasia

Case 138: Proximal Femoral Focal Deficiency

a) Turner syndrome presents in females with short limbs, scoliosis, developmental dysplasia of the hip, genu valgum, depression of the medial tibial plateau and enlargement of the overlying medial femoral condyle. Bony coalitions are also frequently noted.

b) Proximal femoral focal deficiency: Correct! The radiograph of the pelvis and bilateral legs of the newborn infant demonstrates a congenital partial absence of the proximal end of the bilateral femur. On the right side, the dysplastic femur is centered towards a hypoplastic acetabulum. There is an associated right fibular hemimelia. On the left side, the acetabulum is absent, and the femur is dislocated laterally and superiorly. Note also multiple segmentation anomalies of the lumbar spine and sacrum as well as agenesis of the distal sacrum.

c) Campomelic means "bent bones." Campomelic dysplasia presents with a bell-shaped narrow chest, dislocated hip, and knee joints, bowing (but not shortening) of the the long bones and hypoplastic fibulae. More than 95% of patients die within the first few months of life.

d) Achondroplasia presents with squared iliac wings with horizontal acetabular roof and short sacroiliac notches. The proximal fibula is unusually long and ends at the level of the tibial plateau. Other typical findings include posterior vertebral scalloping and decreasing interpedicular distance of the lumbar spine.

Patient 139: A male patient with prominent forehead
Author: Heike E. Daldrup-Link, M.D.

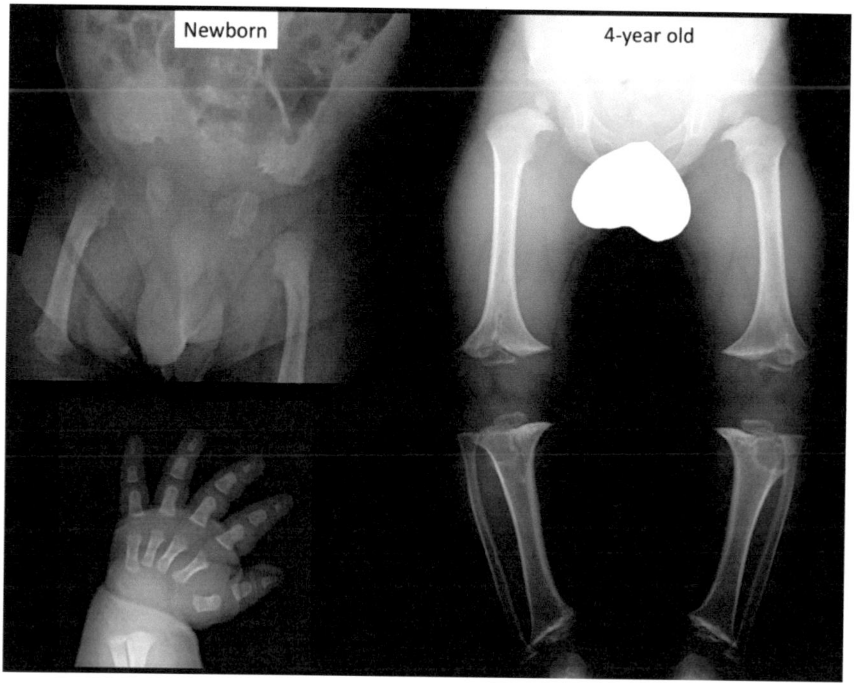

What is the most likely diagnosis:

a) Turner Syndrome
b) Hurler syndrome
c) Campomelic Dysplasia
d) Achondroplasia

Case 139: Achondroplasia

a) Turner syndrome presents in females with short limbs, cubitus valgus, brachymetacarpia, Madelung deformity, shortening of the fourth metacarpal, scoliosis, developmental dysplasia of the hip, genu valgum, depression of the medial tibial plateau and enlargement of the overlying medial femoral condyle. Bony coalitions are also frequently noted.

b) Hurler syndrome is one of the mucopolysaccharidoses and presents with short stature, macrocephaly, anterior inferior vertebral beaking, wide ribs with proximal narrowing, flared iliac wings with increased (rather than decreased) acetabular angles, coxa valga and wide metacarpals with proximal tapering.

c) Campomelic means "bent bones." Campomelic dysplasia presents with a bell-shaped narrow chest, dislocated hip, and knee joints, bowing (but not shortening) of the the long bones and hypoplastic fibulae. More than 95% of patients die within the first few months of life.

d) Achondroplasia. Correct! The radiograph of the pelvis of the newborn infant demonstrates small squared squared iliac wings with horizontal acetabular roof and short sacroiliac notches. The radiograph of the hand demonstrates shortened metacarpals and phalanges, with separation between the third and fourth finger, the so-called "trident hand". There is also mild metaphyseal flaring of the distal radius and ulna. The radiograph of the lower extremities at age four demonstrates characteristic flaring of the metaphyses of the femur and tibia, with a typical "Chevron sign", an inverted V-shape of the metaphysis. The proximal fibula is unusually long and ends at the level of the tibial plateau. Other typical findings include a relatively large cranial vault with frontal bossing, posterior vertebral scalloping and decreasing interpedicular distance of the lumbar spine.

Patient 140: 5-year-old male, palpable masses over both wrists

Author: Heike E. Daldrup-Link, M.D.

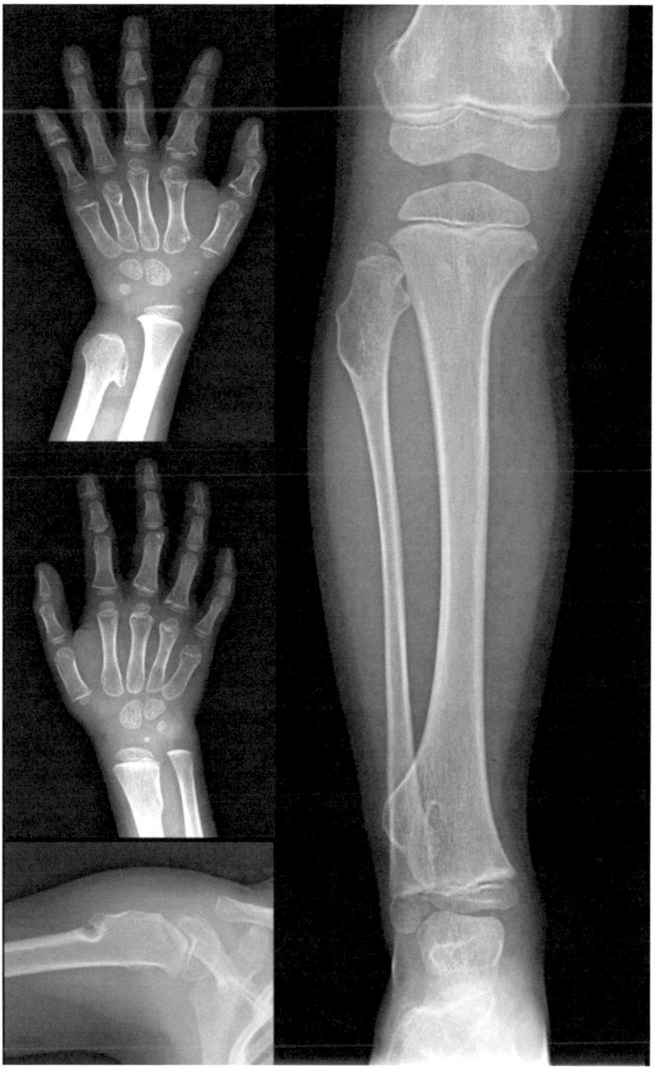

What is the most likely diagnosis:

a) Trevor disease
b) Ollier disease
c) Metachondromatosis
d) Multiple hereditary exostoses

Case 140: Multiple Hereditary Exostoses

a) Trevor disease is characterized by osteochondromas of the epiphyses, which grow towards the joint. It is due to asymmetric overgrowth of cartilage in the epiphyses.

b) Ollier disease refers to multiple enchondromas, well-defined benign cartilaginous neoplasms which present on bone x-rays as lucent lesions within the medullary cavity of the bone.

c) Metachondromatosis is characterized by the presence of both enchondromas and osteochondromas. The images here show multiple osteochondromas, but no enchondromas.

d) Multiple hereditary exostoses: Correct! Multiple exostoses are classified as a skeletal dysplasia. Most cases are inherited with an autosomal dominant trait. The radiographs here demonstrate bilateral symmetric sessile and lobulated outgrowths of bone, which extend from the metaphysis outwards and are pointing away from the joint. The lesions are covered by a cartilage cap, which can have a thickness of 1 to 3 cm in children due to the ongoing growth process and sometimes cause an indentation of the adjacent cortex, as seen with the lesion of the proximal humerus. Cap thickness exceeding 2 cm in an adult and more than 3 cm in a child should raise suspicion for malignancy.

Patient 141: 10-year-old female patient with precocious puberty and multiple café au lait spots on the back

Author: Heike E. Daldrup-Link, M.D.

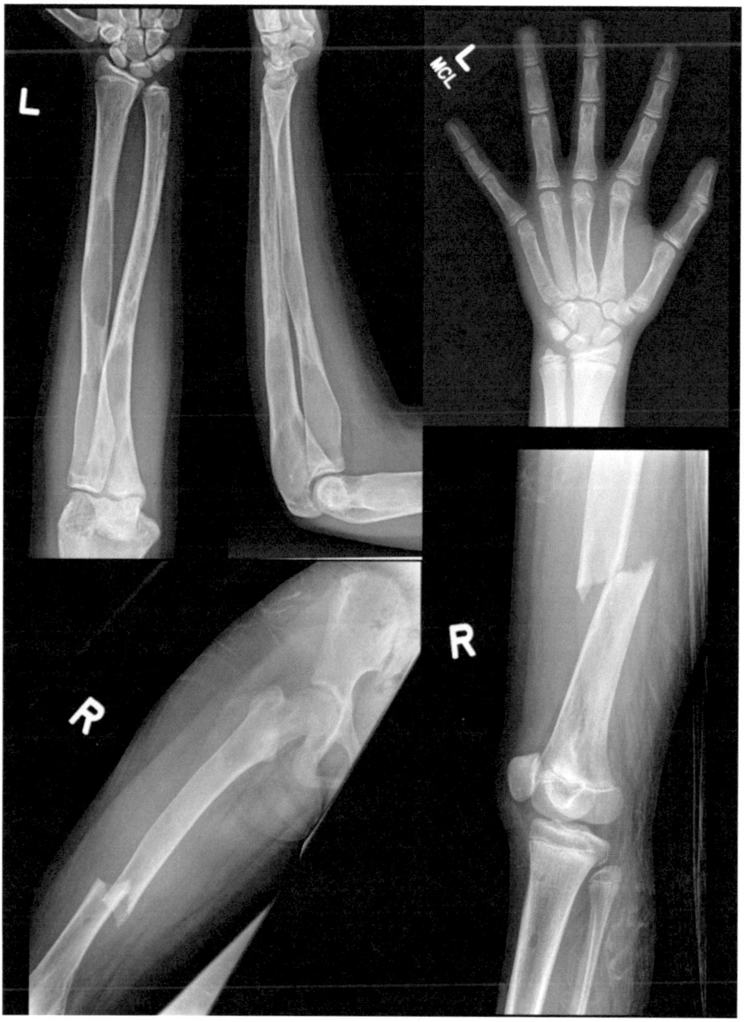

What is the most likely diagnosis:

a) Turner Syndrome
b) Hurler syndrome
c) McCune Albright Syndrome
d) Campomelic Dysplasia

Case 141: McCune Albright Syndrome

a) Turner syndrome presents in females with short limbs, cubitus valgus, brachymetacarpia, Madelung deformity, shortening of the fourth metacarpal, scoliosis, developmental dysplasia of the hip, genu valgum, depression of the medial tibial plateau and enlargement of the overlying medial femoral condyle. Bony coalitions are also frequently noted.

b) Hurler syndrome (Mucopolysaccharidoses type 1) presents with short stature, macrocephaly, anterior inferior vertebral beaking, wide ribs with proximal narrowing, flared iliac wings with increased (rather than decreased) acetabular angles, coxa valga and wide metacarpals with proximal tapering.

c) McCune Albright Syndrome: Correct! The radiograph demonstrates multiple expansile lytic intramedullary lesions in the left radius and ulna, the 2nd – 5th metacarpal bone and the second phalanx of the left hand as well as the right femur. There is a pathologic fracture through a lytic lesion in the mid shaft of the right femur. The intramedullary lesions have a ground glass matrix and expand the underlying bone without significant periosteal reaction. The findings are consistent with multiple fibrous dysplasias. The combination of clinically described precocious puberty, irregular café-au-lait skin pigmentations ("coast of Maine") and polyostotic fibrous dysplasia is consistent with the diagnosis of McCune Albright Syndrome.

d) Campomelic ("bent bones") dysplasia presents with a bell-shaped chest, dislocated hip, and knee joints, bowing (but not intramedullary ground glass lesions) of the the long bones and hypoplastic fibulae. More than 95% of patients die within the first few months of life.

GI, GU, and Interventional

1) Esophagus and Stomach

Patient 142: Four-day-old premature infant, respiratory distress
Author: Heike E. Daldrup-Link, M.D.

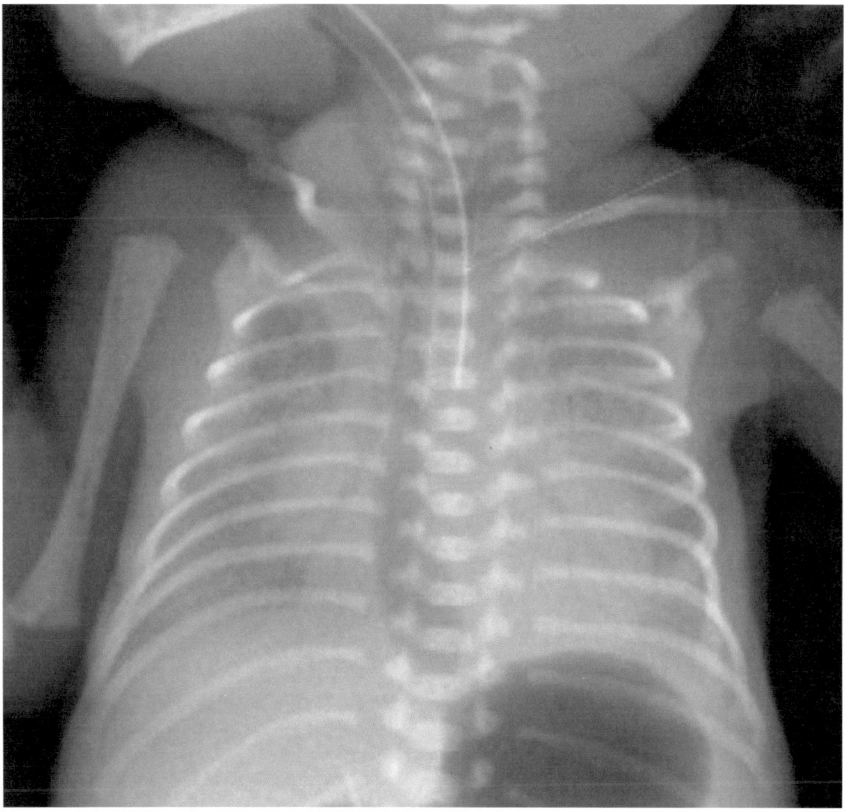

What is the most likely diagnosis:

a) Pneumomediastinum
b) Hiatal Hernia
c) Esophageal Intubation
d) Open Chest

Case 142: Esophageal Intubation

a) Pneumomediastinum. The air seen here localizes to the esophagus. The ETT tube is misplaced.

b) Hiatal Hernia: The radiograph shown here demonstrated an ETT tube projecting on the esophagus. The stomach is noted under the left diaphragm.

c) Esophageal Intubation: Correct! The radiograph of the neck shows the ETT tube projecting posterior to the air-filled trachea. The esophagus and stomach are gas distended because they are being ventilated. The lungs demonstrate diffuse hazy opacities bilaterally, consistent with bilateral microatelectases.

d) Open Chest: There are no lines and tubes to suggest a recent surgery. The longitudinal shape of the mediastinal lucency seen here is consistent with the location of the esophagus.

Patient 143: 2-week-old infant with vomiting

Authors: Marcello Chang, Jayne M. Seekins, D.O.

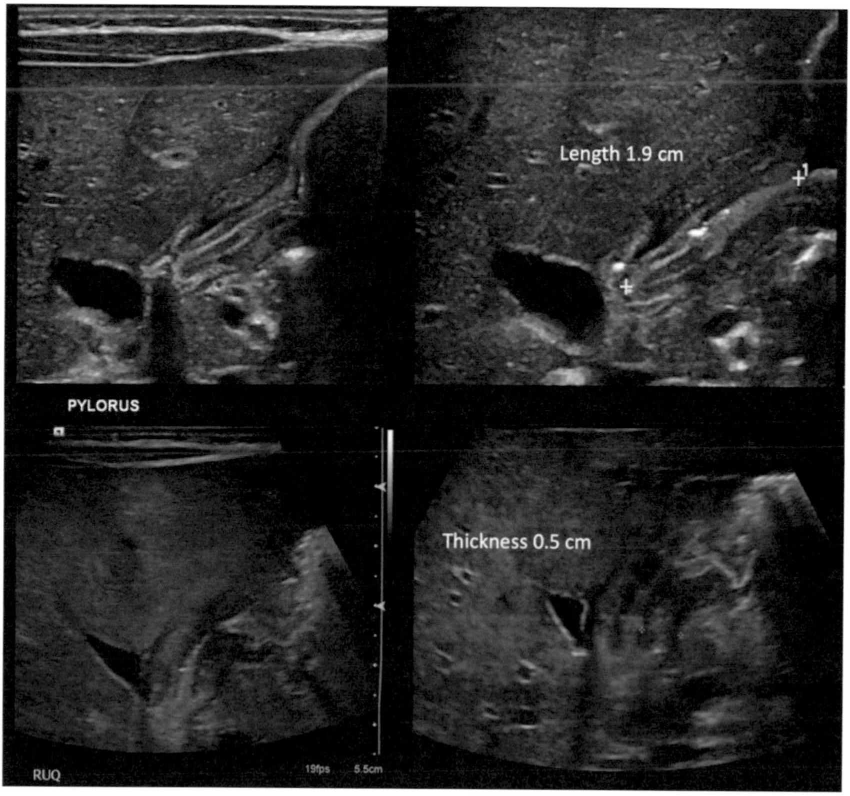

What is the most likely diagnosis:

a) Hypertrophic Pyloric Stenosis
b) Midgut Volvulus
c) Duodenal Atresia
d) Duodenal web

Case 143: Hypertrophic Pyloric Stenosis

a) Hypertrophic Pyloric Stenosis: Correct! The ultrasound scan shows an elongated and hypertrophied muscle of the pylorus leading to gastric outlet obstruction. The pylorus length is measured at 18 mm and muscle thickness is measured at 5 mm. In this case, there is also mucosal hypertrophy that protrudes into the antrum of the stomach. Measurements of pyloric length of more than 15 mm and muscle wall thickness of more than 3 mm help confirm the diagnosis. In this case since the US is diagnostic, further imaging is not required.
Hypertrophic pyloric stenosis is the most common cause of gastric outlet obstruction in infants and involves hypertrophy and hyperplasia of the pyloric sphincter. The condition is managed with pyloromyotomy and initial supportive treatment in preparation for surgery.

b) A midgut volvulus typically presents with a whirl sign on ultrasound reflecting bowel rotating around the mesentery and associated vasculature. Color doppler ultrasound may show an inversion of the usual position of the SMA or SMV, with the SMA located to the right of the SMV. In addition, an enlarged proximal duodenum might ne noted, indicating an upper small bowel obstruction. An enlarged pylorus would not be expected.

c) Duodenal atresia typically presents with a double bubble sign on conventional x-rays and ultrasound with a dilated stomach and dilated duodenum. An enlarged pylorus would not be expected.
Note the doubly bubble sign is mostly seen and described on plain film radiography. However, a double bubble sign can also be seen on ultrasound, including preterm ultrasound, leading to an early diagnosis.

d) A duodenal web typically presents with a dilation of the duodenum and stomach proximal to the obstruction. It may also show the membranous web or diverticulum. An enlarged pylorus would not be seen in this condition.

Patient 144: Two-year-old male
Author: Heike E. Daldrup-Link, M.D.

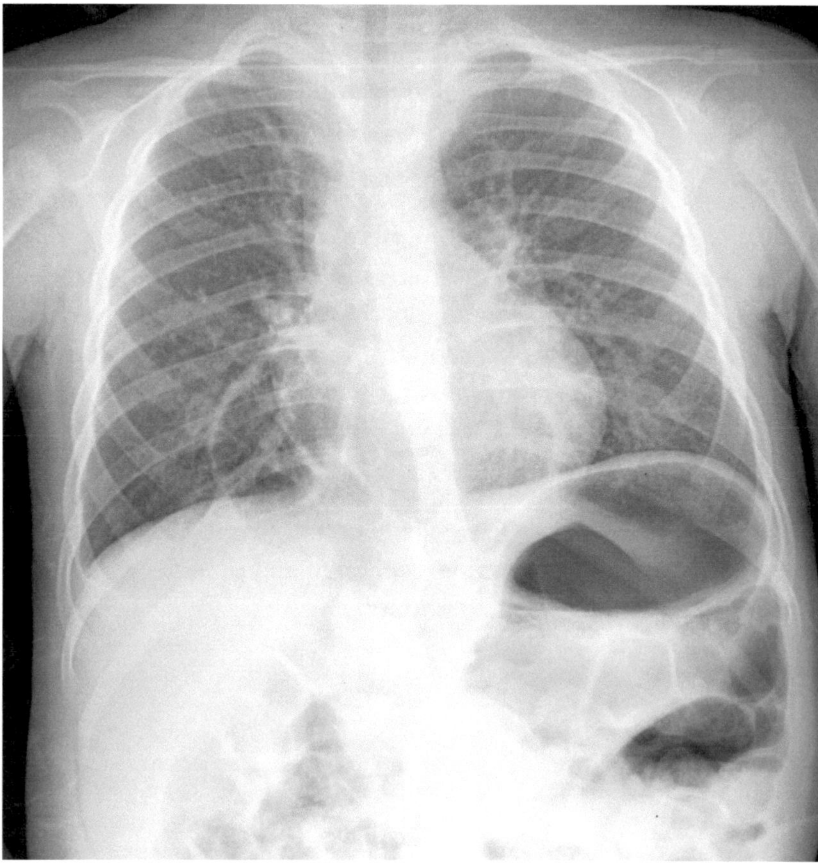

What is the most likely diagnosis:

a) Pneumomediastinum
b) Hiatal Hernia
c) Morgagni Hernia
d) Bochdalek Hernia

Case 144: Morgagni Hernia

a) Pneumomediastinum. The air seen here demonstrates bowel signature with haustrae.

b) Hiatal Hernia: The radiograph shown here demonstrated a bowel signature with haustrae. The stomach is noted under the left diaphragm.

c) Morgagni Hernia: Correct! The radiograph demonstrates a gas-filled bowel loop with haustrae projecting on the right anteromedial mediastinum. The bowel loops seem to connect with the gas-filled transverse colon. Morgagni hernias typically involve the anterior diaphragm, and the majority of hernias are right sided. A Morgagni hernia is often asymptomatic and presents several months or few years after birth.

d) Bochdalek Hernia: A Bochdalek hernia is a diaphragmatic defect that typically presents on fetal ultrasound or shortly after birth. It typically affects the left-posterior diaphragm and presents with bowel loops projecting on the left hemithorax.

Patient 145: Child with abdominal pain

Author: Heike E. Daldrup-Link, M.D.

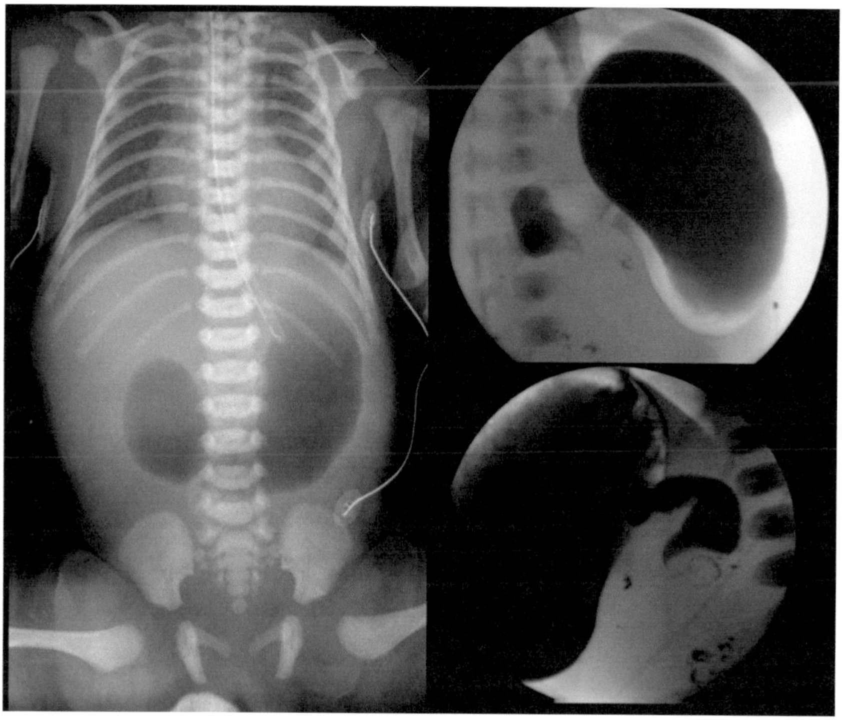

What is the most likely diagnosis:

a) Duodenal Atresia
b) Midgut volvulus
c) Small bowel intussusception
d) Free abdominal air

Case 145: Midgut Volvulus

a) A duodenal atresia can present with a double bubble sign, as noted on the radiograph here. However, the upper GI fluoroscopy images suggest a different diagnosis.

b) Midgut volvulus: Correct! The radiograph demonstrates a "double bubble sign", a gas-distended stomach and proximal duodenum with lack of air in distal bowel loops, suggesting an upper GI obstruction. The upper GI fluoroscopy images after oral administration of barium solution redemonstrate a dilated stomach and proximal duodenum. The duodenum demonstrates a "beak sign", a tapered distal end due to its rotation around the mesenteric axis. There is also a "corkscrew sign", a corkscrew-shaped small track of barium contrast material in the twisted proximal small bowel. Instant diagnosis of this condition is important to minimize the time of bowel ischemia and enable surgical decompression with rescue of ischemic bowel.

c) Small bowel intussusception: There is no evidence for an intussusception on the provided images. The imaging modality of choice for evaluation of a suspected intussusception would be an ultrasound.

d) Free abdominal air: There is free air noted on this radiograph.

Patient 146: Newborn Baby Girl

Author: Heike E. Daldrup-Link, M.D.

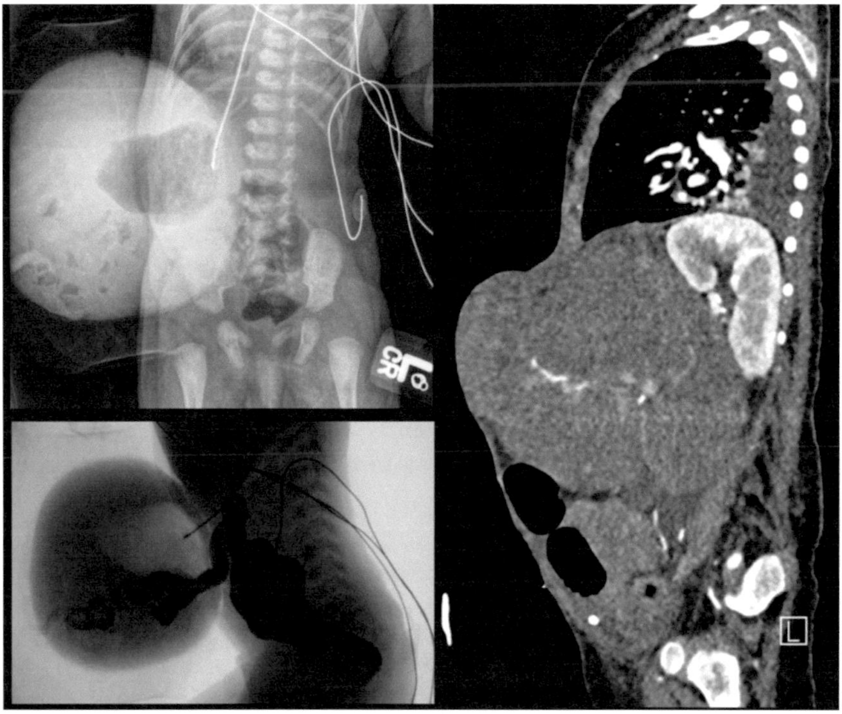

What is the most likely diagnosis:

a) Gastroschisis
b) Omphalocele
c) Physiological bowel herniation
d) Pentalogy of Cantrell

Case 146: Omphalocele

a) A gastroschisis presents as a para-median anterior wall defect with herniation of abdominal contents, most commonly bowel loops. There is no membrane that covers the herniated abdominal structures. The alpha-fetoprotein (AFP) is often elevated.

b) Omphalocele: Correct! The radiograph demonstrates a gas-filled stomach and bowel loops in a membrane covered anterior wall hernia. The underlying pathology is a herniation of abdominal contents into the umbilical cord. The sagittal CT scan confirms a midline abdominal wall defect with herniation of liver into the omphalocele. The upper GI fluoroscopy image after rectal administration of barium solution demonstrates the dilated gas-filled stomach and contrast-filled colon within the omphalocele. Omphaloceles are associated with multiple genetic anomalies, such as Wiedemann-Beckwith syndrome, Turner syndrome, Klinefelter syndrome as well as trisomy 13, 18 and 21, among others. There is also an association with bladder exstrophy and congenital heart diseases.

c) Normal physiologic herniation of the fetal bowel occurs between 8 and 12 weeks of gestation and is typically noted on a first trimester sonogram.

d) Pentalogy of Cantrell describes five congenital midline birth defects that encompass a lower sternal defect, congenital heart disease, absence of the diaphragmatic pericardium, anterior diaphragmatic defect, and an abdominal wall defect.

GI, GU, and Interventional

2) Duodenum and Small Bowel

Patient 147: 17-year-old female with abdominal pain

Author: Heike E. Daldrup-Link, M.D.

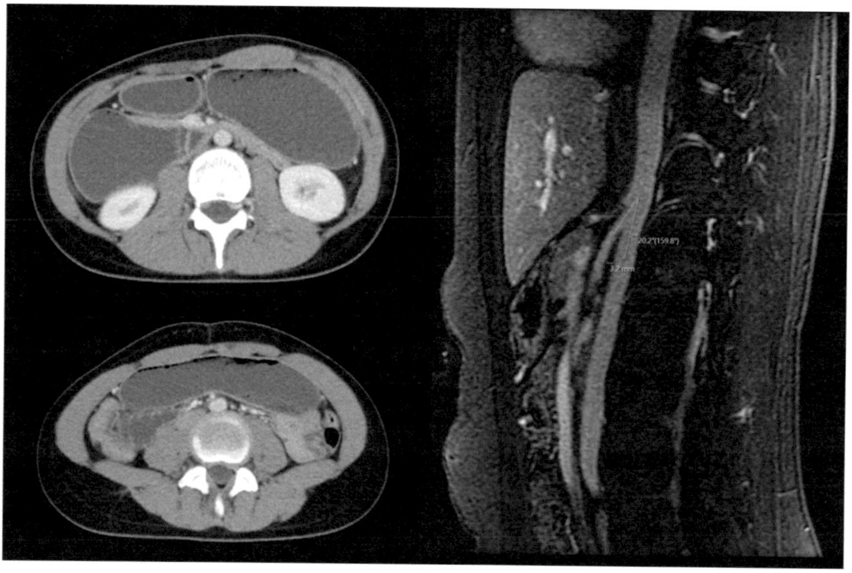

What is the most likely diagnosis:

a) Nutcracker syndrome
b) SMA syndrome
c) Lemierre syndrome
d) Diabetic gastroparesis

Case 147: SMA syndrome

a) Nutcracker syndrome describes the compression of the left renal vein between the abdominal aorta and the superior mesenteric artery.

b) Superior mesenteric artery (SMA) syndrome: Correct! On CT/MRI scans, the aortomesenteric angle measures less than 28 degrees and the aortomesenteric distance measures less than 10 mm. Cross-sectional imaging and upper GI fluoroscopy show dilatation of the first and second part of the duodenum in the right abdomen and collapsed small bowel in the left abdomen.

c) Lemierre syndrome: Thrombophlebitis of the internal jugular veins after oropharyngeal infection, which can lead to pulmonary septic emboli.

d) Diabetic gastroparesis: In this case, the stomach and the duodenum are dilated. The small bowel in the left abdomen is not dilated. This is typical of SMA syndrome.

Patient 148: Three-year old male, abdominal pain

Author: Heike E. Daldrup-Link, M.D.

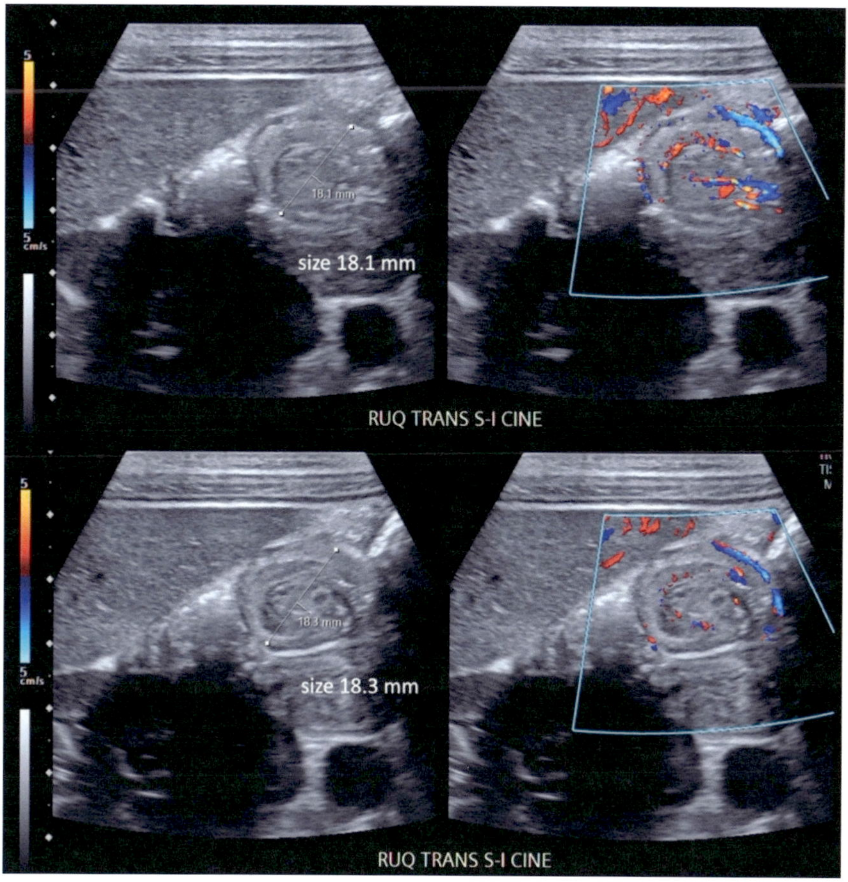

What is the most likely diagnosis:

a) Colocolic intussusception
b) Midgut volvulus
c) Small bowel intussusception
d) Duodenal hematoma

Case 148: Small Bowel Intussusception

a) A colocolic intussusception is rare. It would also present with a target sign, but the affected bowel loop would be much larger with a diameter of more than 2 cm (typically around 4-6 cm).

b) Midgut volvulus: The ultrasound would show a "whirlpool sign" on color doppler ultrasound as well as an inversion of the superior mesenteric vein (SMV) and mesenteric artery (SMA) with the SMA located to the right of the SMV. The whirlpool sign is seen as a swirling appearance of the SMV and mesentery around the SMA.

c) Small bowel intussusception: Correct! The Ultrasound demonstrates an abnormal bowel loop with a target or doughnut sign in the right upper abdominal quadrant. The target sign is created by two components: the inner intussusceptum (the donor loop) and the outer intussuscipiens (the receiving bowel loop). A diameter of less than 2 cm strongly favors a small bowel intussusception. The doughnut sign describes the alternating echogenic mucosa/muscularis and hypoechoic submucosa of the two bowel loops. The crescent-in-doughnut sign describes a doughnut sign with eccentrically located hyperechoic mesentery in the intususceptum. Additional signs that favor a small bowel intussusception (not shown here) include a length of less than 3 cm and preserved bowel wall motility. Small bowel intussusceptions are more commonly found in the periumbilical region or left upper abdominal quadrant. But they can also be found in the right abdomen. A small bowel intussusception is usually transient and resolves spontaneously. However, if it does not resolve spontaneously, a surgery may be rarely required.

d) Duodenal hematoma: A duodenal hematoma would present with a thickened bowel wall with hyperechogenic intramural and intraluminal components, consistent with intramural and intraluminal blood. The hematoma would not demonstrate internal flow on color Doppler ultrasound.

Patient 149: 15-year-old male, palpable mass above belly button

Author: Heike E. Daldrup-Link, M.D.

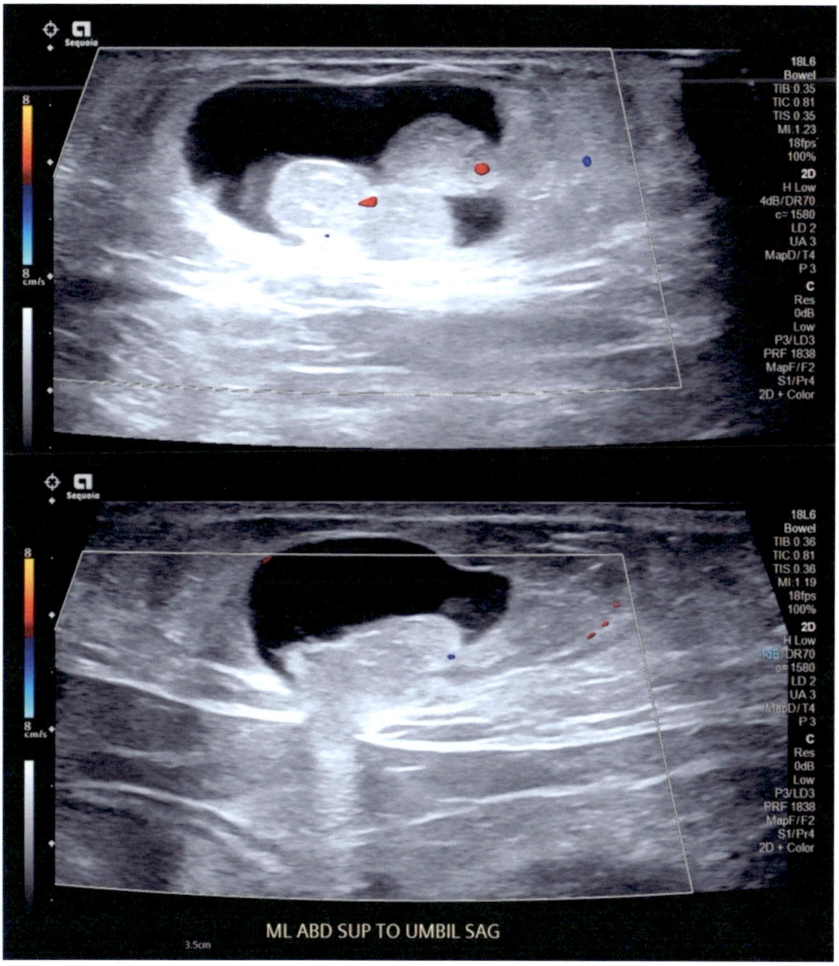

What is the most likely diagnosis:

a) Epigastric hernia
b) Richter hernia
c) Spigelian hernia
d) Littre hernia

Case 149: Epigastric hernia

a) Epigastric hernia. Correct! There is midline hernia in the epigastric region containing a bowel lop and free fluid. The bowel loop shows minimal to absent perfusion on the doppler ultrasound. A dynamic exam did not show any peristalsis of the trapped bowel. These features, along with the relatively large amount of surrounding free fluid are concerning for bowel loop strangulation and warrant an immediate surgical consult.

b) A Richter hernia describes the protrusion of only part of the circumference of the intestine's antimesenteric border through a rigid small defect of the abdominal wall. In most cases, because less than two-thirds of the circumference of the bowel wall is involved, the lumen of the intestine remains free, and obstruction or incarceration does not occur.

c) A Spigelian hernia is a hernia through a *lateral* abdominal wall defect, between the rectus muscle and the lateral oblique muscle. Most Spigelian hernias occur in the lower abdomen.

d) A Littre hernia is a hernia which contains a Meckel diverticulum. Usual sites of Littre hernia are inguinal, umbilical, and femoral.

Patient 150: 5-year-old male with abdominal distention

Author: Heike E. Daldrup-Link, M.D.

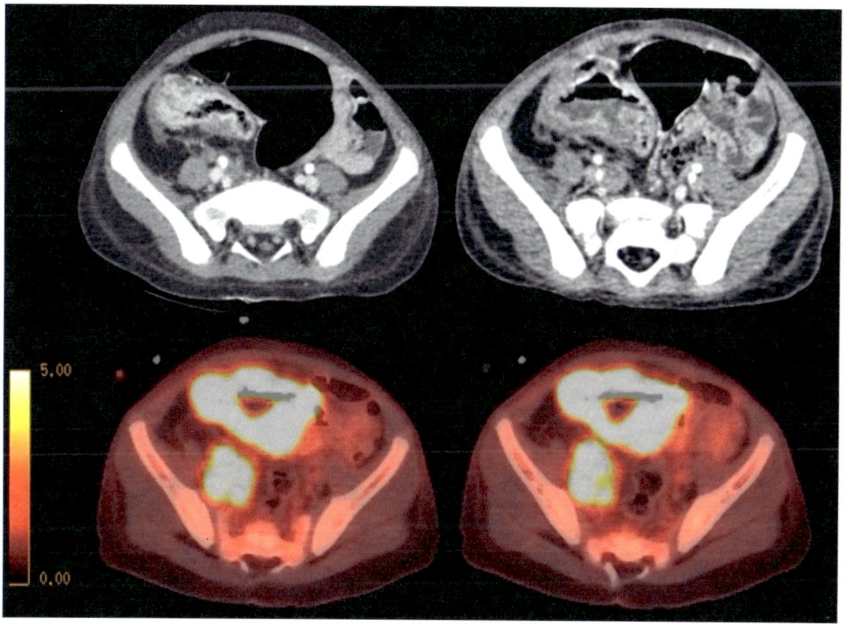

What is the most likely diagnosis:

a) Meckel's diverticulum
b) Rhabdomyosarcoma
c) Appendicitis
d) Lymphoma

Case 150: Small Bowel Lymphoma

a) Meckel's diverticulum refers to an ileal outpouching due to persistence of the omphalomesenteric or vitelline duct. A CT would typically show a fluid- or air-filled blind ending pouch, which arises from the distal ilium. If it is inflamed, there can be mural thickening of the diverticulum and adjacent small bowel. A 99m-Tc-Na-pertechnetate scan can aid in the diagnosis of typical gastric mucosa in the diverticulum. An 18F-FDG-PET scan would not usually be done.

b) A rhabdomyosarcoma can present as a centrally necrotic soft tissue mass. However, the abnormality shown here has bowel signature.

c) Appendicitis would present with an enlarged, bling ending tubular structure and/or an associated abscess. The abnormality shown here has bowel signature.

d) Lymphoma: Correct! There is a single abnormal loop of ilium in the right lower abdominal quadrant, which shows marked circumferential bowel wall thickening and significant aneurysmal dilation on the CT scan. The abnormal bowel loop demonstrates marked hypermetabolic activity on the 18F-FDG-PET scan. Taken together, these findings are most consistent with a small bowel lymphoma. The terminal ilium is the most common location. The bowel dilation is due to tumor infiltration of the muscularis propria and destruction of the autonomic nerve plexus. By contrast, carcinomas typically cause an obstruction due to a desmoplastic reaction.

GI, GU, and Interventional

3) Colon and General Abdominal Problems

Patient 151: One day old baby with distended abdomen
Author: Heike E. Daldrup-Link, M.D.

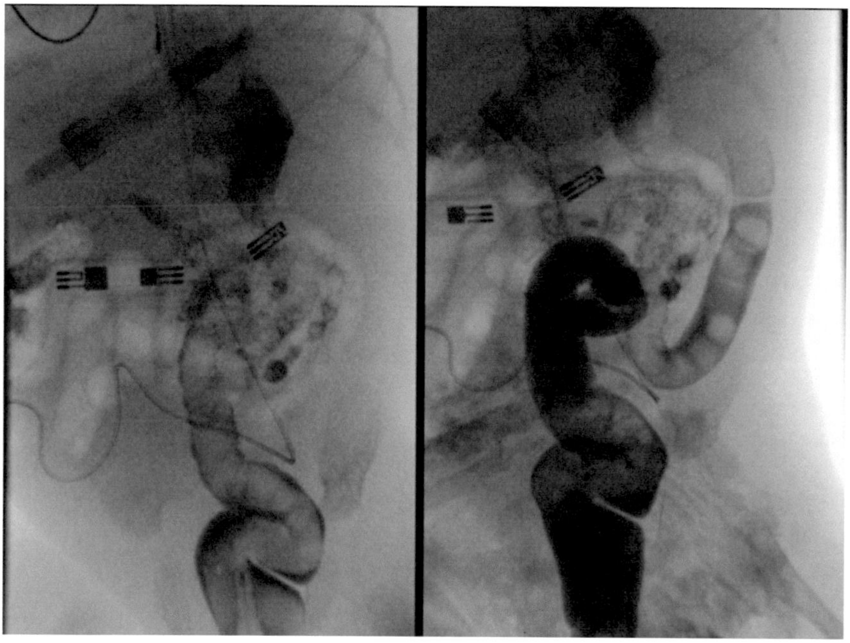

What is the most likely diagnosis on this contrast enema:

a) Meconium ileus
b) Ileal atresia
c) Meconium plug syndrome
d) Hirschsprung disease

Case 151: Meconium plug syndrome

a) Meconium ileus: The fluoroscopy images here do not show an obstruction of the distal ileum.

b) Ileal atresia: The fluoroscopy images here do not show a stenosis or obliteration of the distal ileum.

c) Meconium plug syndrome: Correct! The contrast enema demonstrates filling defects in the rectum and small caliber left colon, consistent with retained meconium. It is associated with maternal diabetes. An enema with water soluble contrast material is both diagnostic and therapeutic, leading to evacuation of meconium.

d) Hirschsprung disease: The contrast enema demonstrates a normal caliber colon, which would be unusual in patients with Hirschsprung disease.

Patient 152: 17-year-old adolescent, acute abdominal pain

Author: Lisa Adams, M.D.

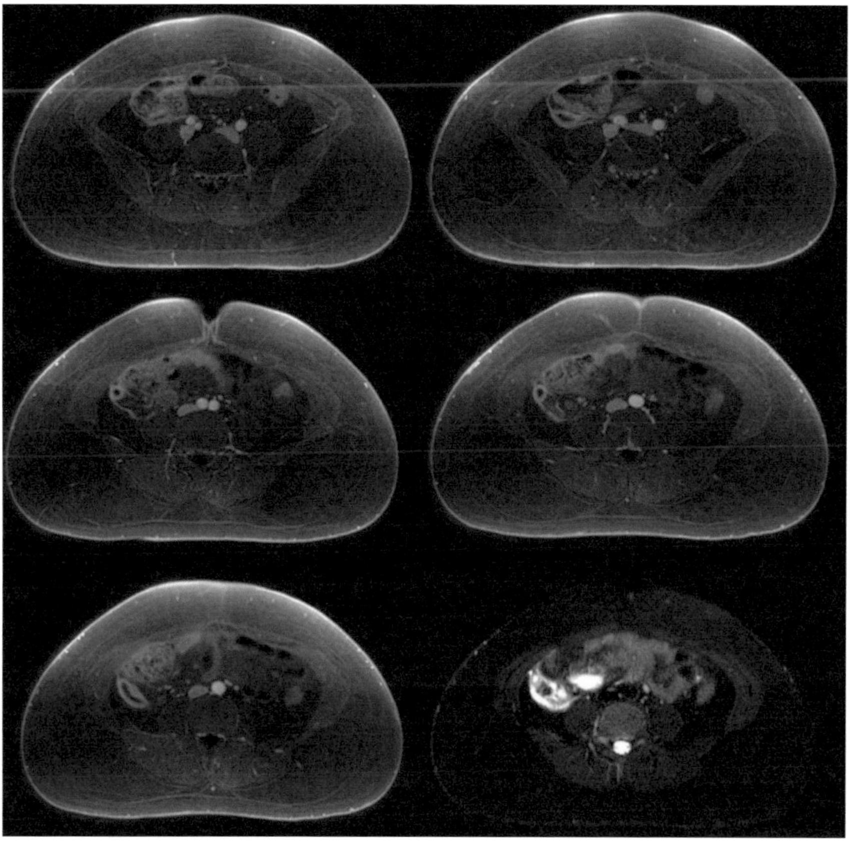

What is the most likely diagnosis:

a) Small bowel obstruction
b) Appendicitis
c) Meckel's diverticulum
d) Cecal diverticulitis

Case 152: Appendicitis

a) A small bowel obstruction would be associated with an abrupt transition from dilated to nondilated bowel. There is no transition point noted on the images shown. In addition, the localized free abdominal fluid in the right lower abdominal quadrant would not be expected.

b) Appendicitis – Correct! The appendix is enlarged, the wall of the appendix is thickened and hyperenhancing on contrast-enhanced T1-weighted MRI images. The T2-weighted MRI scans demonstrates fee fluid around the inflamed appendix. These findings are consistent with an acute appendicitis. The appendix is intact. There is no rupture of the appendix.

c) Meckel's diverticulum refers to an ileal outpouching due to persistence of the omphalomesenteric or vitelline duct. MRI would typically show a fluid- or air-filled bling ending pouch, which arises from the distal ilium. If it is inflamed, there can be mural mural thickening of the diverticulum and adjacent small bowel. 99m-Tc-Na-pertechnetate scan can aid in the diagnosis of typical gastric mucosa in the diverticulum.

d) Cecal diverticulitis is extremely rare in pediatric patients. There is no diverticulum noted on the provided MRI images.

Patient 153: Patient with leukemia and neutropenia

Author: Heike E. Daldrup-Link, M.D.

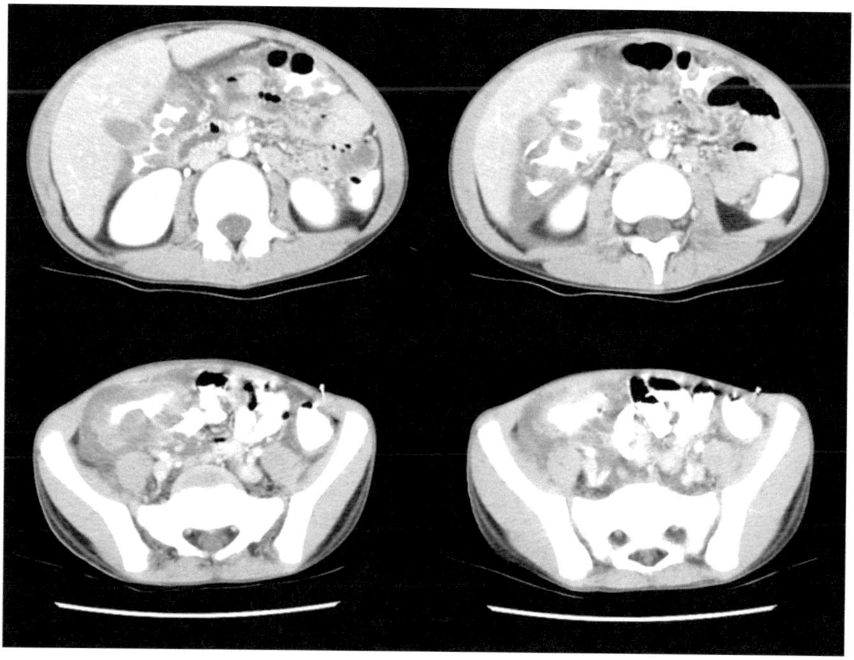

What is the most likely diagnosis:

a) Crohn's disease
b) Appendicitis with periappendiceal abscess
c) Neutropenic Typhlitis
d) Pseudomembranous Colitis

Case 153: Neutropenic Typhlitis

a) Crohn's disease could also present with localized bowel wall thickening and edema. However, the history of leukemia and neutropenia as well as the preferential involvement of the cecum and ascending colon suggest a different diagnosis.

b) The appendix is not noted on the CT scan here. The edematous thickened bowel loop in the right lateral abdomen shows haustrae, identifying it as abnormal colon.

c) Neutropenic Typhlitis: Correct! The CT scan shows marked bowel was swelling and edema of the cecum and ascending colon. Neutropenic typhlitis is due to intramural bacterial invasion without inflammatory reaction due to an underlying neutropenia.

d) Pseudomembranous colitis presents in patients with history of antibiotic therapy, such as clindamycin and cephalosporins, which lead to overgrowth of clostridium difficile, bacterial invasion and bowel wall thickening of the entire colon. A significant amount of ascites might be also present.

Patient 154: 11-month-old male, abdominal pain

Author: Heike E. Daldrup-Link, M.D.

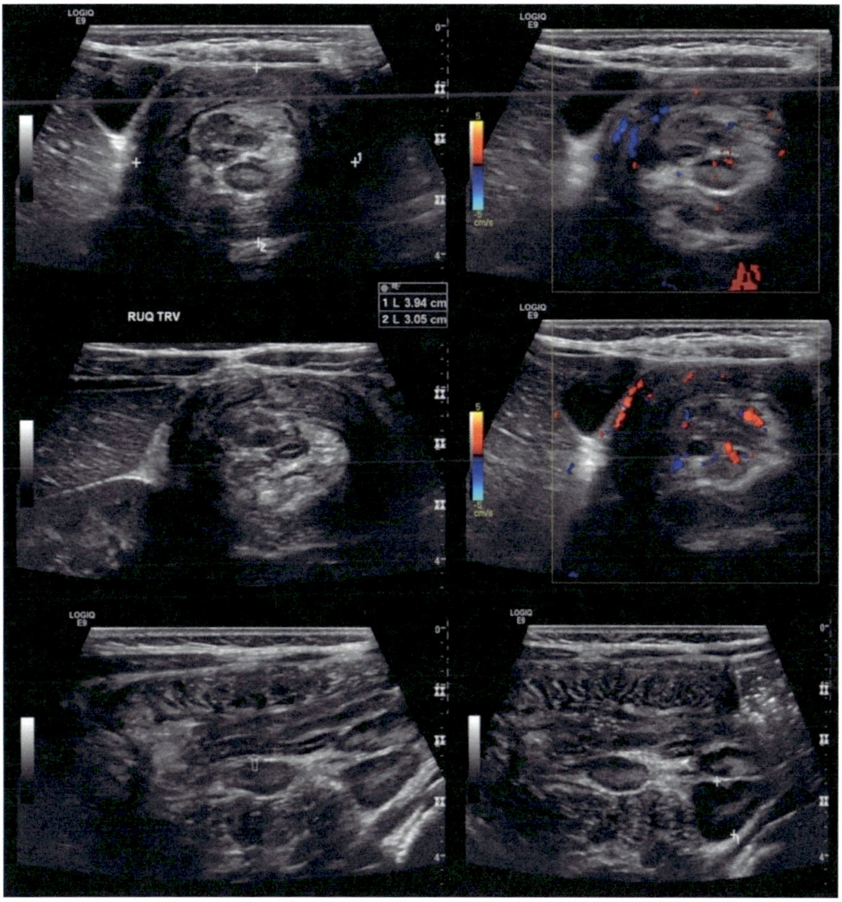

What is the most likely diagnosis:

a) Ileocolic Intussusception
b) Appendicitis
c) Small bowel intussusception
d) Germ Cell Tumor

Case 154: Ileocolic Intussusception

a) Ileocolic Intussusception: Correct! The Ultrasound demonstrates a characteristic target sign, a hypoechoic edematous wall of the intusscipiens around an echo-dense center of the intussuceptum. The diameter of the lesion is relatively large, measuring 3.9 cm. Mesenteric fat and lymph nodes are noted in the center of the intussusception. Multiple enlarged lymph nodes were noted in the lower abdominal quadrant, and likely served as the lead point for the intussusception.

b) Appendicitis: The lower right ultrasound image shows a normal appendix.

c) A small bowel intussusception can also present with a target or doughnut sign. However, the diameter of a small bowel intussusception is typically less than 2 cm. There is usually little no no central fat. Small bowel intussusceptions are more commonly found in the periumbilical region or left upper abdominal quadrant.

d) Germ cell tumor: A germ cell tumor in a male infant would be most found in the testis. It would typically present as an inhomogeneous mass, with areas of soft tissue, cysts, and calcifications. Lymph node metastases of malignant germ cell tumors could be found in the abdomen. But the lymph nodes shown here show a normal fatty hilum and no imaging signs of malignancy (large size, absent fatty hilum, inhomogeneous echotexture).

Patient 155: 11-month-old male, abdominal pain
Author: Heike E. Daldrup-Link, M.D.

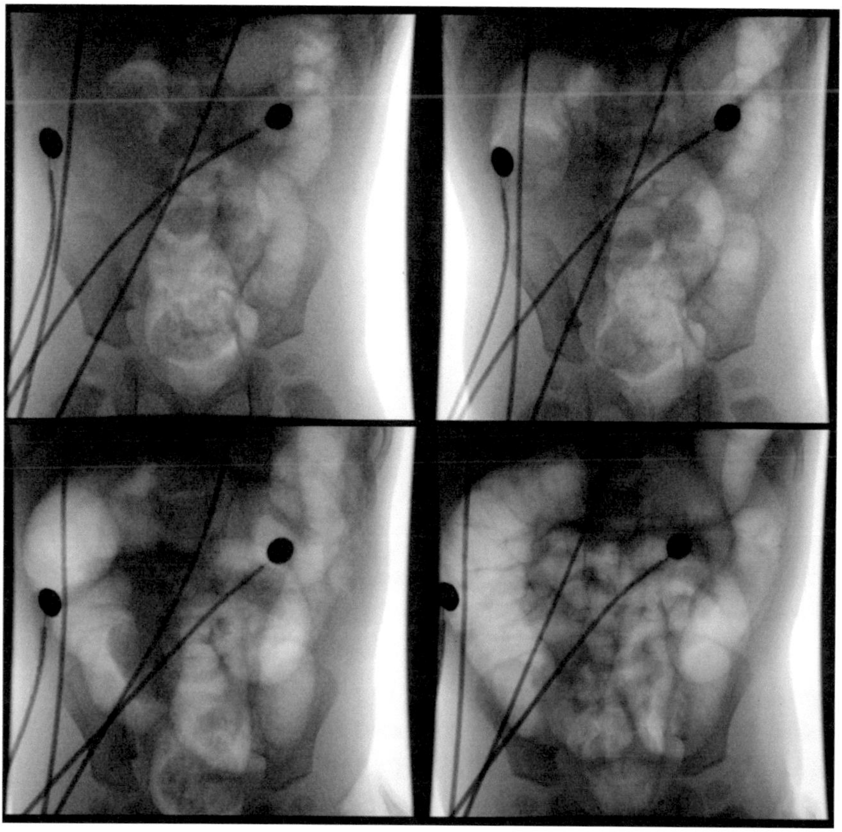

The maximum limit of air pressure applied for a pneumatic air reduction of an ileocolic intussusception is:

a) 60 mm Hg
b) 80 mm Hg
c) 100 mm Hg
d) 120 mm Hg

Case 155: Pneumatic air reduction of an ileocolic intussusception under fluoroscopic guidance

a) A pneumatic pressure of 60 mm Hg would usually not be sufficient to reduce an ileocolic intussusception.

b) A pneumatic pressure of 80 mm Hg would usually not be sufficient to reduce an ileocolic intussusception.

c) A pneumatic pressure of 100 mm Hg can be sufficient to reduce an ileocolic intussusception to the ileocecal valve. However, a slightly higher pressure if often needed to push the intususcipiens across the ileocecal valve.

d) Correct! A pneumatic pressure of 120 mm Hg is considered the upper limit of air pressure for pneumatic air reduction of an ileocolic intussusception under fluoroscopic guidance. The fluoroscopic images shown here demonstrate air insufflation into the ascending and transverse colon. The air outlines the intussusception at the right colonic flexure. The intussusception is gradually removed, as shown by successive air insufflation into the ascending colon. The reduction is followed fluoroscopically until backflow of air into distal small bowel loops is noted. At the end of the exam, air should flow freely from the cecum into the distal small bowel loops to signify complete reduction.

Patient 156: Premature infant with distended abdomen

Author: Heike E. Daldrup-Link, M.D.

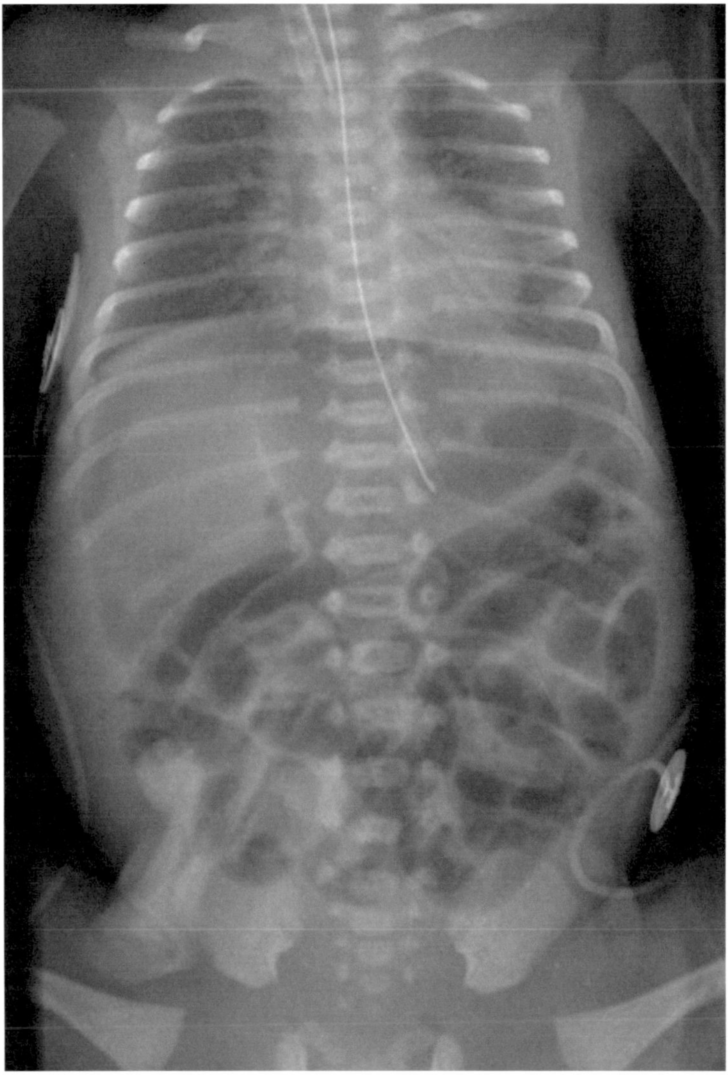

What is the most likely diagnosis:

a) Meconium pseudocyst
b) Free abdominal air
c) Midgut volvulus
d) Rectal atresia

Case 156: Necrotizing Enterocolitis, Free Abdominal Air

a) Meconium pseudocyst: There are no intraabdominal calcifications noted on this radiograph.

b) Free abdominal air: Correct: The radiograph demonstrates focal round and linear lucencies along multiple loops of bowel in the right-lateral, left upper and left lower abdomen, consistent with intramural air and necrotizing enterocolitis (NEC). In addition, there is a lucency projecting on the liver with a central dense linear opacification, consistent with a "football sign", air outlining the falciform ligament. A cross table lateral radiograph confirmed free abdominal air. Bowel rupture is a severe complication of NEC.

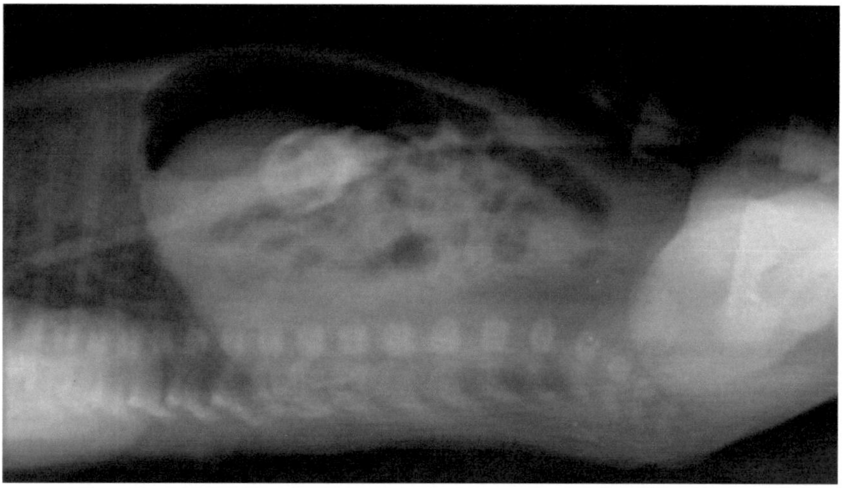

c) Midgut volvulus: A midgut volvulus presents with an upper GI obstruction. An x-ray of the abdomen would classically show a gas filled stomach and first/second portion of the duodenum with a beaked ending and decompressed distal bowel loops. The diagnosis is confirmed with an upper GI fluoroscopy.

d) Rectal atresia. The radiograph shown here does not show air in the rectum. That is a common finding in infants who are laying on their back. The rectum might be filled with fluid or meconium and/or a fluid filled urinary bladder might compress it. A concern for rectal atresia is diagnosed based on a clinical exam and lower GI fluoroscopy, if deemed appropriate.

Patient 157: Term newborn, mother diagnosed with ascites at third trimester of gestation

Author: Wipawee Morakote, M.D.

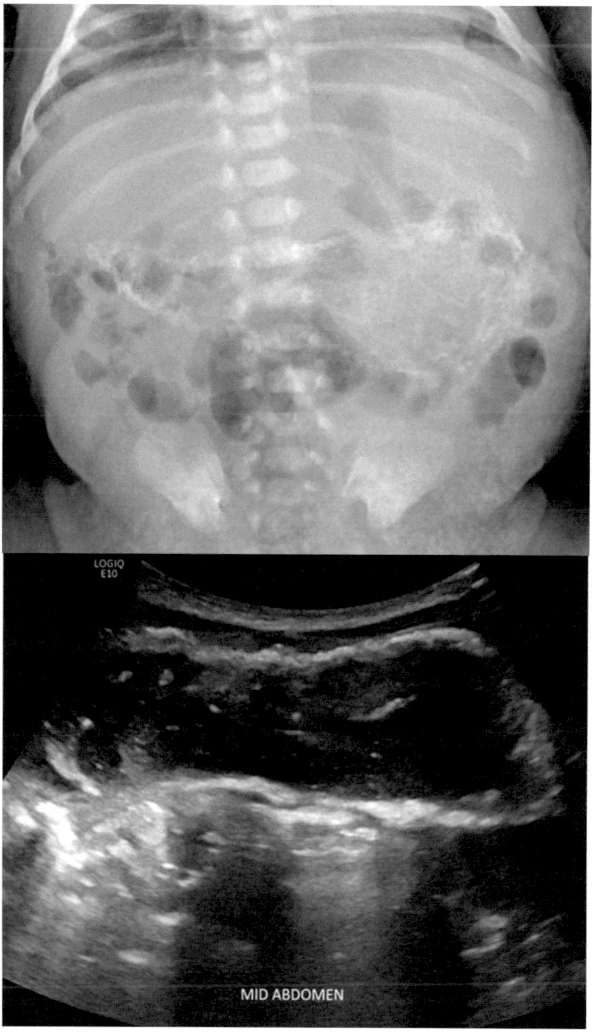

What is the most likely diagnosis:

a) Meconium pseudocyst
b) Enteric duplication cyst
c) Liver abscess
d) Pneumoperitoneum

Case 157: Meconium pseudocyst

a) Meconium pseudocyst: Correct! The abdominal radiograph shows a calcified mass in the mid abdomen, which displaces bowel loops laterally. The ultrasound reveals a cystic lesion with "snow-storm appearance", an echogenic wall with acoustic shadowing due to rim calcifications. These findings are suggestive of a meconium pseudocyst, a complication of intrauterine bowel perforation with formation of a cystic lesion around extruded meconium.

b) Enteric duplication cyst: The wall of the cyst does not show the gut signature sign, which includes five alternating hyperechoic and hypoechoic layers.

c) Liver abscess: The lesion is located in the mid abdomen, below the level of the the liver.

d) Pneumoperitoneum. The radiograph does not demonstrate any evidence of free air.

Patient 158: 8-month-old infant with constipation

Authors: Desiree R. Eshraghi, Soni C. Chawla, M.D.

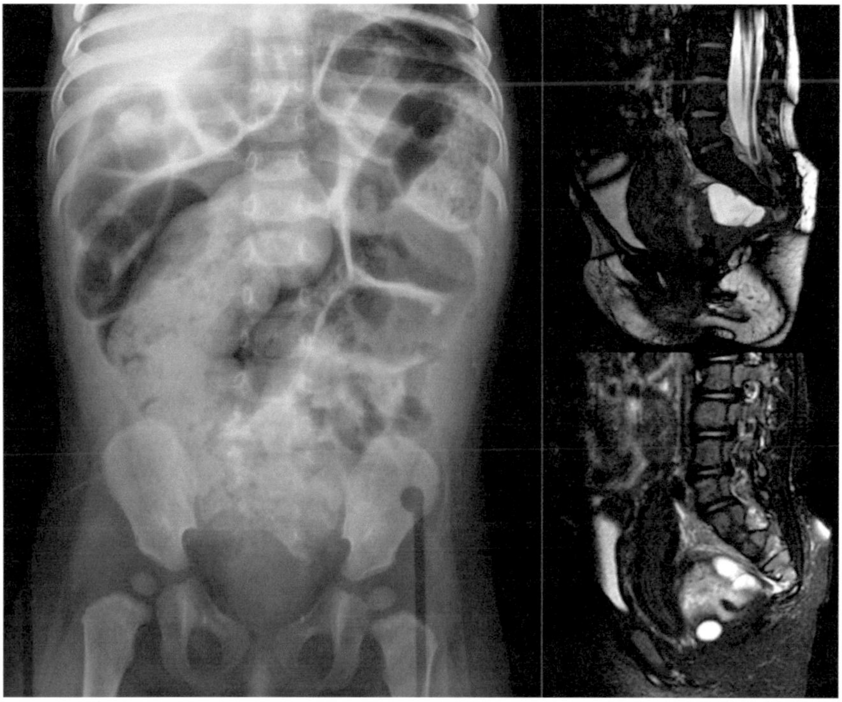

What is the most likely diagnosis:

a) Hirschsprung disease
b) Ovarian teratoma
c) Vanishing bone disease
d) Currarino Triad

Case 158: Currarino Triad

a) Hirschsprung disease. Hirschsprung disease leads to rectal narrowing and upstream colonic impaction. However, a sacral deformity would not be part of this disease.

b) Ovarian teratomas are typically located in front of the rectum. The inhomogeneous, partly solid, and partly cystic lesion shown here is located between the rectum and the sacrum, which is typical for a sacrococcygeal teratoma.

c) In vanishing bone disease, a lymphatic malformation leads to resorption of the bone. There is no lymphatic malformation noted here.

d) **Currarino Triad: Correct! Currarino triad is a rare autosomal dominant syndrome with characteristic findings of partial sacral agenesis, presacral teratoma and constipation. The frontal radiograph of the abdomen and pelvis demonstrates a sickle shaped appearance of the sacrum, consistent with partial agenesis. In addition, excessive and dense fecal material is noted in the sigmoid colon and rectum, consistent with rectal impaction and upstream colonic dilation. Sagittal T2-weighted MRI images of the pelvis demonstrate a large heterogeneous predominantly cystic presacral mass, which compresses and displaces the rectum anteriorly. The distal sacrum is absent, consistent with partial agenesis. A low-lying cord in a patulous spinal canal is consistent with a tethered cord.**

Patient 159: Teenager, abdominal pain

Author: Heike E. Daldrup-Link, M.D.

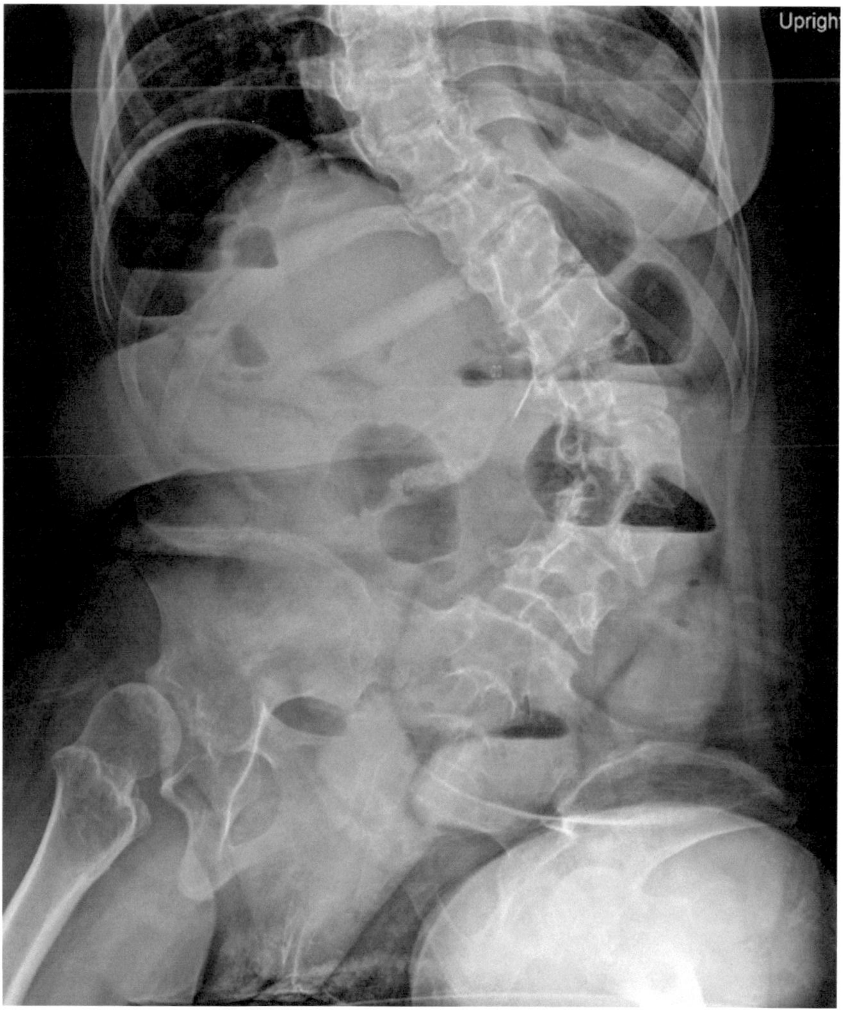

What is the most likely diagnosis:

a) Chilaiditi Syndrome
b) Marfan Syndrome
c) Bile Plug Syndrome
d) Hurler Syndrome

Case 159: Chilaiditi syndrome

a) Chilaiditi Syndrome: Correct! The radiograph demonstrates an interposition of gas-filled colon between the liver and the diaphragm.

b) Marfan Syndrome can present with scoliosis. However, typical skeletal findings of this syndrome are not present here, such as chest wall deformities, gracile ribs, an increased interpedicular distance of vertebral bodies, vertebral scalloping, enlarged sacral foramina and/or acetabular protrusion.

c) Bile plug syndrome represents an obstruction of the common bile duct by bile sludge in full-term infants.

d) Hurler syndrome (mucopolysaccharidosis I) presents with multiple skeletal anomalies, such as shortening and widening of long bones, widened anterior ribs with narrowed posterior parts (paddle ribs), hypoplastic vertebral bodies, especially at the thoracolumbar junction, and anterior inferior vertebral beaking, among others.

Patient 160: 13-year-old teenager, abdominal pain

Author: Heike E. Daldrup-Link, M.D.

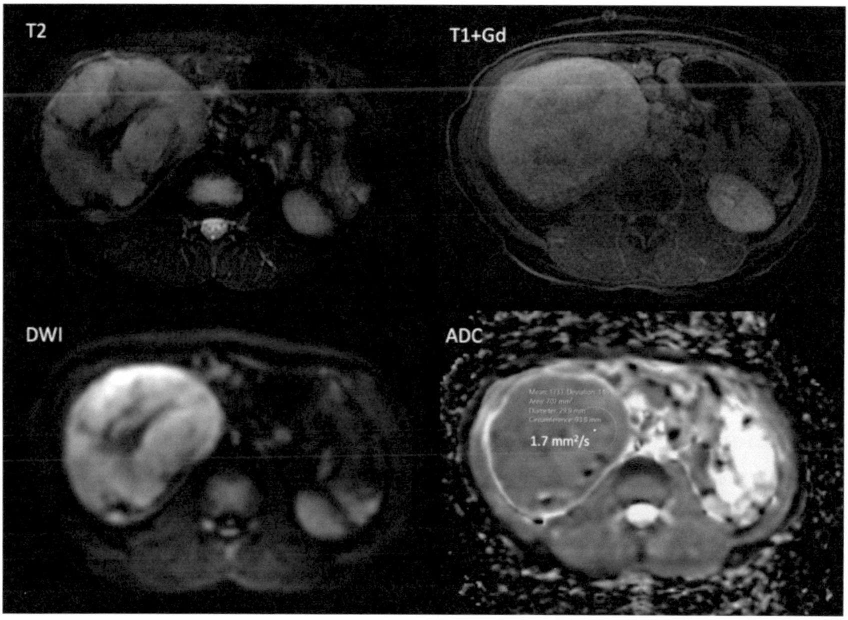

What is the most likely diagnosis:

a) Wilm's tumor
b) Lymphoma
c) Desmoid fibromatosis
d) Sclerosing mesenteritis

Case 160: Desmoid Fibromatosis

a) A Wilms tumor would typically occur in a child less than 3 years of age. The right kidney is not seen on the provided images. It was displaced caudally by the mass (not shown here). There is no claw sign noted. A Wilms tumor typically present with markedly restricted diffusion and ADC value of less than 1.0 mm^2/s.

b) Lymphomas in teenagers typically present with markedly restricted diffusion and ADC value of less than 1.0 mm^2/s. s.

c) Desmoid fibromatosis: Correct! The MRI demonstrates a large, relatively well circumscribed lesion in the right lower abdominal quadrant, which demonstrates markedly hypointense central and peripheral areas on T2 weighted MRI images, consistent with fibrosis. In addition, the lesion shows marked contrast enhancement on delayed Gd-enhanced images and moderately restricted diffusion on diffusion-weighted MRI with an ADC value of 1.733 mm^2/s. Typical malignant tumors in pediatric patients, such as lymphoma, neuroblastoma, Wilm's tumor and sarcomas would typically demonstrate markedly restricted diffusion on diffusion-weighted MRI with an ADC value of less than 1.0 mm^2/s. Mesenteric desmoid tumors can occur sporadically or be associated with familial polyposis coli.

d) Sclerosing mesenteritis typically presents more centrally at the root of the mesentery.

Patient 161: One day old baby with distended abdomen
Author: Heike E. Daldrup-Link, M.D.

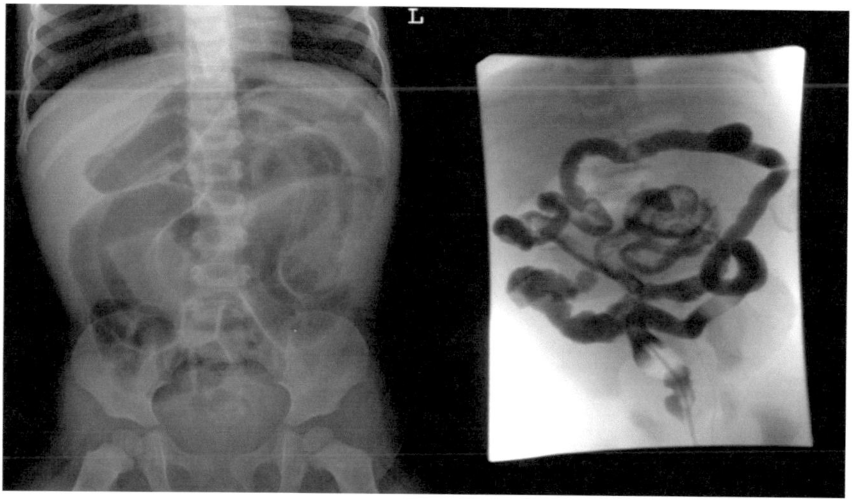

What is the most likely diagnosis on this contrast enema:

a) Meconium ileus
b) Ileal atresia
c) Meconium plug syndrome
d) Hirschsprung disease

Case 161: Meconium Ileus

a) Meconium ileus: Correct! The radiograph demonstrates gas-distended proximal and distal small bowel loops. The contrast enema demonstrates a microcolon and filling defects in the distal ileum. Meconium ileus is highly associated with cystic fibrosis. Water-soluble contrast enema usually clears the impacted meconium.

b) Ileal atresia: The fluoroscopy images here do not show a stenosis or obliteration of the distal ileum.

c) Meconium plug syndrome is diagnosed as a filling defect in the rectum, consistent with retained meconium.

d) Hirschsprung disease: The contrast enema demonstrates a filling defect in the terminal ileum, which would be unusual in patients with Hirschsprung disease.

Patient 162: One week old premature baby

Author: Heike E. Daldrup-Link, M.D.

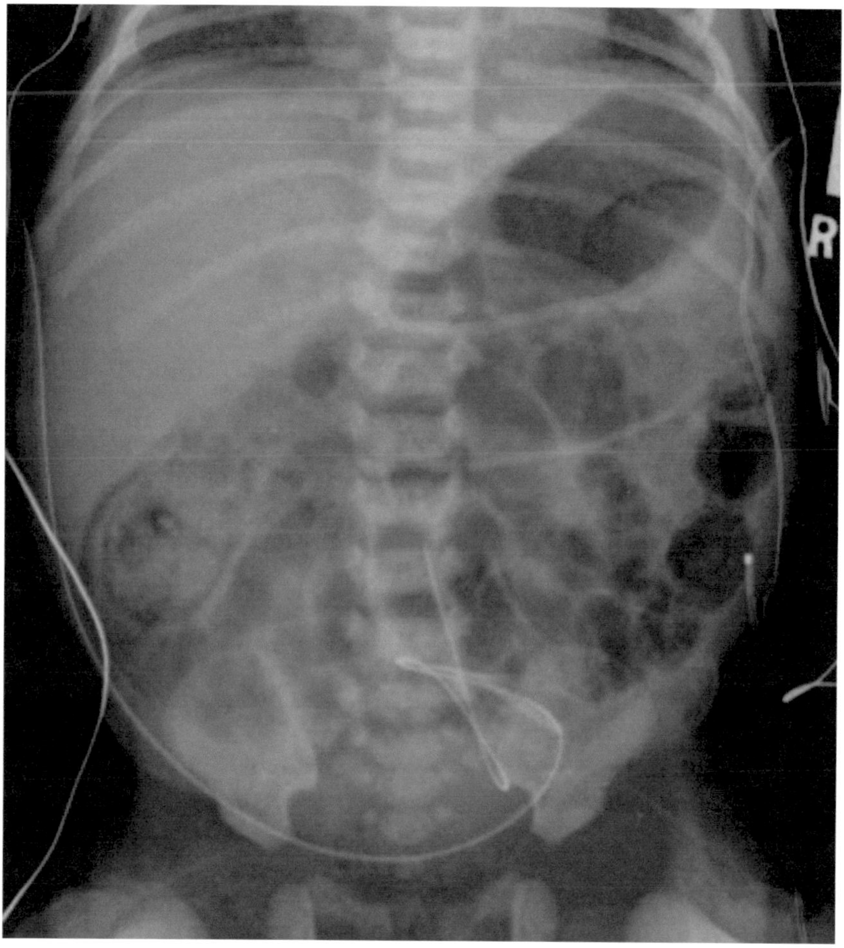

What is the most likely diagnosis:

a) Bezoar
b) Pneumoperitoneum
c) Intussusception
d) Necrotizing enterocolitis

Case 162: Necrotizing Enterocolitis

a) Bezoars would be very unusual at this early age. A trichobezoar, a bezoar consisting of ingested hair, would be most commonly located in the stomach. A phytobezoar, a bezoar consisting of indigestible food material, would not be expected in a baby which is typically fed with milk. A lactobezoar, a bezoar consisting of milk curds can be seen in premature infants and typically localizes to the stomach.

b) Pneumoperitoneum: The radiograph does not show free abdominal air. The air seen here localizes to the bowel wall.

c) Intussusception: The ring-like lucency in the right lower abdomen, shown here, is very low in density, consistent with pneumatosis. Sometimes, mesenteric fat between an intussusceptum and the recipient colon can also create a ring-like lucency. However, it is much more subtle than the linear lucency shown here.

d) Necrotizing enterocolitis (NEC): Correct! The abdominal radiograph demonstrates linear lucencies outlining the colonic wall in the right lower abdomen, mid abdomen and left upper abdomen. In addition, there are focal round lucencies, projecting on bowel loops in the left lower abdomen. These findings are typical for pneumatosis intestinalis. In a premature infant, the most common underlying diagnosis is an NEC.

Patient 163: Newborn baby, bulging flanks

Author: Heike E. Daldrup-Link, M.D.

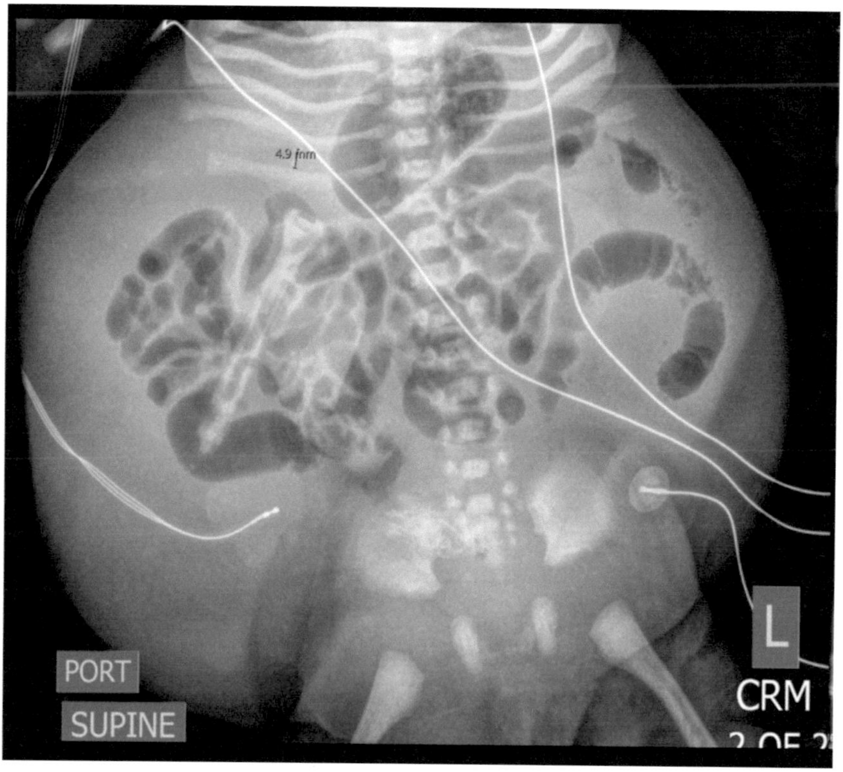

Prune Belly syndrome is characterized by the following triad:

a) Anterior abdominal wall defect, hydroureteronephrosis, microcolon
b) Deficient or absent abdominal wall musculature, hydroureteronephrosis, cryptorchidism
c) dilated non-obstructed urinary bladder, very small colon, decreased or absent intestinal movements
d) Necrotizing enterocolitis

Case 163: Prune Belly / Eagle-Barrett syndrome

a) Prune Belly syndrome is not associated with a microcolon. Other anomalies associated with Prune Belly Syndrome are congenital heart defects, malrotation of the bowel and imperforate anus.

b) Prune belly syndrome / Eagle Barret syndrome: Correct! The radiographs demonstrate markedly bulging flanks due to absence of the abdominal wall musculature and marked bilateral hydronephrosis. The syndrome is associated with undescended testes.

c) The triad of dilated non-obstructed urinary bladder (megacystis), very small colon (microcolon), and decreased or absent intestinal movements (intestinal peristalsis) describes the megacystis microcolon intestinal hypoperistalsis syndrome.

d) There are no signs of intramural gas, portal venous gas or free abdominal air to suggest a necrotizing enterocolitis.

Patient 164: One week old male infant

Author: Heike E. Daldrup-Link, M.D.

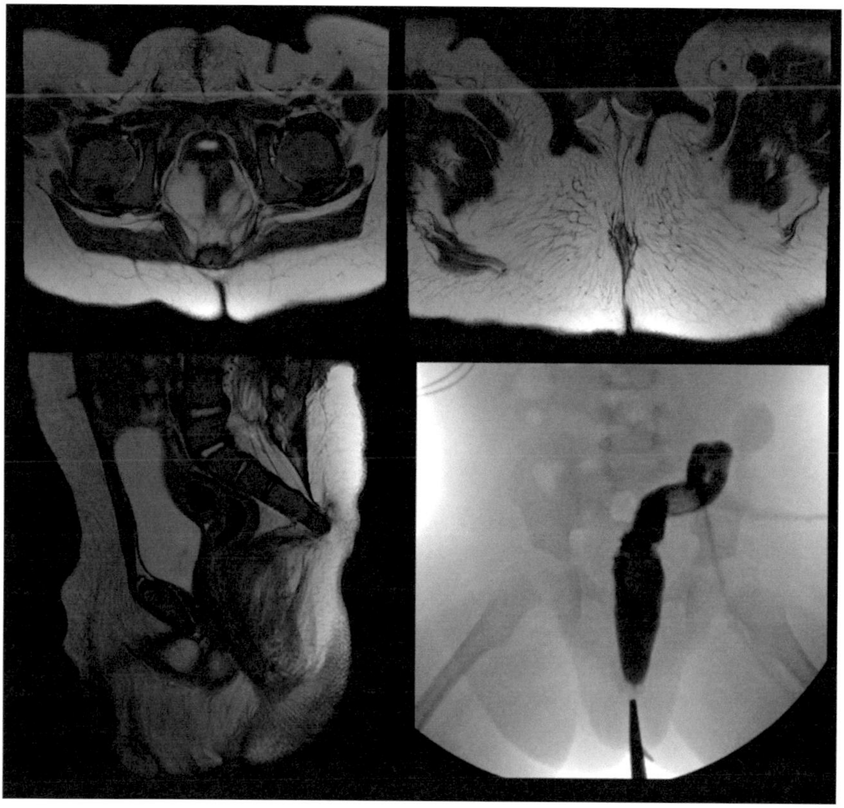

What is the most likely diagnosis:

a) Anal Atresia
b) Herlyn Werner Wunderlich Syndrome
c) Patent Urachal Duct
d) Currarino Triad

Case 164: Anal Atresia

a) Anal Atresia: Correct! The axial and sagittal T2-weighted MRI shows a blind-ending, anteriorly displaced distal rectum. The anus cannot be identified, and the levator ani musculature is atretic. The anal atresia is located below the level of the levator musculature, with a distance of less than 2 cm to the perineal surface, characterizing it as a low atresia. The sagittal MRI also shows an associated partial agenesis of the sacrum. The patient was treated with a colonostomy. The fluoroscopy images show contrast material, which has been injected through the colonostomy into the descending colon and rectum. A forceps marks the location of the skin surface. The short distance between the distal rectum and the perineal surface confirms the low atresia.

b) Herlyn Werner Wunderlich Syndrome is a Mullerian Duct Anomaly, characterized by an obstructed hemivagina, uterus didelphys and ipsilateral renal agenesis. The patient here is male. If you do not know an answer on a multiple-choice list, focus on the remaining options and check if you can rule out the others. If not, you got the correct answer.

c) A patent urachal duct refers to a patent connection between the dome of the urinary bladder and the umbilicus. The structure shown here is a blind ending rectum.

d) Currarino triad is defined by partial sacral agenesis, presacral teratoma and constipation. There is no teratoma or constipation noted on the images here.

Patient 165: 4-year-old female with abdominal pain

Author: Heike E. Daldrup-Link, M.D., Shelby Payne, M.D.

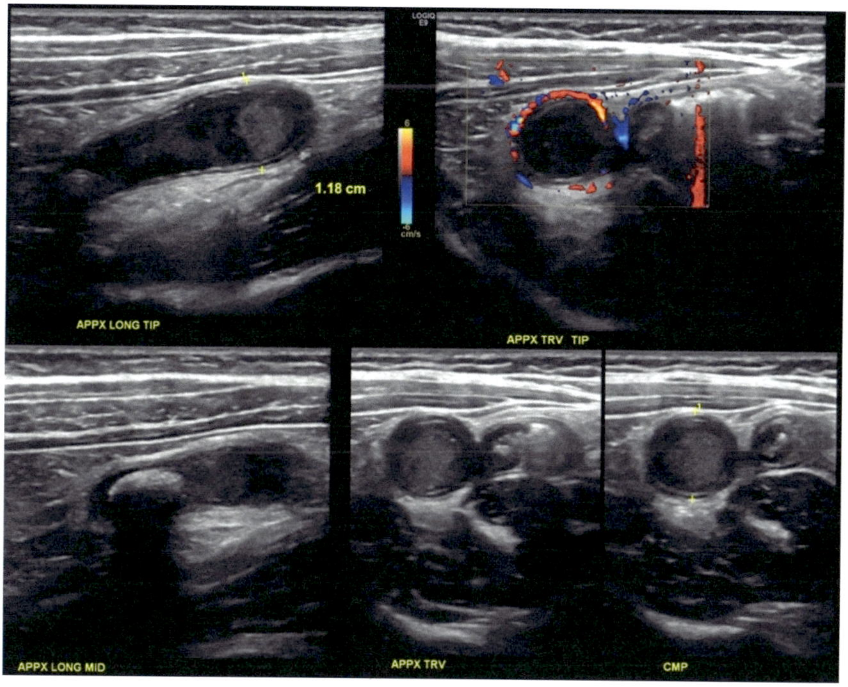

What is the most likely diagnosis:

a) Meckel's diverticulum
b) Rhabdomyosarcoma
c) Acute Appendicitis
d) Lymphoma

Case 165: Acute Appendicitis

a) Meckel's diverticulum refers to an ileal outpouching. Most diagnoses are made based on cross-sectional and/or radionuclide imaging. A CT scan would typically show a fluid- or air-filled blind ending pouch, which arises from the distal ilium. A 99m-Tc-Na-pertechnetate scan can aid in the diagnosis of typical gastric mucosa in the diverticulum. The appendicolith as seen here would be unusual in a Meckel's diverticulum.

b) A rhabdomyosarcoma can present as a centrally necrotic soft tissue mass. However, the abnormality shown here has bowel signature.

c) Acute Appendicitis: Correct! The ultrasound demonstrates an enlarged, bling ending tubular structure, which has a diameter of more than 6 mm, is not compressible and markedly hyperemic on color doppler ultrasound. A hyperechogenic lesion is noted in the proximal lumen and shows posterior acoustic shadowing, consistent with an appendicolith.

d) Bowel lymphoma typically presents with marked circumferential bowel wall thickening and significant aneurysmal dilation of the affected bowel loop. Most diagnoses are made based on cross-sectional and/or radionuclide imaging. An 18F-FDG-PET scan shows an abnormal bowel loop with marked hypermetabolic activity.

GI, GU, and Interventional

4) Liver, Spleen and Pancreas

Patient 166: 14-year-old female, history withheld
Author: Heike E. Daldrup-Link, M.D.

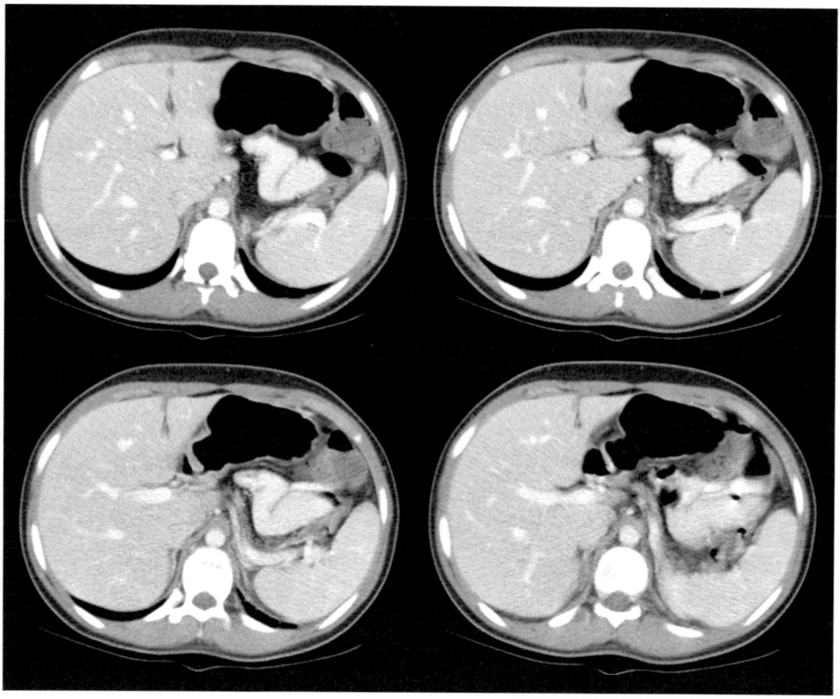

What is the most likely diagnosis:

a) Cushing syndrome
b) Cystic fibrosis
c) Dorsal pancreatic agenesis
d) Lonely spleen syndrome

Case 166: Cystic Fibrosis

a) Cushing syndrome can lead to pancreatic lipomatosis and overall increased visceral fat. The latter is not seen here.

b) Cystic fibrosis: Correct! The CT scan demonstrates hypodense parenchyma of the pancreas with negative attenuation values, consistent with lipomatosis. The normal dense pancreatic parenchyma has been completely replaced by low density fat.

c) An agenesis of the dorsal pancreas is a rare congenital malformation in which either the entire dorsal pancreas or part of the dorsal pancreas fails to develop.

d) Lonely spleen syndrome: I hope this fictitious name made you smile!

Patient 167: Newborn with abdominal distension

Authors: Desiree R. Eshraghi, Soni C. Chawla, M.D.

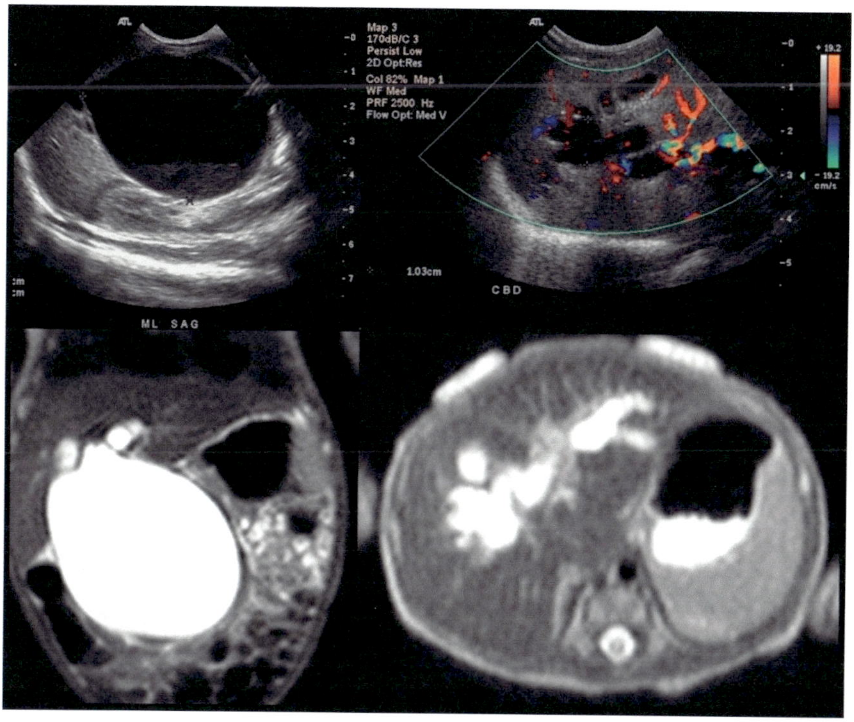

What is the most likely diagnosis:

a) Choledochal cysts
b) Hepatic cysts
c) Duodenal atresia
d) Gallbladder duplication

Case 167: Choledochal Cyst

a) Choledochal cysts: Correct! The ultrasound images demonstrate severe intrahepatic biliary ductal dilation and a large cystic dilation of the extrahepatic common bile duct. Coronal and axial T2 haste images of the abdomen demonstrate severe fusiform dilation of the common bile duct consistent with a type I choledochal cyst.

b) Hepatic cysts are common benign liver lesions. They have well-defined margins with thin walls and no malignant potential. The lesion shown here is centered outside of the liver and branches into dilated right and left intrahepatic bile ducts, which is consistent with a dilated common bile duct.

c) A duodenal atresia would present with a double bubble sign on conventional radiographs and ultrasound. It would not usually be associated with a dilation of the intra-hepatic bile ducts.

d) A gallbladder duplication represents an accessory gallbladder. It would not usually be associated with a dilation of the intra-hepatic bile ducts.

Patient 168: Two-month-old male with jaundice, pale stool, and dark urine.

Author: Wipawee Morakote, M.D.

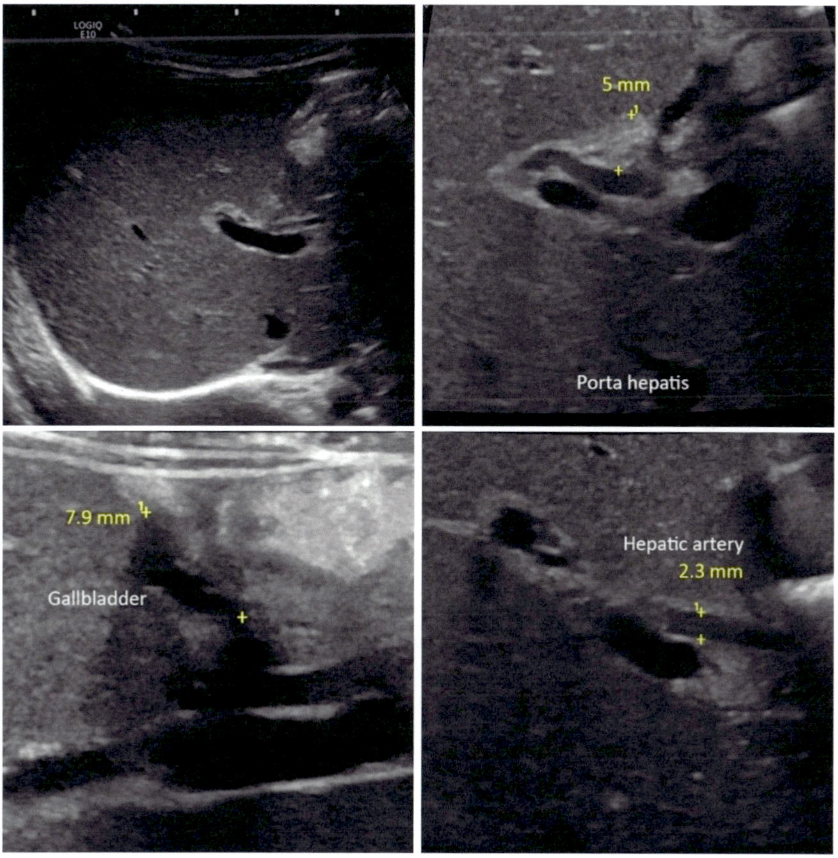

What is the most likely diagnosis:

a) Choledochal Cyst
b) Neonatal Hepatitis
c) Biliary Atresia
d) Congenital Hepatic Fibrosis

Case 168: Biliary Atresia

a) A choledochal cyst is a congenital hepatobiliary anomaly characterized by dilatation of the extrahepatic and/or intrahepatic bile duct(s). The Todani classification divides choledochal cysts into five major types. The most common type 1 is a fusiform dilatation of the common bile duct. The images shown here do not show a dilatation of the bile duct.

b) Neonatal hepatitis is an inflammation of the liver in the first 1-2 months of live due to various causes, such as a viral infection. The ultrasonographic findings in neonatal hepatis can include an inhomogenous, abnormal hepatic parenchymal echogenicity (increased or decreased). The biliary system is normal including normal size of the gallbladder and normal common bile duct.

c) Correct! The ultrasound of the liver demonstrates a triangular cord sign, an abnormal gallbladder, and an enlarged hepatic artery, which are highly suspicious of biliary atresia. The triangular cord sign describes triangular echogenic tissue with a thickness of 4 mm or more anterior to the right portal vein or portal bifurcation. It represents the fibrous remnant of the obliterated bile duct. An abnormal gallbladder is defined based on small size (<15 mm in length), irregular shape, and irregular wall. In some cases of biliary atresia, the gallbladder may be absent. Another important finding of biliary atresia is an enlargement of the hepatic artery greater than 1.5 mm in axial diameter. Increased subcapsular flow and splenomegaly (not shown) can also be seen. The hepatobiliary scan of this patient showed no excretion of the radiotracer into the gallbladder and small bowel, confirming the diagnosis of biliary atresia.

d) Congenital hepatic fibrosis is associated with autosomal recessive polycystic kidney disease (ARPKD). The ultrasonographic findings include increased hepatic echogenicity and poorly defined portal vessels.

Patient 169: 14-year-old female with abdominal pain

Author: Heike E. Daldrup-Link, M.D.

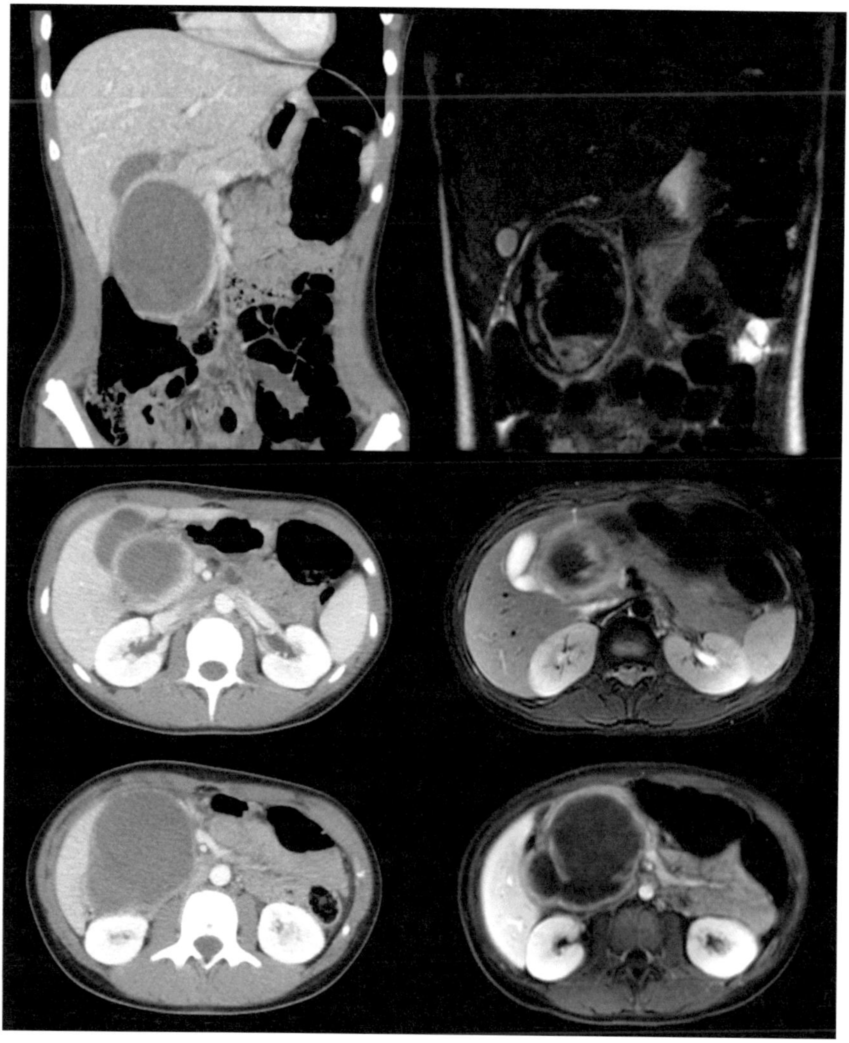

What is the most likely diagnosis:

a) Choledochal cysts
b) Hepatic cyst
c) Duodenal atresia
d) Solid Pseudopapillary Tumor of the Pancreas

Case 169: Solid Pseudopapillary Tumor of the Pancreas

a) Choledochal cyst: A choledochal cyst is characterized by a dilation of the extrahepatic common bile duct, often associated with intrahepatic biliary ductal dilation. There is no biliary duct dilation noted here.

b) Hepatic cysts are common benign liver lesions. They have well-defined margins with thin walls and no malignant potential. The lesion shown here is centered outside of the liver. Coronal CT and MRI scans demonstrate a claw sign of the pancreas, suggesting pancreatic origin of the lesion.

c) A duodenal atresia would present with a dilated stomach and proximal duodenum. Coronal CT and MRI scans here demonstrate a non-dilated stomach. Air is noted in multiple distal bowel loops.

d) Solid Pseudopapillary Tumor of the Pancreas: Correct! The CT and MRI images demonstrate a focal, well-demarcated, inhomogeneous, partially cystic, and partially solid, contrast-enhancing lesion in the head of the pancreas. The coronal images show a claw sign of the pancreatic head around the apex of the lesion. The T2-weighted MRI demonstrates non-enhancing hypointense components, consistent with hemorrhagic degeneration. Note that some pseudopapillary tumors can present as completely solid masses. Approximately 85% of solid pseudopapillary tumors are benign and 15% are malignant.

Patient 170: 10-year-old male

Author: Heike E. Daldrup-Link, M.D.

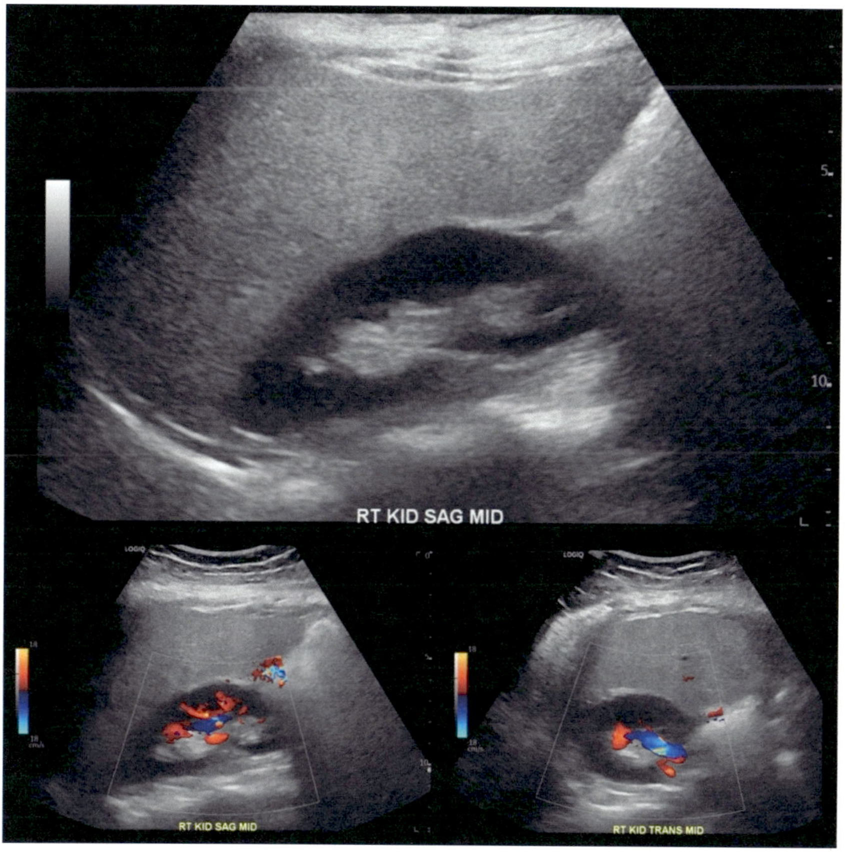

What is the most likely diagnosis:

a) Chronic kidney disease
b) Medullary Nephrocalcinosis
c) Oxalosis
d) Hepatic Steatosis

Case 170: Hepatic Steatosis

a) Chronic kidney disease presents with variable findings on ultrasound, such as echogenic kidneys, small size, reduced cortical thickness, renal cysts and reduced renal vascularity on doppler ultrasound. None of these findings are noted here.

b) Medullary nephrocalcinosis usually presents with hyperechogenic pyramids which demonstrate posterior acoustic shadowing. The ultrasound shown here demonstrates prominent fat in the area of the renal pelvis, consistent with clinically diagnosed obesity.

c) Oxalosis leads to calcium oxalate deposition in the kidneys with ultrasound findings of renal stones and cortical nephrocalcinosis.

d) Hepatic Steatosis: Correct! The ultrasound shows a markedly hyperechogenic liver when compared to the renal cortex as an internal reference standard. The most common etiologies in children and young adults are obesity and diabetes mellitus. An elastography exam could be added to determine the presence and degree of an associated fibrosis of the liver parenchyma.

Patient 171: A child with acute abdominal pain

Authors: Wipawee Morakote, M.D., Pannee Visrutaratna, M.D.

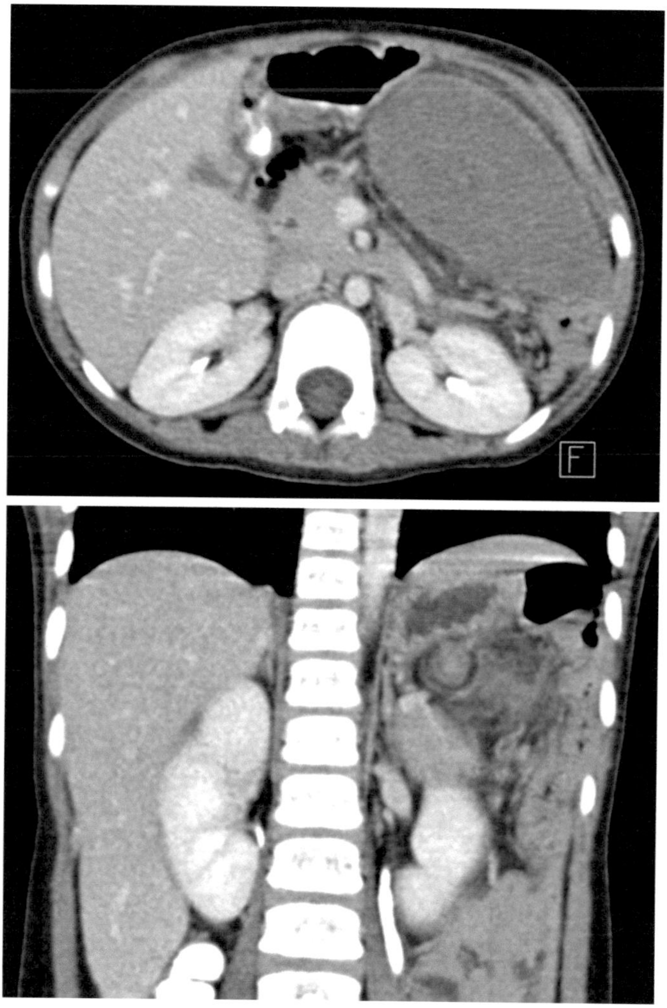

What is the most likely diagnosis:

a) Acute pancreatitis
b) Wandering spleen with torsion
c) Small bowel intussusception
d) Intra-abdominal abscess

Case 171: Wandering Spleen with Splenic Pedicle Torsion

a) Pancreatitis: The pancreas is normal enhancement and contour. No peripancreatic fluid is demonstrated.

b) Wandering spleen with torsion: Correct! The axial CT scan shows the spleen in an unusually low location in the mid abdomen. The spleen demonstrates poor enhancement. The coronal CT scan shows a typical whirlpool sign of the splenic pedicle, consistent with torsion.

c) Small bowel intussusception: the round lesion above the left kidney on the coronal CT scan shows a typical whirlpool sign, consistent with torsion of the splenic pedicle.

d) Intra-abdominal abscess: the lesion shown here demonstrates soft tissue attenuation and the shape of the spleen. And abscess would present with central fluid and a thick, contrast enhancing rim.

Patient 172: 2-year-old child, increased abdominal girth
Author: Heike E. Daldrup-Link, M.D.

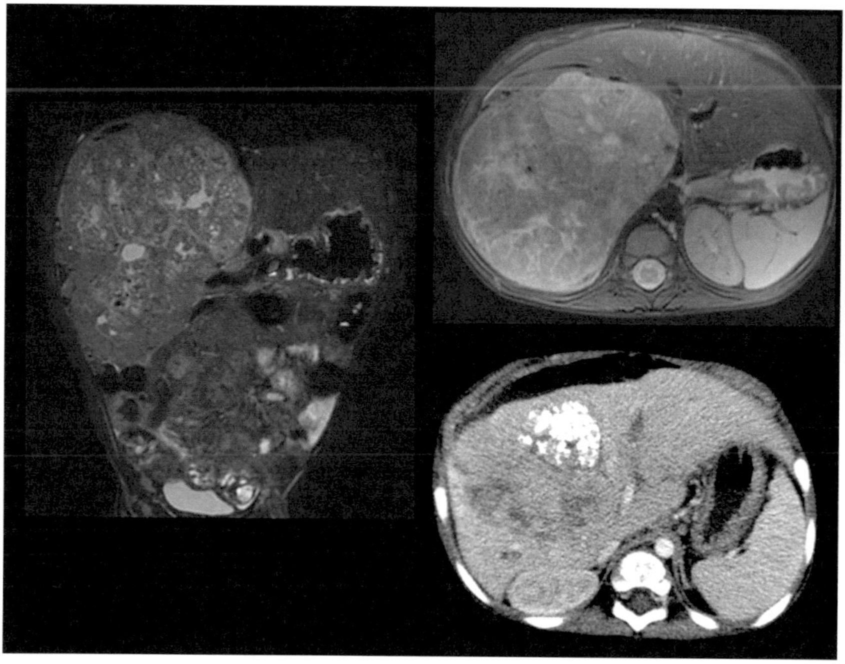

What is the most likely diagnosis:

a) Mesoblastic Nephroma
b) Mesenchymal Hamartoma
c) Embryonal Carcinoma
d) Hepatoblastoma

Case 172: Hepatoblastoma

a) Mesoblastic Nephroma originates from the kidney. The CT scan demonstrates a fat plane between the lesion and the right kidney. The lesion shown here originates from the liver.

b) A mesenchymal hamartoma is a predominantly cystic mass with thin and thick, soft tissue septations. It can rarely present with more prominent soft tissue components. But these would still contain many large cystic spaces, leading to a "Swiss cheese" appearance.

b) An embryonal sarcoma (not carcinoma) typically occurs in teenagers and is composed of large cystic or necrotic spaces, which demonstrate fluid equivalent signal on T2 weighted MRI sequences and are hypodense on CT scans. Soft tissue septations or nodules within the lesion show slow contrast media accumulation with enhancement on delayed postcontrast scans.

c) Hepatoblastoma: Correct! The coronal and axial T2-weighted MRI scans demonstrates a large, ill defined, inhomogeneous soft tissue mass in the right liver lobe. The CT scan shows calcifications in the mass. Considering the age of the patient, this is a hepatoblastoma until proven otherwise.

Patient 173: Three-month-old male with multiple bright red lesions on the skin.

Author: Wipawee Morakote, M.D.

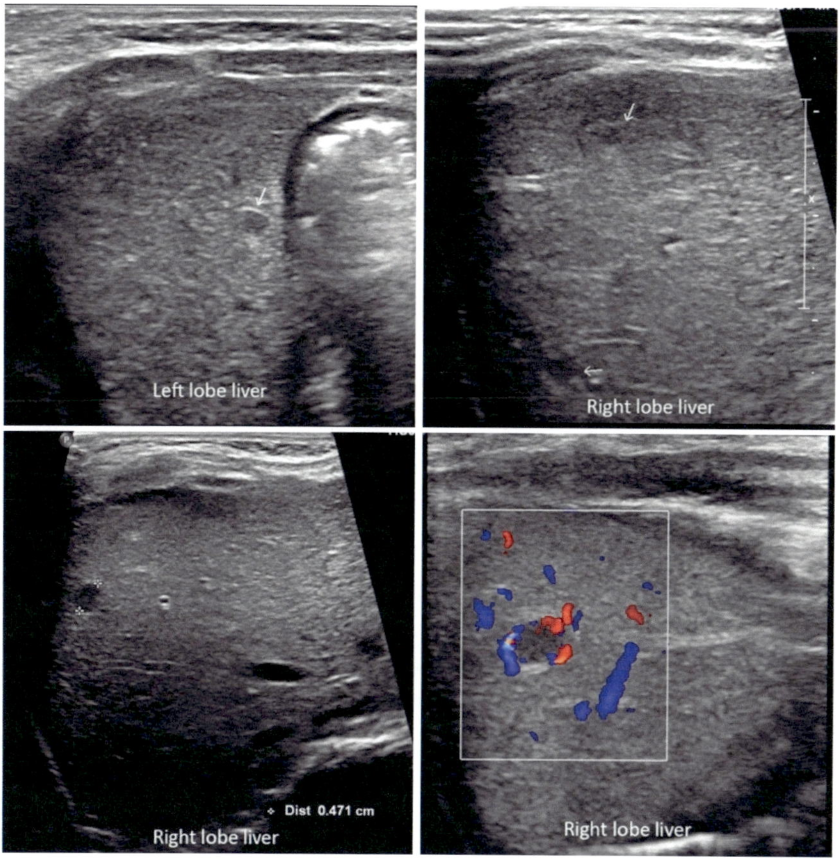

What is the most likely diagnosis:

a) Von Meyenburg complex
b) Caroli disease
c) Hepatoblastoma
d) Hepatic hemangioma

Case 173: Hepatic hemangiomas

a) Von Meyenburg complex or biliary hamartomas are caused by ductal plate malformations of the small bile ducts and lead to cystic dilation of the bile duct with surrounding fibrous tissue. Biliary hamartomas present on ultrasound as numerous small (usually 1-5 mm) hyperechoic foci throughout the liver. The lesions can appear hypoechoic if they are larger than 1 cm.

b) Caroli disease is a Todani type V cystic dilation of intrahepatic bile ducts. The pathognomonic finding of Caroli disease is the "central dot" sign, which represents dots of intrahepatic portal vein branches surrounded by dilated intrahepatic bile ducts.

c) Hepatoblastoma is the most common malignant hepatic tumor in young children. It usually appears as a large heterogeneous hyperechoic mass with areas of necrosis or calcification. Vascular invasion is an important feature of hepatoblastoma.

d) Corrected! The ultrasonography of the liver demonstrates multiple small hypoechoic lesions in both hepatic lobes. Color Doppler ultrasonography demonstrate peripheral vascular flow of a representative lesion. These are typical appearances of hepatic hemangiomas in infant. Hepatic hemangioma is the most common benign hepatic neoplasm in children. They may be associated with cutaneous hemangiomas. Larger intrahepatic hemangiomas can show more complex appearances and internal calcifications. Peripheral or central vascularity can be seen on color Doppler ultrasound. Please keep in mind that infantile hepatic hemangioma differs from adult cavernous hemangioma which is typically hyperechogenic on ultrasonography.

Patient 174: 7-year-old child with abdominal pain

Author: Heike E. Daldrup-Link, M.D.

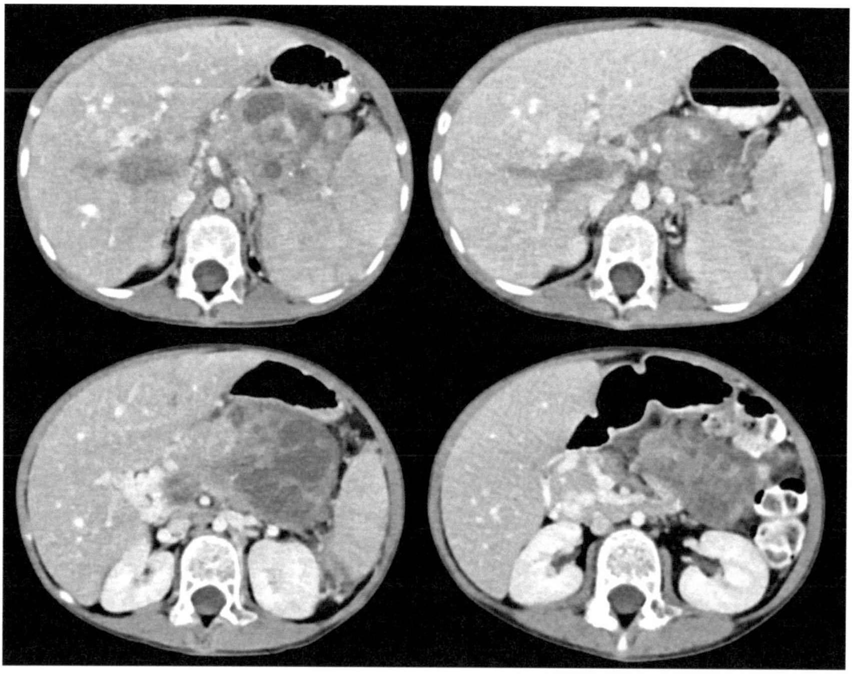

What is the most likely diagnosis:

a) Wilms Tumor
b) Neuroblastoma
c) Hepatoblastoma
d) Pancreatoblastoma

Case 174: Pancreatoblastoma

a) Wilms Tumor: The tumor shown here does not originate from the kidney. There is no "claw sign".

b) Neuroblastoma: The adrenal glands are normal. Children with neuroblastoma are usually younger. A thrombus in the portal vein would be unusual.

c) Hepatoblastoma: The CT scan demonstrates a hypodense mass in the porta hepatis. There are multiple venous collaterals. This suggests an extension of the mass in the portal vein. The large extrahepatic mass in the left upper abdomen would be unusual for a hepatoblastoma. Lymph node metastases can occur, this lesion would be unusually large for a lymph node metastasis.

d) Pancreatoblastoma: Correct! The CT scan demonstrates a large, inhomogeneous mass in the pancreas with fine calcifications and a tumor thrombus in the portal vein. Multiple venous collaterals are noted at the porta hepatis.

Patient 175: Two-week-old female with jaundice and massively increased liver enzymes

Author: Heike E. Daldrup-Link, M.D.

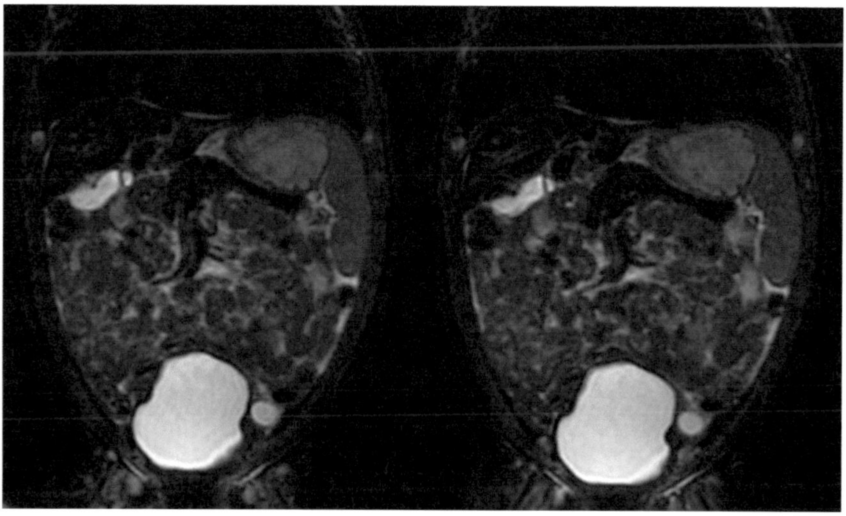

What is the most likely diagnosis:

a) Biliary Atresia
b) Wilson Disease
c) Hemosiderosis
d) Neonatal hemochromatosis

Case 175: Neonatal Hemochromatosis

a) Biliary atresia is characterized by diminished bile ducts and a small or absent gallbladder. In this case, the gallbladder is normal.

b) Wilson disease is a rare autosomal recessive metabolic disorder which leads to abnormal copper deposition in the liver, brain, and other organs. Copper does not cause specific signal changes on MRI. Clinical symptoms develop slowly over time and are very rare in the first few years of live. Teenagers and young adult patients can present with liver cirrhosis.

c) Hemosiderosis represents iron deposition in the reticuloendothelial system, i.e., liver, spleen, and bone marrow. Underlying causes are hemolytic anemias and/or repeated iron transfusions.

d) Neonatal hemochromatosis: Correct! The T2-weighted MRI scan demonstrates abnormally low T2-signal of the liver and pancreas, while the T2-signal of the spleen is normal. The liver is also abnormally small. These findings are consistent with neonatal hemochromatosis, which is characterized by iron deposition in liver, pancreas, and heart muscle. In this case, the underlying cause was gestational alloimmune liver disease (GALD), a maternal-fetal alloimmune disorder where maternal immune cells attack fetal hepatocytes, resulting in progressive hepatocyte injury. It is very important to accurately diagnose this condition in order to initiate appropriate treatment and prevent patient death.

Patient 176: 9-year-old child with abdominal pain and fever

Author: Lisa Adams, M.D., Shakthi Kumaran Ramasamy, M.D.

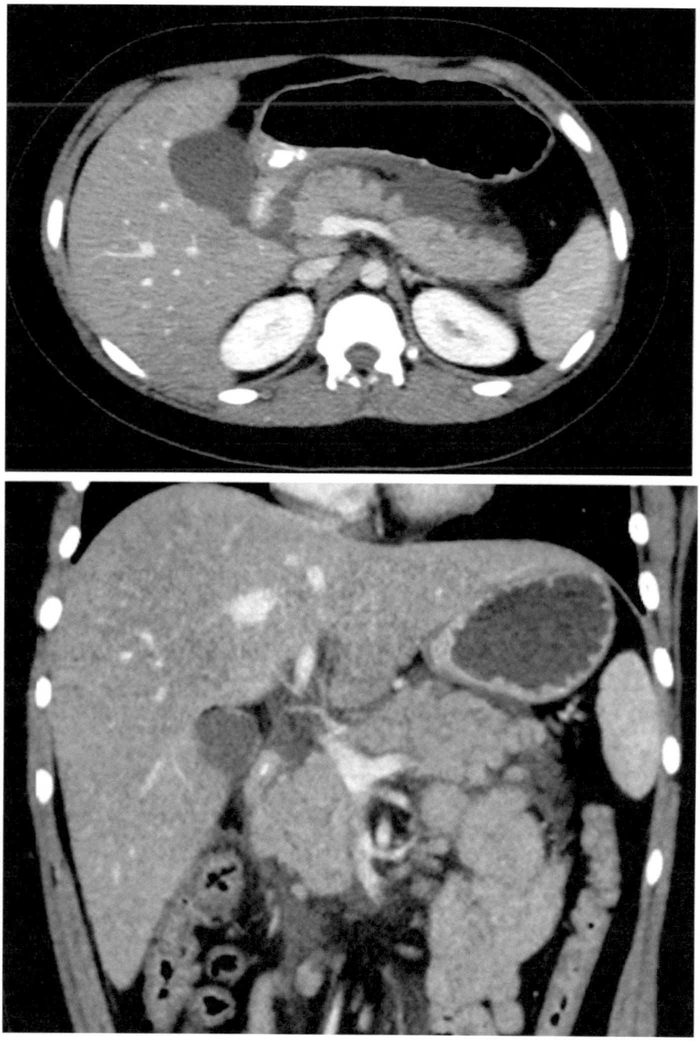

What is the most likely diagnosis:

a) Lymphoma
b) Shock pancreas
c) Acute pancreatitis
d) Acute cholecystitis

Case 176: Acute Pancreatitis

a) Lymphoma of the pancreas is rare and would present as a discrete homogeneous soft tissue mass with little contrast enhancement. It is usually not accompanied by pancreatic or biliary ductal obstruction. There is often peripancreatic lymphadenopathy, along with other sites of lymphomatous involvement.

b) Shock pancreas occurs due to profound hypotension, most commonly due to hypovolemic shock after major trauma. Shock pancreas is characterized by heterogeneous organ enhancement with higher-than-normal density values of peripancreatic fluid (< 20 HU). The aorta and inferior vena cava are typically small in caliber and the spleen demonstrates hypo-enhancement.

c) Acute pancreatitis – Correct! The CT scan shows pancreatic enlargement with homogeneous enhancement, consistent with interstitial edematous pancreatitis. In addition, there is homogeneous peripancreatic fluid without signs of organ necrosis or loculated fluid collections.

d) An acute cholecystitis is characterized by an enlarged gallbladder, gallbladder wall thickening and pericholecystic fluid. It is often accompanied by gallstones.

Patient 177: 9-year-old female with congenital heart disease

Author: Heike E. Daldrup-Link, M.D.

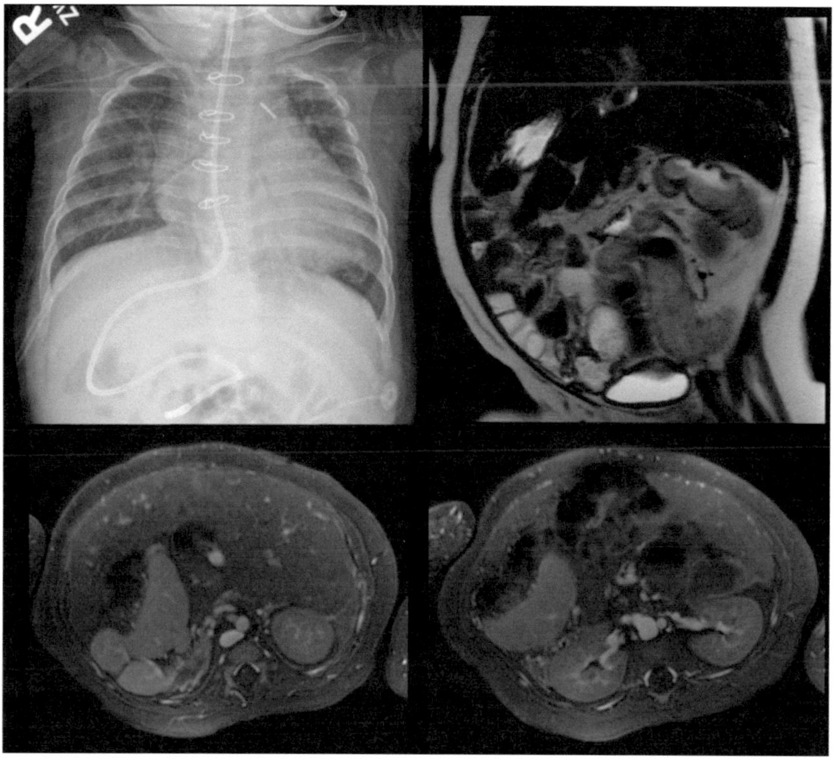

What is the most likely diagnosis:

a) Situs inversus
b) Asplenia
c) Polysplenia
d) Situs solitus

Case 177: Polysplenia

a) Situs inversus describes a reversed/mirrored position of visceral organs in the abdomen with reversed/mirrored position of the heart (situs inversus totalis) or with levocardia (situs inversus partialis). Situs inversus can be associated with Kartagener syndrome (situs inversus, bronchiectasis, sinusitis due to ciliary dyskinesis).

b) Asplenia is characterized by bilateral right isomerism and an absent spleen. The condition is associated with congenital (often cyanotic) heart disease.

c) Polysplenia: Correct! Polysplenia is characterized by bilateral left isomerism and multiple splenules. The x-ray of the chest demonstrates cardiomegaly with prominent pulmonary vessels, consistent with a history of anomalous pulmonary venous return. There is no minor fissure in the right or left lung, suggesting bilateral bilobed lungs. An enteric tube can be followed to the right upper abdomen, suggesting a right-sided stomach. The coronal T2-weighted MRI confirms a right sided stomach and demonstrates a midline liver. The axial contrast-enhanced MRI scans demonstrate multiple splenules in the right upper abdomen. The splenules are typically found in the left abdomen, but can be also located in the right abdomen, as shown here. There is also an enlarged azygos vein due to an interrupted inferior vena cava.

d) Situs solitus describes the normal anatomy of visceral organs, including a left-sided heart, left-sided systemic atrium, left sided cardiac apex, right sided pulmonary atrium, and right sided minor fissure. Within the abdomen, the stomach is on the left, the spleen is on the left and the liver is on the right side.

Patient 178: 3-year-old child, car accident one month ago

Authors: Desiree R. Eshraghi, Soni C. Chawla, M.D.

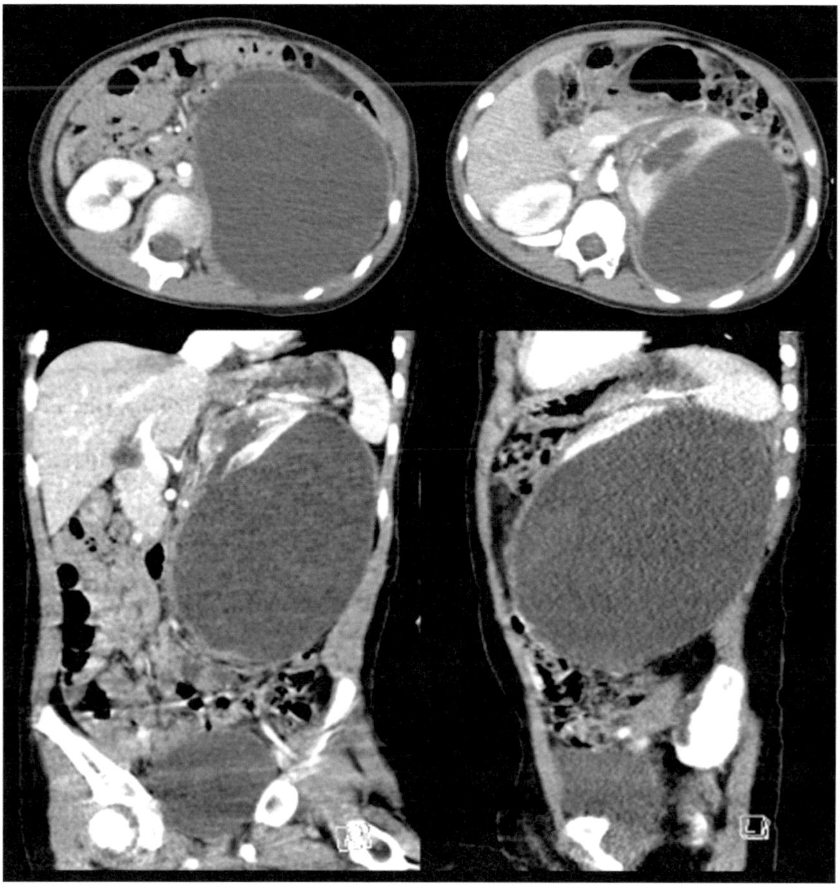

What is the most likely diagnosis:

a) Incidental finding of a renal cyst
b) Multicystic dysplastic kidney (MCKD)
c) Laceration of the left kidney with urinoma
d) Acute tubular necrosis (ATN)

Case 178: Laceration of the left kidney with urinoma

a) Renal cysts can be of varying sizes, single or multiple with thin imperceptible walls. They can be located in the renal cortex, medulla or para-pelvic. However, the degree of renal parenchymal distortion shown here would be unusual for a simple cyst.

b) A multicystic dysplastic kidney is typically composed of multiple non-communicating cysts of varying sizes. The renal parenchyma is diminutive and nonfunctional.

c) Laceration of the inferior pole of the left kidney: Correct! The CT scan demonstrates a large hypodense fluid collection with a cranio-caudal diameter of 13.5 cm, which communicates with the left renal pelvis. The findings are compatible with extravasated urine/urinoma and AAST grade 4 renal laceration. No definite evidence of an active contrast media extravasation to suggest a vascular injury. The urinoma displaces the spleen cranially and bowel loops to the right and lower abdomen. The spleen and right kidney are intact.

d) An acute tubular necrosis is characterized by damage or death of renal tubular cells. A typical CT scan would reveal a delayed nephogram without excretion of contrast material into the collecting system. A large fluid collection would be unusual.

Patient 179: 6-year-old female with abdominal pain

Author: Heike E. Daldrup-Link, M.D.

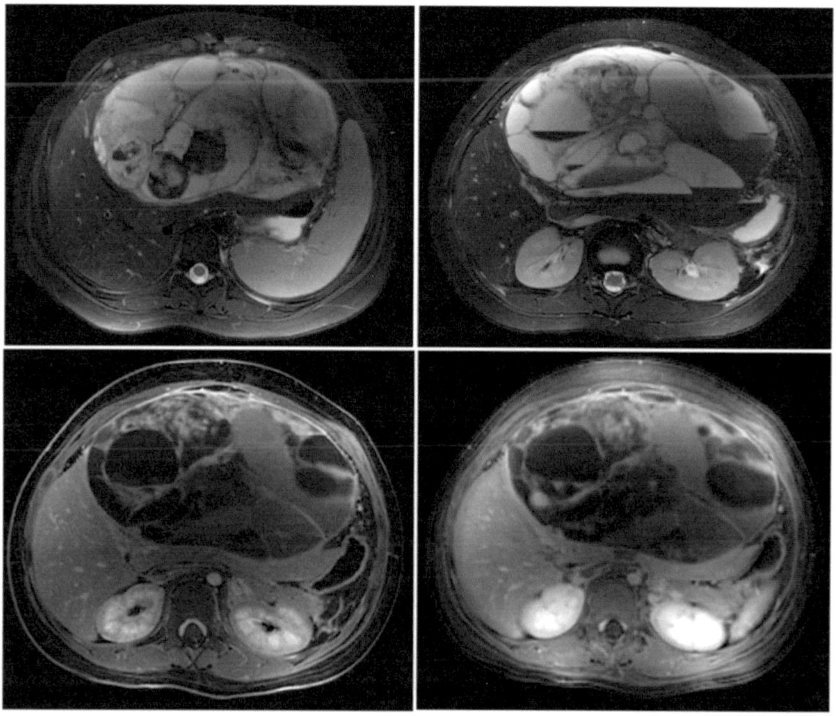

What is the most likely diagnosis:

a) Hydatid Cyst
b) Mesenchymal Hamartoma
c) Embryonal Carcinoma
d) Hepatoblastoma

Case 179: Embryonal Sarcoma

e) A hydatid cyst or Echinococcus cyst is a cyst that develops after infection with the Echinococcus tapeworm. MRI scans typically show a T2-hyperintense multicystic mass with multiple internal daughter cysts. The MRI signal can vary based on the degree of living material or debris in the cysts. After contrast media administration, the cyst wall and septae enhance. But there are usually not large enhancing soft tissue nodules in the mass as shown here.

b) A mesenchymal hamartoma typically occurs in very young children, 1-3 years of age, and presents as a predominantly cystic mass with thin and thick soft tissue septations. It can rarely present with more prominent soft tissue components and well-defined cysts, leading to a "Swiss cheese" appearance.

c) Embryonal sarcoma: Correct! The MRI scan demonstrates a large, in homogenous mass in the left liver lobe, which is composed of large cystic or necrotic spaces, which demonstrate fluid equivalent signal on T2 weighted MRI sequences. Soft tissue septations or soft tissue nodules within the lesion show slow contrast media accumulation with increasing enhancement on delayed postcontrast scans. The patient is relatively young for this diagnosis. Embryonal sarcomas typically occur in teenagers. If an ultrasound has been obtained, there is a typical mismatch of a predominantly solid mass on ultrasound and mostly cystic mass on CT or MRI.

d) A hepatoblastoma typically presents in young children, less than five years of age, as a large, ill defined, inhomogeneous soft tissue mass. Hepatoblastoma can contain necrosis. However, usually, most of the mass is composed of soft tissue. Since hepatoblastomas arise from hepatocytes, the T2-signal of the mass is typically very similar to that of the surrounding liver parenchyma.

Patient 180: Four-year old with abdominal pain
Author: Heike E. Daldrup-Link, M.D.

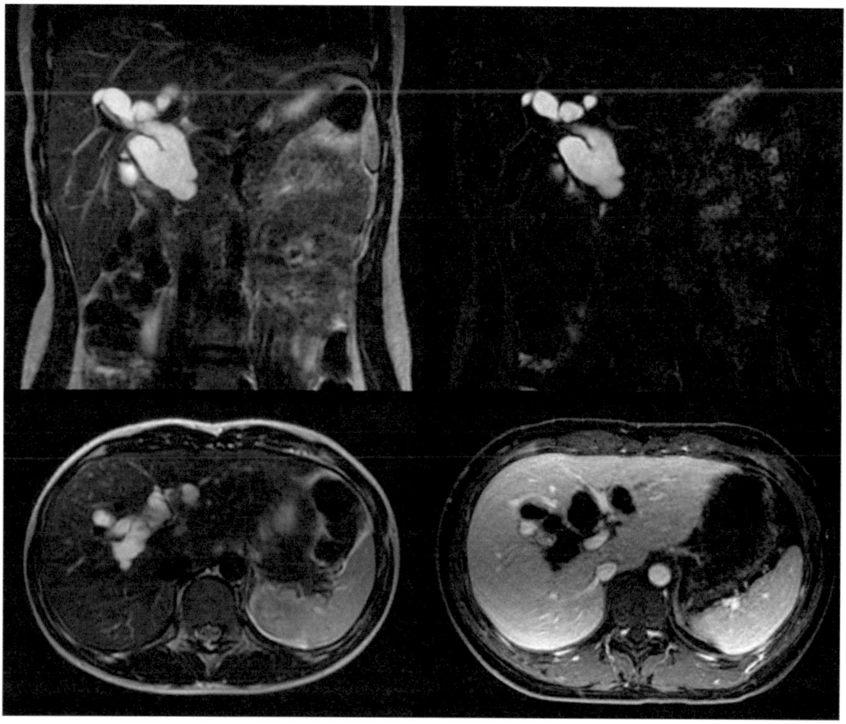

What is the most likely diagnosis:

a) Type 1 Choledochal Cyst
b) Impacted Gallstone
c) Type 4 Choledochal Cyst
d) Biliary Atresia

Case 180: Choledochal Cyst

a) A type 1 choledochal cyst is characterized by a cystic dilation of the extrahepatic common bile duct.

b) Gallstones are rare in the first few years of life. There is no gallstone noted on the MRI images.

c) **Type 4 choledochal cyst: Correct! The MR images demonstrate a large cystic dilation of both intra- and extra-hepatic bile ducts. A type 4 choledochal cyst is the second most common type. Todani classification of choledochal duct cysts:**
Type 1 – cystic dilation of the extrahepatic bile duct only
Type 2 – diverticulum of the extrahepatic bile duct
Type 3 – dilation of the distal extrahepatic bile duct, within the duodenal wall
Type 4 – cystic dilation of intra- and extrahepatic bile ducts
Type 5 – multiple cystic dilations of intrahepatic bile ducts (Caroli disease)

d) Biliary atresia is defined as absence or severe narrowing (not dilation) of extrahepatic bile ducts. The gallbladder is atretic or absent.

GI, GU, and Interventional

5) Kidney

Patient 181: 3-year-old child with increased abdominal girth
Author: Heike E. Daldrup-Link, M.D.

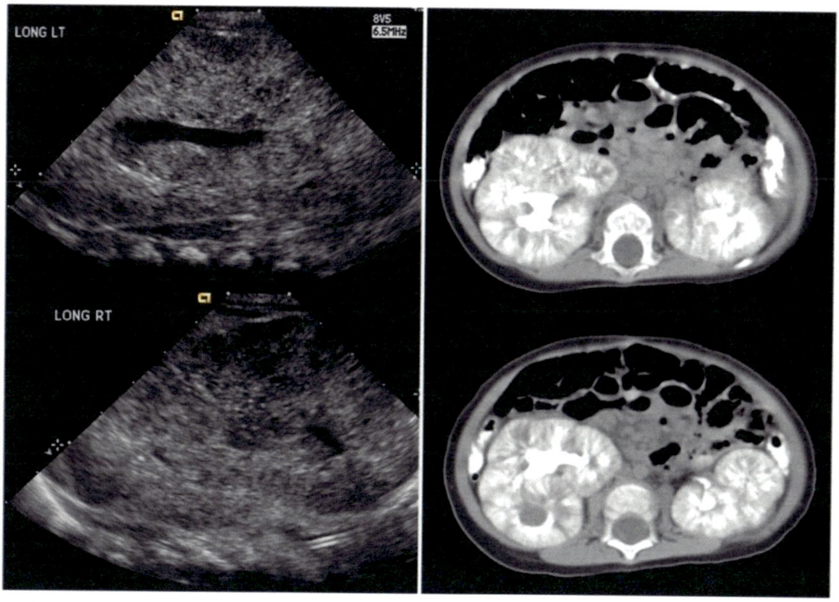

What is the most likely diagnosis:

a) Nephroblastomatosis
b) Autosomal Dominant Polycystic Kidney Disease
c) Autosomal Recessive Polycystic Kidney Disease
d) Pyelonephritis

Case 181: Autosomal Recessive Polycystic Kidney Disease

a) Nephroblastomatosis or embryonic rests represent focal lesions in the kidney. If the entire kidney parenchyma is composed of embryonic rests, it can be enlarged. However, embryonic rests demonstrate minimal contrast enhancement. The striated nephrograms shown here would not be consistent with this diagnosis.

b) Autosomal Dominant Polycystic Kidney Disease (ADPKD) typically manifests in older children or young adults with macroscopic cysts in the bilateral kidneys, liver, and pancreas. 5-10% of patients with ADPKD have cerebral berry aneurysms.

c) Autosomal Recessive Polycystic Kidney Disease (ARPKD). Correct! The ultrasound scan demonstrates enlarged, hyperechogenic kidneys bilaterally. The CT scan demonstrates enlarged kidneys with striated nephrograms. These findings are consistent with early imaging signs of autosomal recessive polycystic kidney disease. The disease is due to an abnormal proliferation and dilatation of collecting tubules resulting in 1-2 mm cysts. In early stages of the disease, these lead to the findings shown here. When the patients get older, the cysts may be seen on imaging studies. ARPKD is associated with fibrosis of the liver and pancreas.

d) Pyelonephritis: The CT scan demonstrates striated nephrograms which can ne seen in patients with pyelonephritis. However, the kidneys are markedly enlarged, which would not be consistent with an acute pyelonephritis. There is no history of fever or clinical signs of an infection.

Patient 182: 6-month-old child with a renal mass

Author: Heike E. Daldrup-Link, M.D.

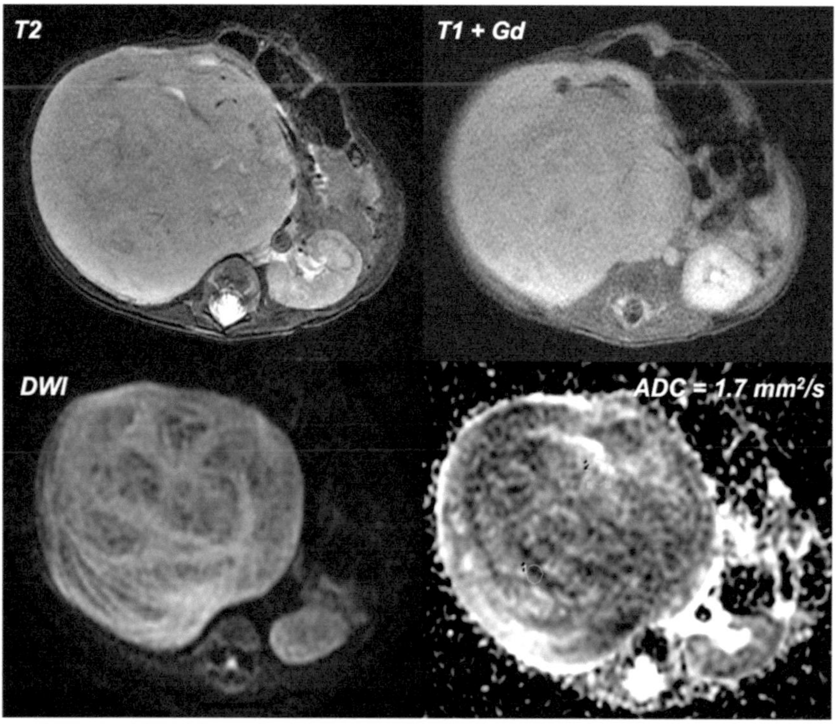

What is the most likely diagnosis:

a) Nephroblastomatosis
b) Mesoblastic Nephroma
c) Autosomal Recessive Polycystic Kidney Disease
d) Nephroblastoma

Case 182: Mesoblastic Nephroma

a) Nephroblastomatosis or nephrogenic rests present as focal or diffuse T1-hypointense and T2-hyperintense lesions compared to the surrounding kidney parenchyma. The lesions show minimal contrast enhancement, less than that of the surrounding kidney parenchyma.

b) Mesoblastic Nephroma: Correct! The CT scan demonstrates a large, relatively well-defined mass in the right kidney with limited restricted diffusion on diffusion-weighted MRI and an ADC value of more than 1.3 mm^2/s. This is characteristic of a benign lesion. Mesoblastic nephroma is the most common solid kidney mass in children less than one year of age. There are different histological and subtypes. The classical type typically presents as a homogeneous lesion. The less common cellular type presents as a more inhomogeneous mass, which may demonstrate aggressive features and restricted diffusion.

c) Autosomal Recessive Polycystic Kidney Disease (ARPKD) in young children presents with bilaterally enlarged kidneys and striated nephrograms on CT scans. When the patients get older, sub-centimeter cysts may be seen on imaging studies. ARPKD is associated with fibrosis of the liver and pancreas.

d) Nephroblastoma (Wilms tumor) is the most common solid kidney mass in children older than one year of age. It presents at a large, very inhomogeneous soft tissue mass with multiple areas of cysts and necrosis. Wilms tumors typically demonstrate markedly restricted diffusion on diffusion-weighted MRI with ADC values of less than 1.2 mm2/s.

Patient 183: **16-year-old adolescent, multiple episodes of hematuria**
Author: Lisa Adams, M.D.

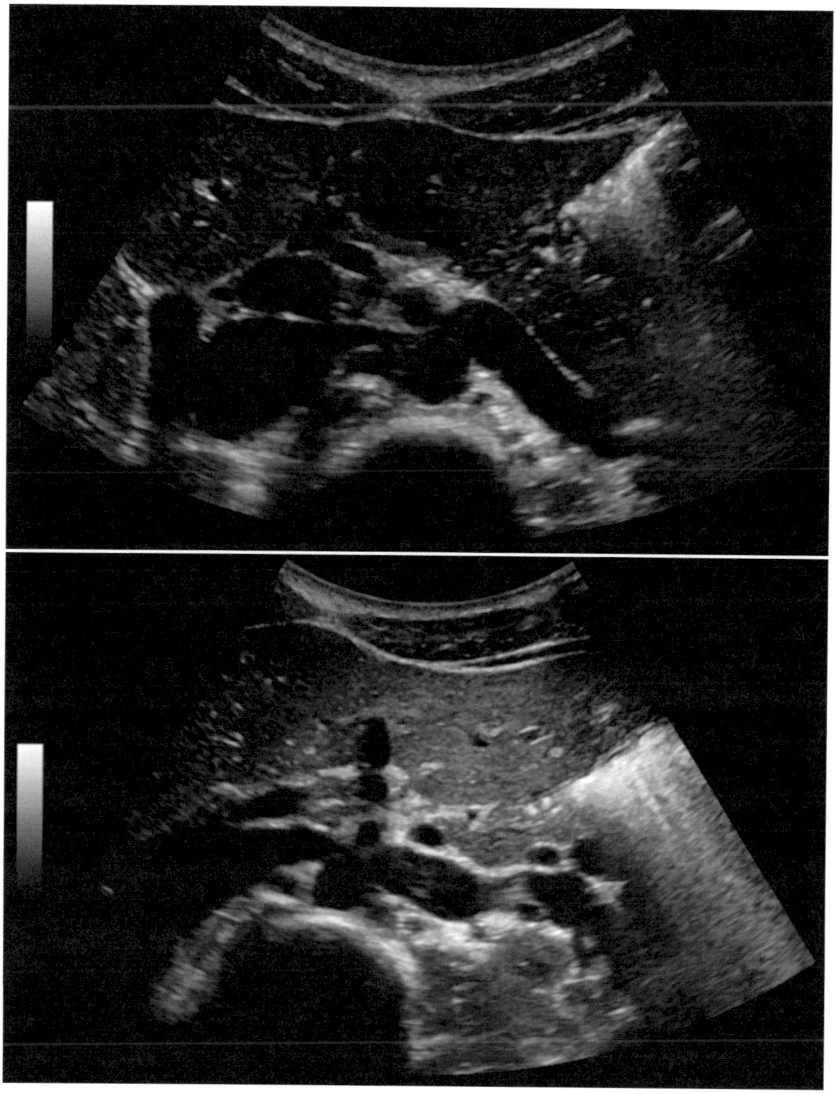

What is the most likely diagnosis:

a) Renal vein thrombosis
b) Renal arteriovenous fistula
c) Median arcuate ligament syndrome
d) Nutcracker syndrome

Case 183: Nutcracker syndrome

a) Renal vein thrombosis is diagnosed based on an intraluminal filling defect, which is not seen here. The kidneys may demonstrate a hypoechogenic renal edema in the acute phase and hyperechogenic areas of hemorrhage or necrosis after approximately 2 weeks.

b) A renal arteriovenous fistula presents with a communication between an artery and a renal vein, as confirmed by an arterialized flow pattern in the draining vein on Color Doppler imaging.

c) Median arcuate ligament syndrome refers to an atypically low insertion of the median arcuate ligament. As a result, there is compression on the proximal celiac axis which results in abdominal pain, nausea, and weight loss. Gray-scale ultrasound typically demonstrates an upward angulation of the proximal celiac artery and post stenotic dilation.

d) Nutcracker syndrome with compression of the left renal vein – Correct! Gray-scale US in supine and upright position at the epigastric level shows marked compression of the left renal vein between the superior mesenteric artery and the aorta. The pre-stenotic renal vein is dilated to more than 1 cm. The findings are most evident in the supine position, while symptoms are more pronounced in the upright position. Nutcracker syndrome can cause a left renal vein outflow obstruction, left renal venous hypertension and hematuria.

Patient 184: 18-year-old female with van Hippel Lindau disease
Author: Heike E. Daldrup-Link, M.D.

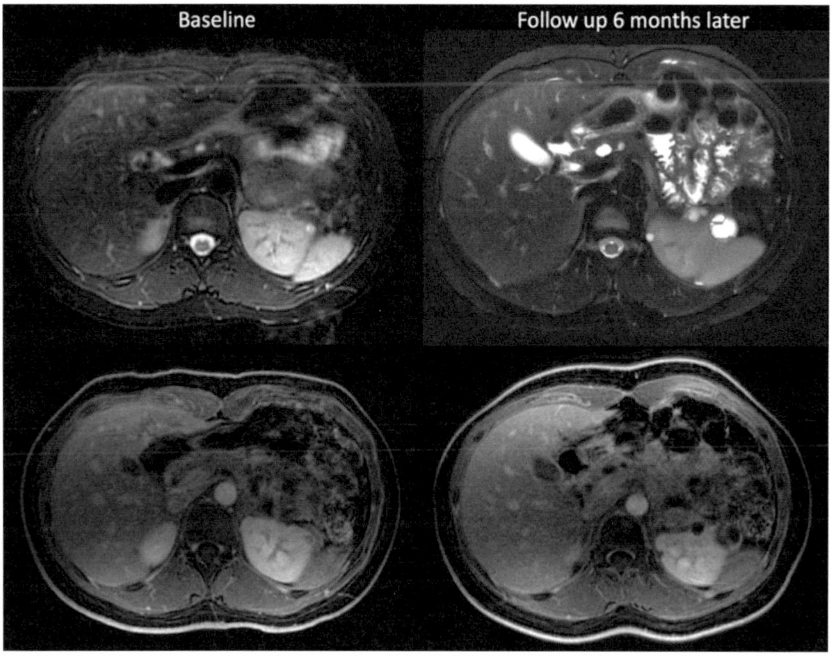

What is the most likely diagnosis:

a) Angiomyolipoma
b) Hemangioblastoma
c) Clear cell renal cell carcinoma
d) Cystadenoma

Case 184: Renal Cell Carcinoma in van Hippel Lindau Disease

a) Angiomyolipomas are typically found in patients with Tuberous Sclerosis. They are not usually seen in patients with van Hippel Lindau disease. The lesion shown here does not contain fat.

b) Hemangioblastomas are benign tumors typically found in the brain and spinal cord in patients with van Hippel Lindau disease. They can occur in the kidney but are rare in this location. Since they are benign, they would not be expected to show rapid interval growth.

c) Clear cell renal cell carcinoma: Correct! The baseline T2- and contrast-enhanced T1-weighted MRIs show a complex, slightly exophytic cystic lesion in the anterolateral cortex of the upper pole of the left kidney. The lesion demonstrates significant interval growth on the 6 month follow up scan, in addition to thick contrast-enhancing septae and soft tissue nodules along the posterior rim of the lesion. About 70% of patients with van Hippel Lindau disease develop renal cell cancers, most commonly clear cell renal cell carcinoma. The renal cysts in these patients contain a lining of preneoplastic cells, which leads to the development of renal cancers within pre-existing cysts due to VHL gene inactivation and constitutive activation of the transcription factor hypoxia-inducible factor 2α (HIF-2α). It is therefore very important to carefully evaluate renal cysts in these patients for interval changes. Note that this patient has additional cysts in the left kidney and pancreas.

d) Cystadenomas typically occur in the pancreas in patients with van Hippel Lindau disease. Since these are benign lesions, they would not demonstrate rapid interval growth.

Patient 185: Child with increasing abdominal girth
Author: Heike E. Daldrup-Link, M.D.

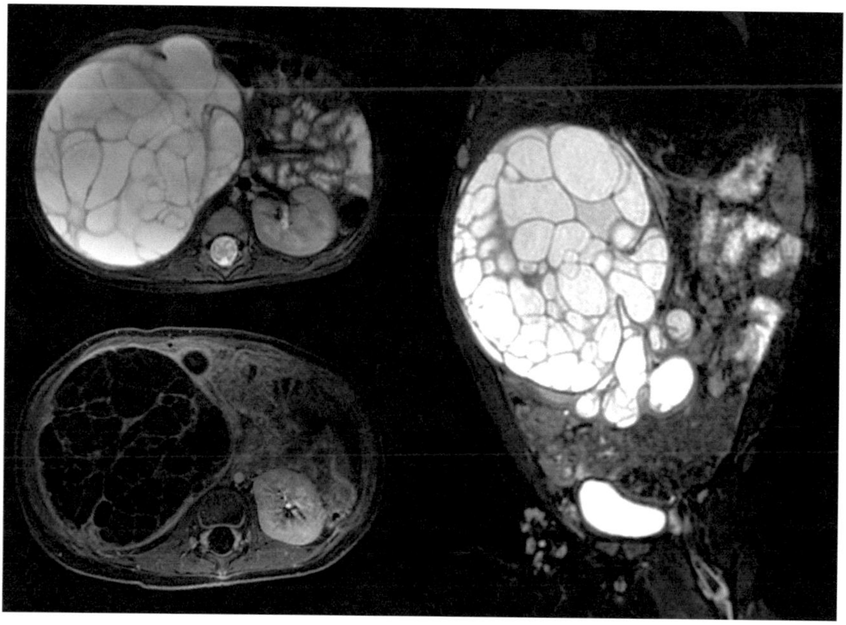

What is the most likely diagnosis

a) Multilocular Cystic Nephroma
b) Mesoblastic Nephroma
c) Clear Cell Sarcoma
d) Polycystic Kidney Disease

Case 185: Multilocular Cystic Nephroma

a) Multilocular Cystic Nephroma: Correct! The T2-weighted MRI demonstrates a large, well defined multi-cystic mass in the right kidney. The coronal MRI demonstrates a thin rim of renal tissue below the lower border of the lesion. The contrast-enhanced T1-weighted MRI demonstrates contrast enhancement of the rim and septae of the lesion. There are no soft tissue nodules noted. Recently, multilocular cystic nephromas in children have been renamed "pediatric cystic nephromas".

b) Mesoblastic Nephroma: A mesoblastic nephroma typically presents in the first year of live as a relatively homogenous soft tissue mass.

c) A clear cell sarcoma of the kidney typically presents as an inhomogeneous soft tissue mass. While a clear cell sarcoma can contain cystic and necrotic areas, it would also contain enhancing soft tissue.

d) Autosomal Dominant Polycystic Kidney Disease (ADPKD) can present with multiple large, non-communicating cysts in both kidneys in older children. The images here show one large, multiseptated cystic mass rather than multiple cysts. Only the right kidney is involved. The left kidney appears to be normal.

Patient 186: 2-year-old child with increased abdominal girth

Author: Heike E. Daldrup-Link, M.D.

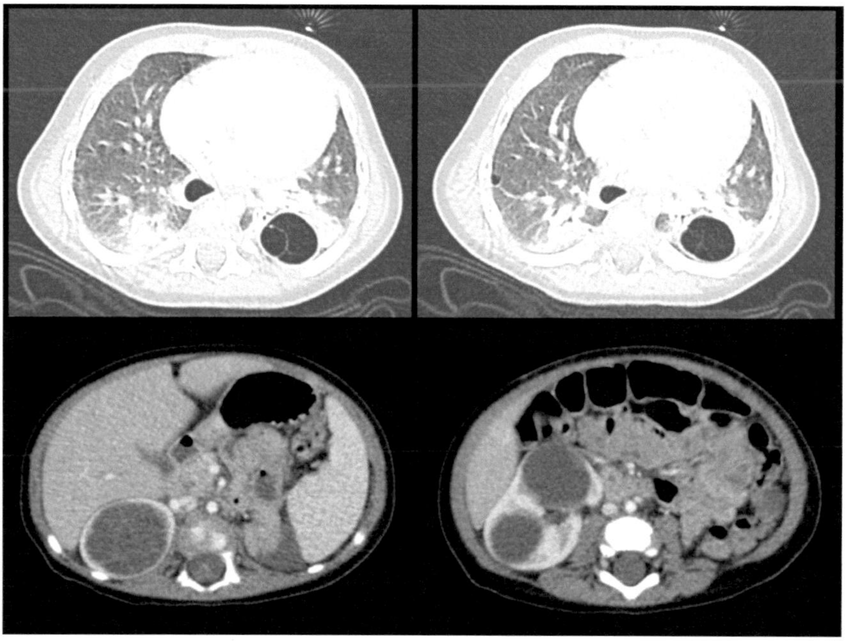

For which possible genetic syndrome should this patient be tested:

a) Beckwith Wiedemann Syndrome
b) Dicer 1 Syndrome
c) Autosomal Recessive Polycystic Kidney Disease
d) Autosomal Dominant Polycystic Kidney Disease

Case 186: Dicer 1 Syndrome

a) Beckwith-Wiedemann Syndrome or BW Spectrum describes an autosomal dominant or sporadic cancer predisposition syndrome, which can manifest with hemihypertrophy, macroglossia, organomegaly (typically on the side of extremity overgrowth) and associated malignancies, such as Wilms tumor, hepatoblastoma, neuroblastoma, rhabdomyosarcoma, and several others.

b) Dicer 1 Syndrome: Correct! Dicer 1 Syndrome describes an autosomal dominant or sporadic cancer predisposition syndrome, which is typically associated with cystic lesions in the kidneys and lungs, as shown here. The CT scan demonstrates three large, relatively well-defined masses in the right kidney, which are concerning for multilocular cystic nephroma. In addition, there is a complex multi-cystic lesion in the left lower lung, which is concerning for a pleuropulmonary blastoma. An additional simple appearing cyst is noted in the periphery of the right lower lung. Additional tumors that may be seen in patients with Dicer 1 Syndrome include ovarian Sertoli-Leydig cell tumor, thyroid cancer, pineoblastoma and Wilms tumor, among a few others.

c) Autosomal Recessive Polycystic Kidney Disease (ARPKD) in young children presents with bilaterally enlarged kidneys and striated nephrograms on CT scans. When the patients get older, sub-centimeter cysts may be seen on imaging studies. ARPKD would not be expected to be associated with lung cysts.

d) Autosomal Dominant Polycystic Kidney Disease (ADPKD) can present with large cysts in older children. ADPKD would not be expected to be associated with lung cysts.

Patient 187: 3-year-old child with increased abdominal girth
Author: Heike E. Daldrup-Link, M.D.

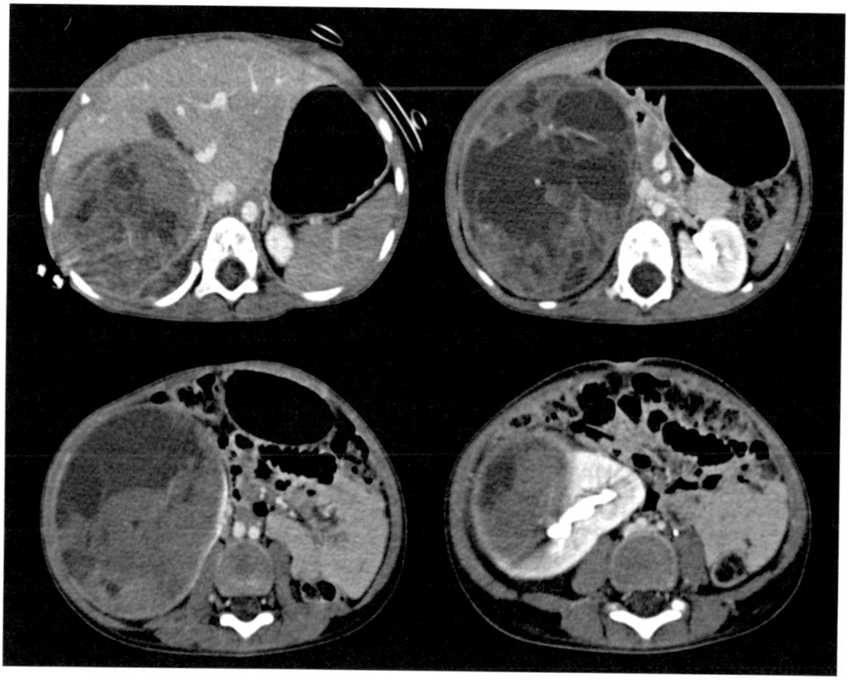

What is the most likely diagnosis:

a) Mesoblastic Nephroma
b) Wilms Tumor
c) Embryonal Carcinoma
d) Hepatoblastoma

Case 187: Wilms Tumor

a) A mesoblastic nephroma is the most common kidney tumor in children less than one year of age. Most tumors are homogenous on CT scans, although cellular subtypes can have a more inhomogeneous appearance. The presence of hemorrhage and necrosis within the tumor would be unusual.

b) Wilm's Tumor (Nephroblastoma): Correct! The CT scan demonstrates a large, inhomogeneous mass in the right kidney, which contains large areas of enhancing soft tissue, cystic and/or necrotic spaces and punctate calcifications. The origin from the kidney is evident based on the *claw sign*, i.e., enhancing kidney tissue which extends medially around the mass.

c) An embryonal carcinoma of the liver typically occurs in teenagers and is composed of large cystic or necrotic spaces, which are hypodense on CT scans. Soft tissue septations or nodules within the lesion show slow contrast media accumulation with enhancement on delayed postcontrast scans.

d) A hepatoblastoma is located in the liver. Just lesion here originates in the right kidney.

Patient 188: 3-year-old child with increased abdominal girth

Author: Heike E. Daldrup-Link, M.D.

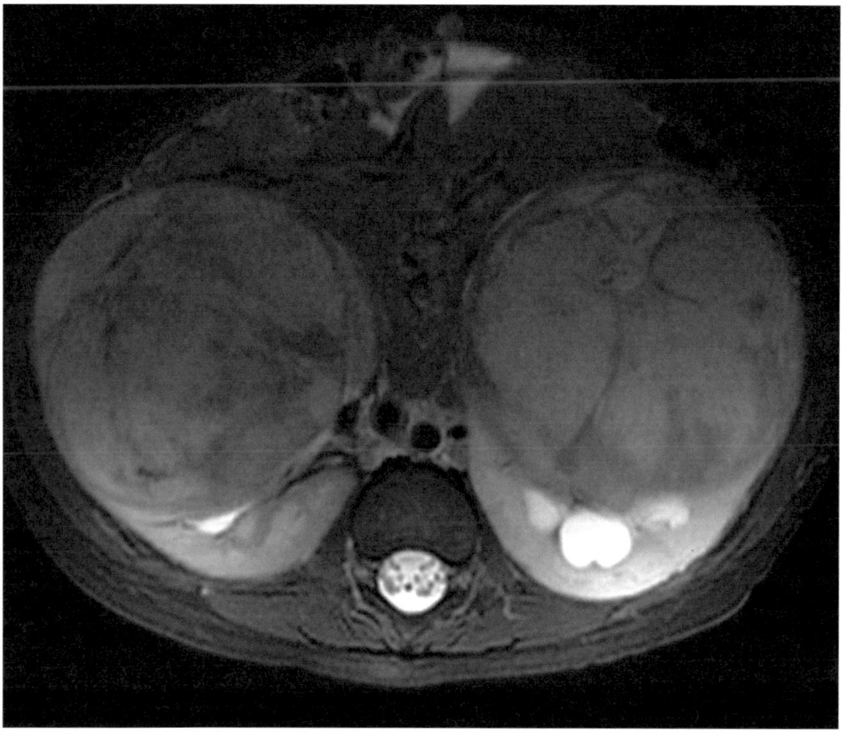

Which genetic syndrome is associated with Wilms Tumor:

a) Tuberous Sclerosis
b) RB1 Gene Mutation
c) WAGR Syndrome
d) Van Hippel Lindau

Case 188: WAGR Syndrome

a) Patients with tuberous sclerosis have a predisposition to develop renal cell carcinomas, in addition to angiomyolipomas and renal cysts, liver adenomas, pancreatic adenomas, cardiac rhabdomyomas and cerebral cortical hamartomas and subependymal giant cell tumors. About 1-2% of patients develop renal cell carcinomas.

b) The retinoblastoma gene (RB1) was the first tumor suppressor gene cloned. It has been associated with a risk of developing retinoblastoma, pineoblastoma, osteosarcoma and soft tissue sarcomas.

c) WAGR Syndrome: Correct! WAGR is an abbreviation for Wilms tumor, aniridia, genitourinary malformation and mental retardation. Other syndromes and clinical signs associated with Wilm's tumors include Beckwith-Wiedemann syndrome, Aniridia, Hemihypertrophy, DICER 1, Denys Drash Syndrome and Trisomy 18. Patients with these predisposition syndromes have a risk of developing unilateral or bilateral Wilms tumors. The MRI scan shown here demonstrates bilateral Wilms tumors.

d) Patients with van Hippel Lindau disease have an increased risk of developing adrenal pheochromocytomas, renal and pancreatic cysts, islet cell tumors and serous cystadenomas. The renal cysts contain a neoplastic cell lining, which can give rise to renal clear cell carcinomas. A significant number of patients die from clear cell carcinomas.

Patient 189: 3-year-old child with PKD1 mutation
Author: Heike E. Daldrup-Link, M.D.

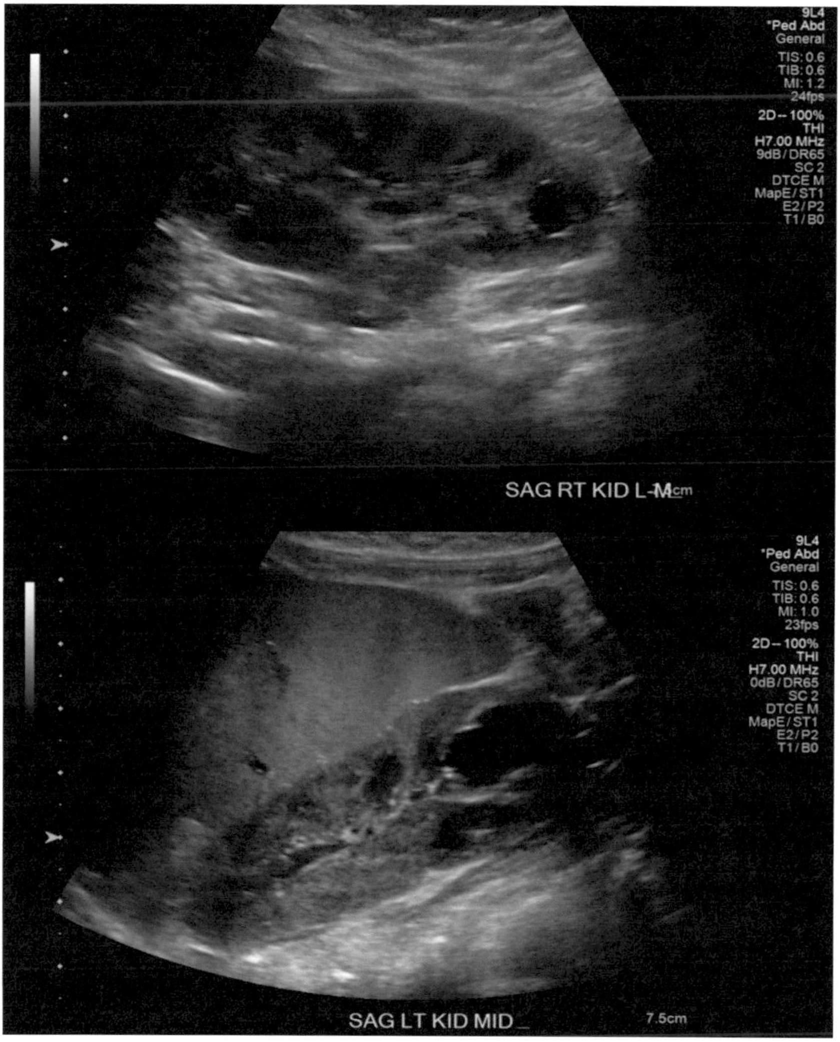

What is the most likely diagnosis:

a) Nephroblastomatosis
b) Autosomal Dominant Polycystic Kidney Disease
c) Autosomal Recessive Polycystic Kidney Disease
d) Multicystic dysplastic kidney (MCDK)

Case 189: Autosomal dominant polycystic kidney disease

a) Nephroblastomatosis or embryonic rests represent focal or diffuse soft tissue lesions in the kidney.

b) Autosomal Dominant Polycystic Kidney Disease (ADPKD): Correct! The ultrasound scan demonstrates a single, well defined simple anechoic lesion in each kidney with posterior acoustic enhancement, consistent with a single cyst. 85% of the patients have a PKD1 mutation, which leads to cystic dilatation of the renal tubules and formation of macroscopic cysts. With increasing age, more cysts develop which ultimately results in renal failure.

c) Autosomal Recessive Polycystic Kidney Disease (ARPKD) present as enlarged, hyperechogenic kidneys bilaterally. The disease is due to an abnormal proliferation and dilatation of collecting tubules resulting in 1-2 mm cysts. ARPKD is associated with fibrosis of the liver and pancreas.

d) Multicystic dysplastic kidney typically presents as unilateral cystic renal disease.

Patient 190: Four-year old female with flank pain
Author: Heike E. Daldrup-Link, M.D.

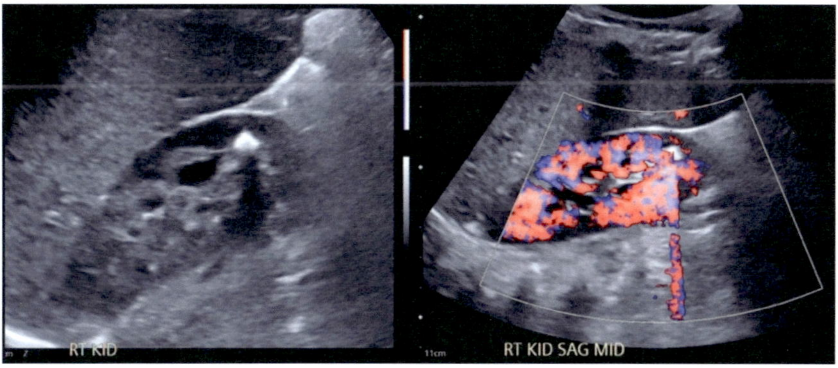

What is the most likely diagnosis

a) Multilocular Cystic Nephroma
b) Angiomyolipoma
c) Renal Stone
d) Polycystic Kidney Disease

Case 190: Renal Stone on Ultrasound

a) A multilocular cystic nephroma would present as a multi-cystic mass in the kidney. There are no cysts noted here.

b) An angiomyolipoma can present as a localized hyperechoic lesion in the parenchyma of the kidney. It can contain echogenic fat. However, it would be unusual to be completely calcified.

c) Renal Stone: Correct! The ultrasound of the right kidney demonstrates a focal hyperechoic lesion in the lower pole with posterior acoustic shadowing. The doppler ultrasound exam demonstrates a twinkling artifact, a string of alternating doppler signals behind a reflective object.

d) Autosomal Dominant Polycystic Kidney Disease (ADPKD) can present with multiple large, non-communicating cysts in both kidneys in older children. The images here do not show any cysts. Note that the renal pyramids in young children can be hypoechoic compared to the renal parenchyma.

Patient 191: 18-year-old male with Sickle Cell disease

Author: Heike E. Daldrup-Link, M.D.

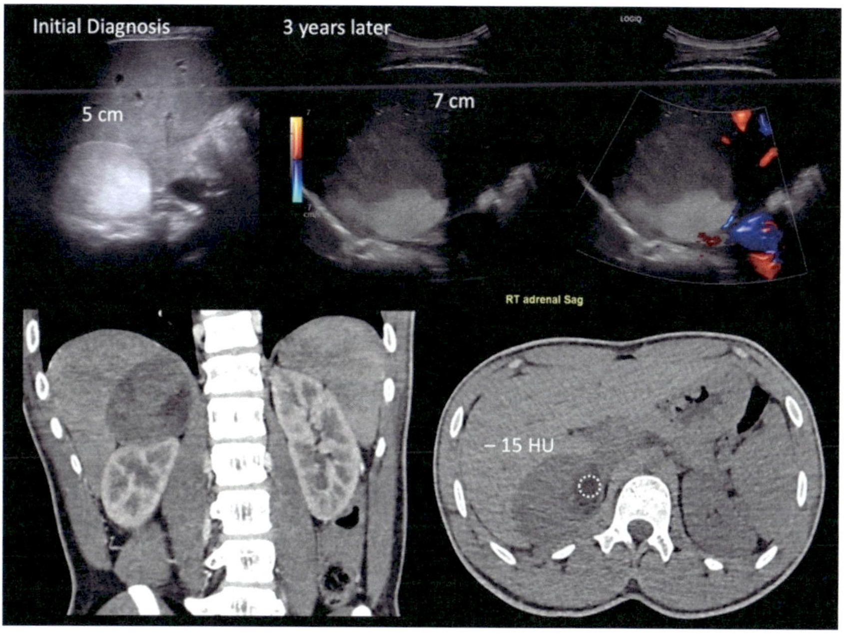

What is the most likely diagnosis:

a) Angiomyolipoma
b) Neuroblastoma
c) Renal medullary carcinoma
d) Adrenal Myelolipoma

Case 191: Adrenal Myelolipoma

a) Angiomyolipomas (AML) are typically found in patients with Tuberous Sclerosis. They are typically located in the kidneys and often demonstrate high vascularity on doppler ultrasound and cross-sectional imaging. Adrenal AMLs are extremely rare.

b) Neuroblastomas are malignant tumors of the adrenal gland which typically present in children younger than 5 years of age, although teenagers can rarely be affected as well. However, the macroscopic fat content and the slow growth of the lesion here suggest a different diagnosis.

c) Patients with Sickle Cell disease have an increased incidence of developing renal medullary carcinomas. However, the tumor noted here is located in the adrenal gland, not the kidney.

d) Adrenal Myelolipoma: Correct! The ultrasound demonstrates a well-defined soft tissue lesion in the area of the right adrenal gland, which contains large echogenic components, suggestive of macroscopic fat. The lesion demonstrates slow growth over time and limited vascularity on doppler ultrasound. The CT scan confirms a well-defined adrenal lesion with macroscopic fat content. Myelolipomas are rare benign tumors of the adrenal gland which contain fat and hematopoietic tissue. There is a documented association between myelolipomas and hemolytic diseases, such as Sickle Cell disease and thalassemia. Adrenal myelolipomas in children and young adults are often asymptomatic, but they can rarely be associated with congenital adrenal hyperplasia, Cushing syndrome and hyperaldosteronism. Adrenal extramedullary hematopoiesis can demonstrate similar features on imaging and histology but is usually associated with other sites of extramedullary hematopoiesis.

GI, GU, and Interventional

6) Ureter and Bladder

Patient 192: 16-year-old female, recurrent urinary tract infections
Author: Heike E. Daldrup-Link, M.D.

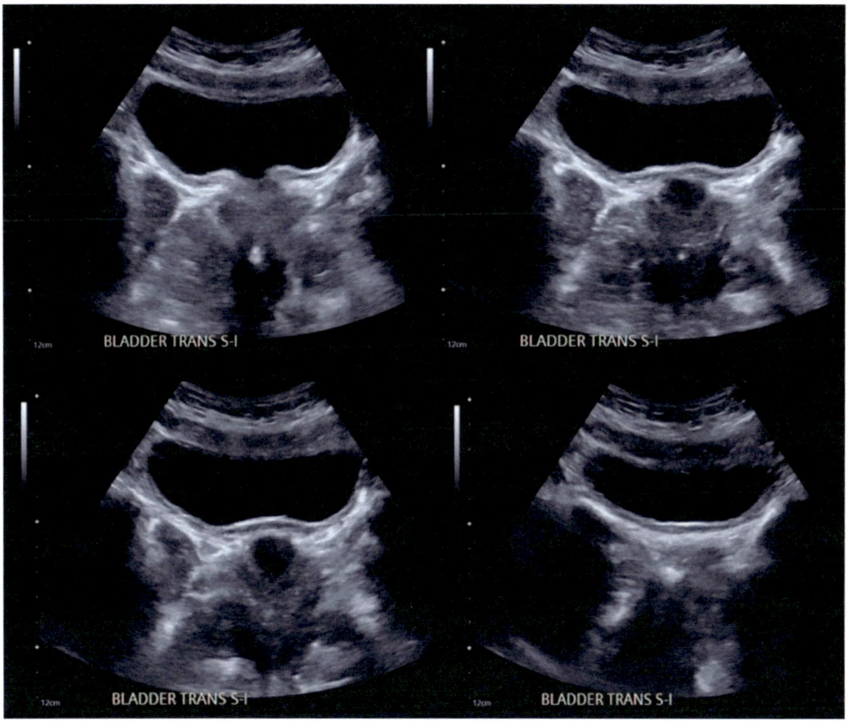

What is the most likely diagnosis:

a) Urachal duct cyst
b) Spinning top urethra
c) Bladder diverticulum
d) Utricle cyst

Case 192: Spinning Top Urethra

a) A urachal duct cyst would be located superior to the urinary bladder. The lesion here is located inferior.

b) Correct! The ultrasound demonstrates a wide bladder neck and dilated posterior urethra. The underlying mechanism is a urodynamic abnormality with voluntary increase in distal sphincter tension so as to prevent leakage of urine. The resulting pressure rise produces distention of the posterior urethra.

c) A bladder diverticulum represents an outpouch of the bladder wall, most commonly at the insertion site of the ureter. This lesion here is located in the midline, at the location of the urethra.

d) A utricle cyst is a rare midline cystic lesion in male patients, which is located within the prostrate gland, between the urinary bladder and the rectum, and connected with the posterior urethra.

Patient 193: Three-week old female, urinary tract infection
Author: Heike E. Daldrup-Link, M.D.

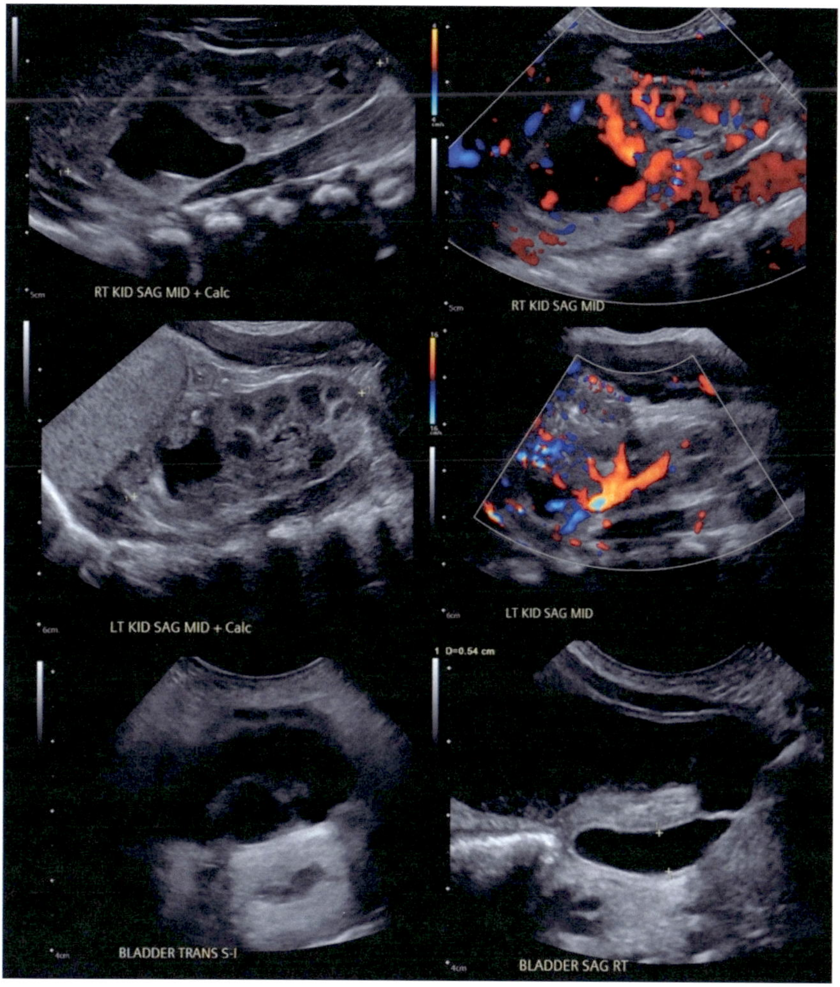

What is the most likely diagnosis:

a) Duplicated renal collecting system bilaterally, ureterocele
b) Bilateral renal abscesses
c) Congenital megacaliyces with hydroureter
d) Ureteropelvic junction obstruction

Case 193: Duplicated renal collecting systems

a) Duplicated renal collecting systems: Correct! The ultrasound demonstrates a markedly dilated renal pelvis of the upper pole of the right kidney. A parenchymal bridge separates the upper pole collecting system from a separate lower pole collecting system. The upper pole collecting system extends into a dilated ureter and a ureterocele. The renal pelvis of the left kidney is similarly duplicated with dilated upper pole collecting system and non-dilated lower pole collecting system.

b) There are no signs of an abscess formation here, such as a localized fluid collection with hypovascularized thick rim. Abscesses often contain complex fluid with internal debris and/or fluid-debris levels.

c) Congenital megacaliyces present with enlarged, flattened, and convex (rather than concave) calices. The renal pelvis may or may not be enlarged as well. Congenital megacaliyces are often associated with a congenital hydroureter.

d) A ureteropelvic junction obstruction is characterized by a dilated, usually single collecting system and a non-dilated ureter.

Patient 194: Two-year old male, recurrent urinary tract infections
Author: Heike E. Daldrup-Link, M.D.

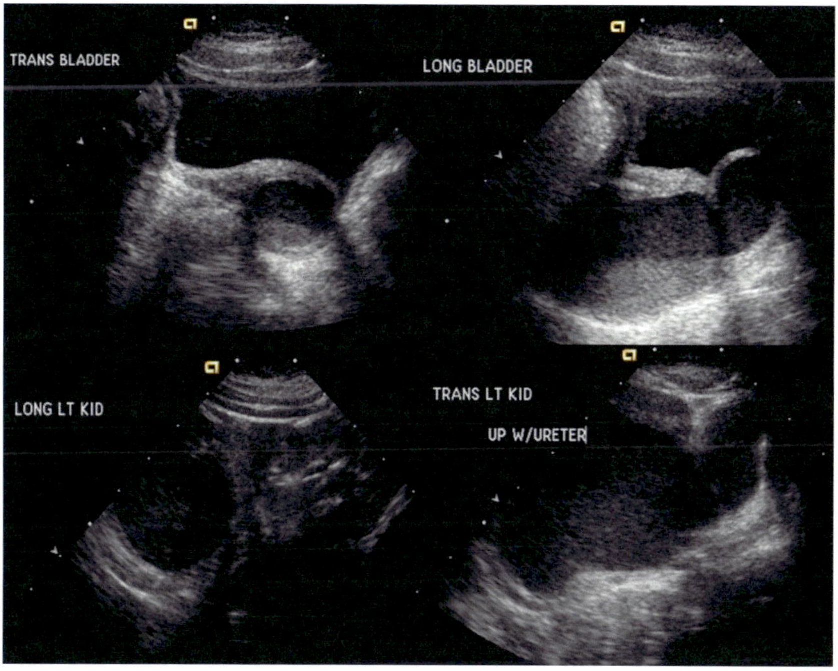

The Weigert Meyer rule states:

a) The lower pole ureter ends mediocaudally into the bladder compared to the upper pole ureter. The upper pole ureter inserts superocranially compared to the lower pole ureter.
b) The upper pole ureter ends mediocaudally into the bladder compared to the lower pole ureter. The lower pole ureter inserts superocranially compared to the upper pole ureter.
c) The lower pole ureter frequently ends in a ureterocele. The upper pole ureter is prone to ureterovesical reflux
d) The lower pole collecting system is usually more dilated compared to the upper pole collecting system.

Case 194: Weigert Meyer Rule

a) The upper pole ureter ends mediocaudally into the bladder compared to the lower pole ureter. The lower pole ureter inserts superocranially compared to the upper pole ureter.

b) In duplicated collecting systems, the ureter of the upper renal moiety often inserts in an ectopic location into the urinary bladder, medial and inferior to the lower pole ureter. The ectopic upper pole ureter frequently ends in a ureterocele, which can lead to an obstruction and dilation of the upper pole ureter and collecting system. The ureter of the lower renal moiety inserts in an orthotopic location into the urinary bladder, lateral and superior to the upper pole ureter. The lower pole ureter is prone to ureterovesical reflux.

c) As seen on the ultrasound shown here, the upper renal moiety ureter frequently ends in a ureterocele. The lower renal moiety is prone to ureterovesical reflux.

d) The upper pole collecting system often ends in a ureterocele, which leads to obstruction. Therefore, the upper pole collecting system is usually more dilated compared to the lower pole collecting system. This is also seen on the ultrasound shown here.

Patient 195: 16-month-old female, urinary tract infection

Author: Heike E. Daldrup-Link, M.D.

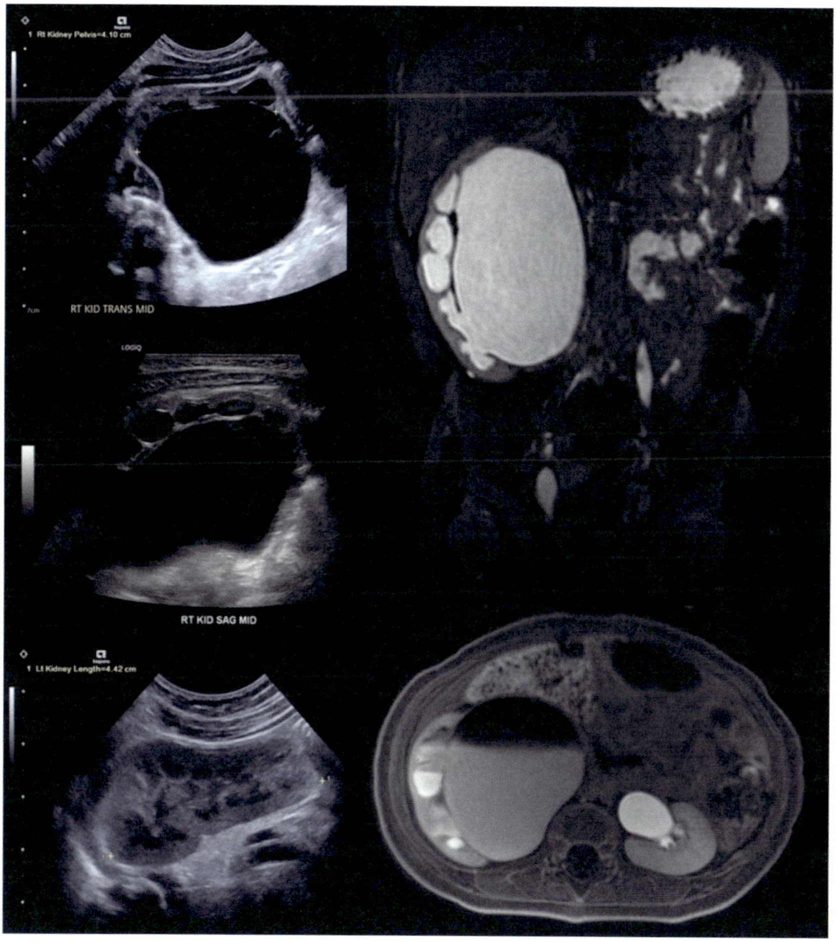

What is the most likely diagnosis:

a) Duplicated renal collecting system bilaterally, ureterocele
b) Multicystic dysplastic kidney
c) Congenital megacaliyces with hydroureter
d) Ureteropelvic junction obstruction

Case 195: Ureteropelvic Junction Obstruction

a) Duplicated renal collecting systems are characterized by a dilated upper pole collecting system of the affected kidney which extends into a hydroureter. A parenchymal bridge separates the upper pole collecting system from a separate lower pole collecting system. The case shown here shows a single dilated collecting system of the right kidney.

b) A multicystic dysplastic kidney is characterized by multiple non-communicating cysts and minimal or absent renal parenchyma.

c) Congenital megacaliyces present with enlarged, flattened, and convex (rather than concave) calices. The renal pelvis may or may not be enlarged as well. Congenital megacaliyces are often associated with a congenital hydroureter.

d) Ureteropelvic junction obstruction: Correct! The ultrasound demonstrates a markedly dilated collecting system of the right kidney and a non-dilated ureter, consistent with an obstruction at the junction between the right renal pelvis and collecting system. The MRI confirms a markedly dilated collecting system of the right kidney on the coronal T2-weighted scan. The surrounding kidney parenchyma is functionally active, as demonstrated by excretion of intravenously administered Gd-chelate in the axial T1-weighted contrast-enhanced MRI scan. The system was decompressed by placement of a stent, followed by pyeloplasty.

GI, GU, and Interventional

7) Urethra, Genital, Adrenal

Case 196: Six-month-old female with precocious puberty
Author: Heike E. Daldrup-Link, M.D.

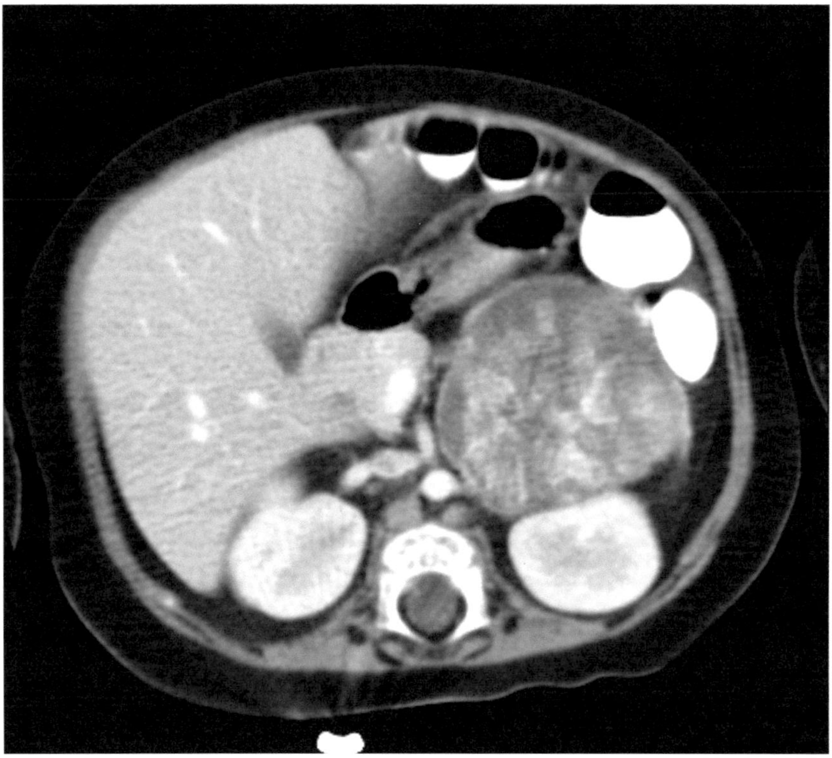

What is the most likely diagnosis:

a) Neuroblastoma
b) Adrenal Hemorrhage
c) Wilms Tumor
d) Adrenocortical Neoplasm

Case 196: Adrenocortical Neoplasm

a) Neuroblastoma: The clinical presentation of precocious puberty is not consistent with a neuroblastoma.

b) Adrenal Hemorrhage: The clinical presentation of precocious puberty is not consistent with an adrenal hemorrhage

c) Wilms Tumor: This lesion is not located in the kidney. There is a fat plane between the lesion and the kidney. There is no "claw sign".

d) Adrenocortical Neoplasm: Correct! The axial CT scan shows a large, inhomogeneous, contrast-enhancing lesion in the left adrenal gland. Together with the clinical presentation of precocious puberty, this finding is consistent with an adrenocortical neoplasm.

Case 197: Teenage female with increasing abdominal girth

Author: Heike E. Daldrup-Link, M.D.

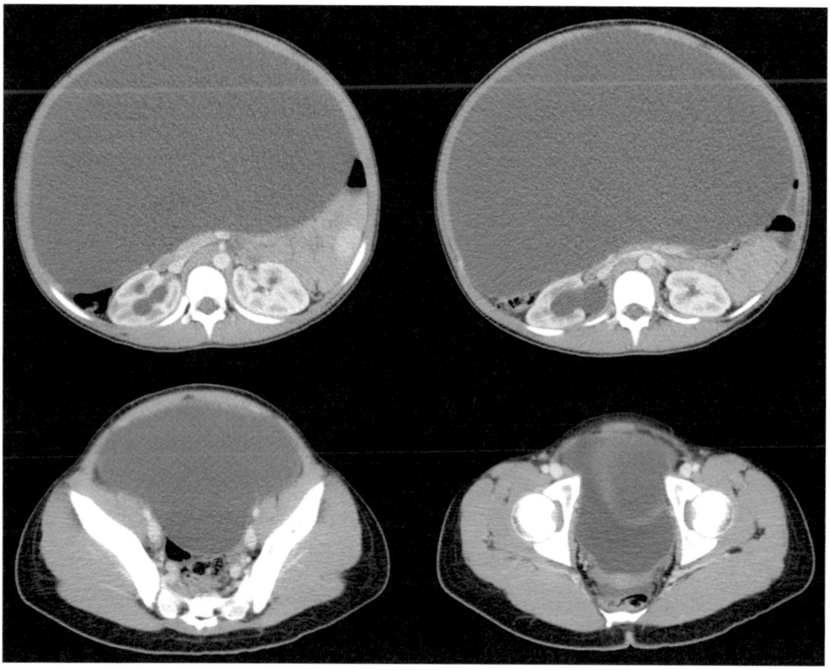

What is the most likely diagnosis:

a) Hydroperitoneum
b) Ovarian Dermoid Cyst
c) Immature Teratoma
d) Hemorrhagic Ovarian Cyst

Case 197: Ovarian Dermoid Cyst

a) Hydroperitoneum is another term for ascites, which usually distributes freely within the abdomen, surrounding visceral organs and extending in between bowel loops.

b) Ovarian Dermoid Cyst: Correct! The CT scan demonstrates a large cystic mass in the abdomen and pelvis, which compresses and displaces bowel loops laterally. The small uterus on the lower right image suggests that this is a pre-pubertal patient. The ovaries are so small that it is difficult to localize the origin of the cystic mass. However, in a pre-pubertal female and in the absence of a relation of the mass to visceral organs or the bowel, a dermoid cyst is the most common differential diagnosis. Histologically, dermoid cysts are composed of ectodermal elements. Mature cystic teratomas can present with identical imaging findings. Histologically, mature cystic teratomas are composed of all three germ layers with ectodermal, mesodermal, and endodermal elements. They can therefore also present as more inhomogeneous lesions, with internal calcifications, bone, teeth, hair, macroscopic fat, etc.

c) An immature teratoma would typically present as an inhomogeneous, cystic, and solid mass with internal areas of fat and calcifications. Immature teratomas can metastasize.

d) Hemorrhagic Ovarian Cyst: There is no evidence of blood products within this lesion. In a pre-pubertal patient, this diagnosis would be highly unlikely. The size of the lesion would also be unusually large.

Patient 198: 5-month-old male with scrotal mass

Author: Marcello Chang, Michael F. Fadell, M.D.

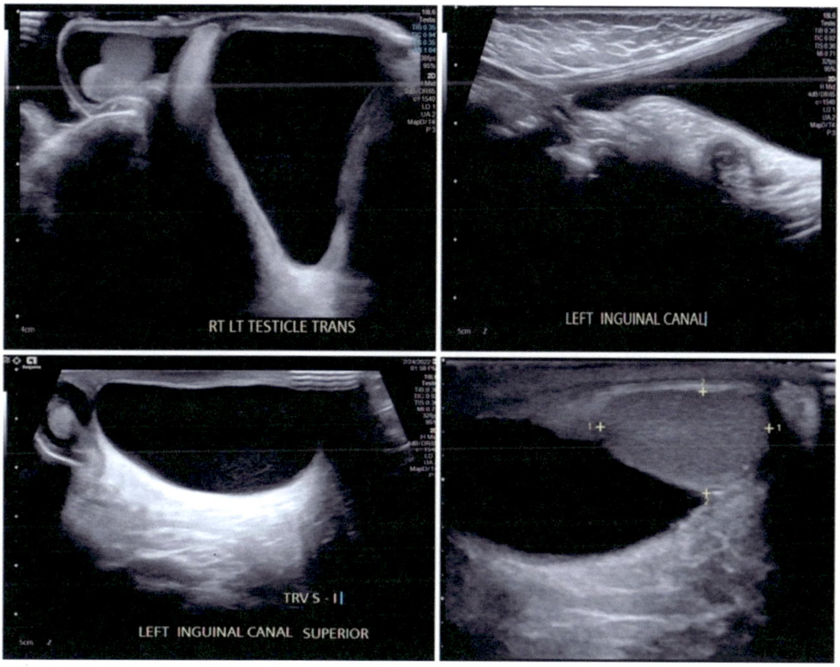

What is the most likely diagnosis:

a) Hydrocele of the cord
b) Inguinal hernia
c) Cryptorchidism
d) Testicular neoplasm

Case 198: Hydrocele of the cord

a) Hydrocele of the cord: Correct! The ultrasound shows an oval, well-defined anechoic fluid collection superior to the left testicle that does not communicate with the peritoneal cavity. The fluid collection contains a small amount of debris but does not contain solid components or bowel. On color Doppler ultrasound (not shown here), the fluid collection is avascular. These findings are consistent with a hydrocele of the spermatic cord. There are two types of hydroceles of the spermatic cord: funicular and encysted. A funicular hydrocoele of the cord communicates with the peritoneal cavity while an encysted hydrocoele of the cord does not. Due to lack of communication with the peritoneal cavity as well as separation from the testicle by a thin fibrous band, these images are most consistent with an encysted hydrocele of the spermatic cord. These are typically painless but may cause symptoms due to mass effect. Encysted hydroceles of the spermatic cord are typically self-limited and involute by 1 year of age and are consequently typically managed conservatively. Funicular hydroceles of the cord are less likely to resolve spontaneously. Surgery may be indicated if either type persists past 12 months or if the hydrocele is growing.

b) An inguinal hernia presents with herniation of peritoneal content into the inguinal canal, particularly bowel and peritoneal fat, neither of which are seen in this ultrasound. In addition, inguinal hernia contents may bulge further with Valsalva maneuvers.

c) Cryptorchidism would show absence of testes in the scrotal sac. The testes are often visualized in the inguinal canal although they can be located anywhere between the lower pole of the kidney and the scrotum. The testicle here is in the scrotum.

d) A testicular neoplasm would manifest as an intra-testicular solid and/or cystic mass, not an extra testicular fluid collection.

Case 199: Pregnant patient (28 weeks), prenatal ultrasound

Authors: Praveen Jayapal, M.D., Ali Rashidi, M.D.

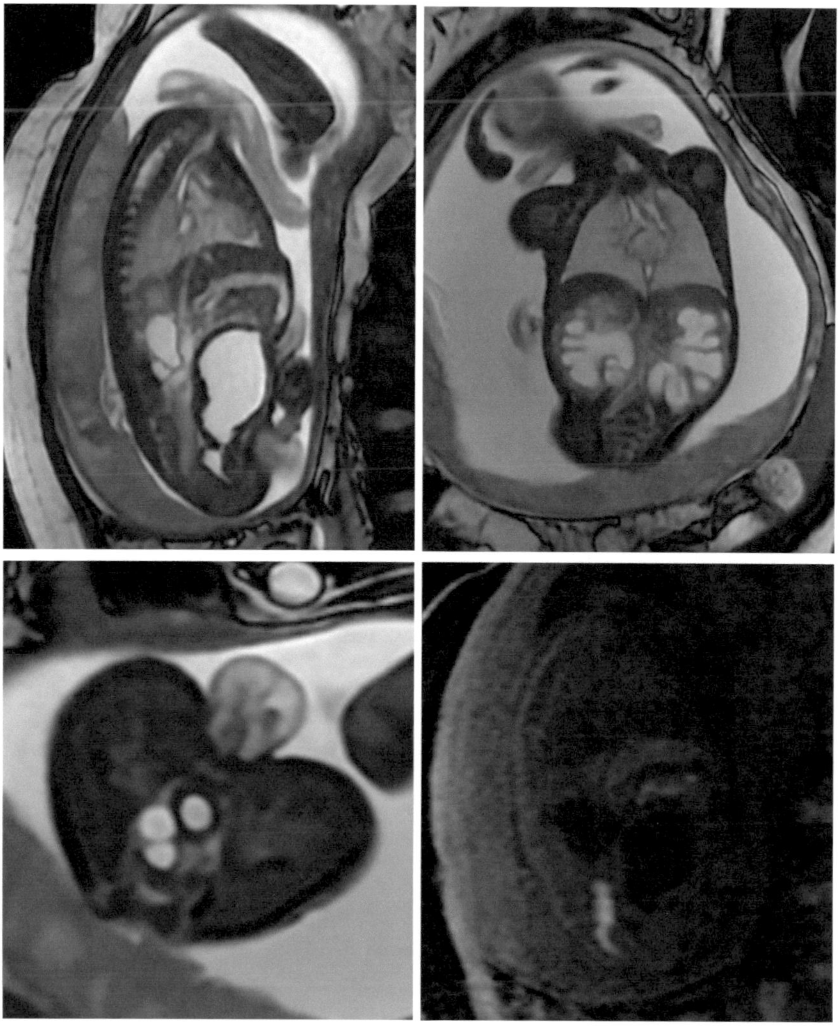

What is the most likely diagnosis:

a) Bilateral multicystic dysplastic kidneys
b) Megacystis microcolon intestinal hypoperistalsis syndrome
c) Posterior urethral valve
d) Cloacal Malformation

Case 199: Posterior urethral valve

a) Bilateral multicystic dysplastic kidneys (MCDK) are characterized by numerous noncommunicating cysts. In most cases, the collecting system and ureter are atretic and the renal parenchyma is markedly diminished or absent. The coronal scan here demonstrates a dilated renal collecting system bilaterally.

b) Megacystis microcolon intestinal hypoperistalsis syndrome (MMIHS) is characterized by a markedly enlarged urinary bladder and a microcolon. This case here demonstrates a normal meconium-filled colon on the sagittal LAVA scan.

c) Posterior urethral valve: Correct! This patient shows characteristic features of lower urinary outflow tract obstruction (LUTO) secondary to a posterior urethral valve. The sagittal (FIESTA) MRI scan demonstrates a dilated urinary bladder with thickened, trabeculated bladder wall and abnormal funneling of the bladder inferiorly into a dilated posterior urethra. The presence of abnormal bladder wall thickening and trabeculation reflects the chronic nature of this obstruction. The coronal T2-weighted MRI scan shows severe bilateral hydroureteronephrosis. The axial fiesta MRI at the level of fetal pelvis demonstrates abnormal funneling of the bladder and a partially visualized tortuous ureter posteriorly. The sagittal T1 weighted image (LAVA) demonstrates a normal meconium filled rectum (tubular structure with high T1 signal) posterior to the bladder and the urinary tract. No communication between the rectum and urinary tract is visualized. The rectal caliber is normal. Patients with severe LUTO usually present with oligohydramnios and pulmonary hypoplasia. However, this patient presented with polyhydramnios due to maternal gestational diabetes; hence the lungs developed normally.

d) Cloacal Malformation is incorrect because a discrete anal canal separate from the urinary tract is noted on the axial MRI scan.

Case 200: 3-year-old male, increased abdominal girth

Author: Heike E. Daldrup-Link, M.D.

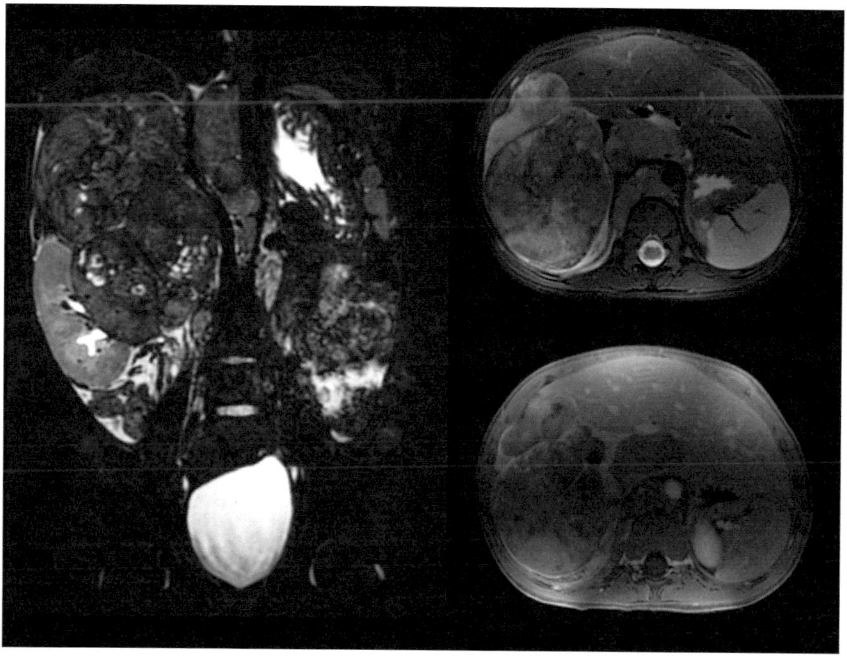

What is the most likely diagnosis:

a) Wilm's Tumor
b) Neuroblastoma
c) Lymphoma
d) Hepatoblastoma

Case 200: Neuroblastoma

a) Wilms Tumor: The tumor shown here extends caudally to the hilum of the kidney. However, there is no typical "claw sign". A Wilms tumor is usually more clearly defined and displaces abdominal vessels rather than encasing them. It would be unusual for a Wilms Tumor to grow behind the aorta.

b) Neuroblastoma: Correct! The coronal and axial T2 weighted MRI demonstrates a large mass, which is centered in the area of the right adrenal gland. The mass encases the IVC and grows behind the aorta. There are multiple associated lymph node metastases. The axial contrast-enhanced T1-weighted MRI demonstrates that the tumor nodules are highly vascularized. All these features are typical for a neuroblastoma.

c) A lymphoma good present with abdominal lymphadenopathy. However, the adrenal mass, shown here, would be unusual. Lymphomas would be more typical in older children.

d) Hepatoblastoma: The lesion shown here does not originate from the liver. While a hepatoblastoma could have an exophytic component, it would displace abdominal vessels rather than encasing them.

Case 201: Teenage female with pelvic pain

Author: Heike E. Daldrup-Link, M.D.

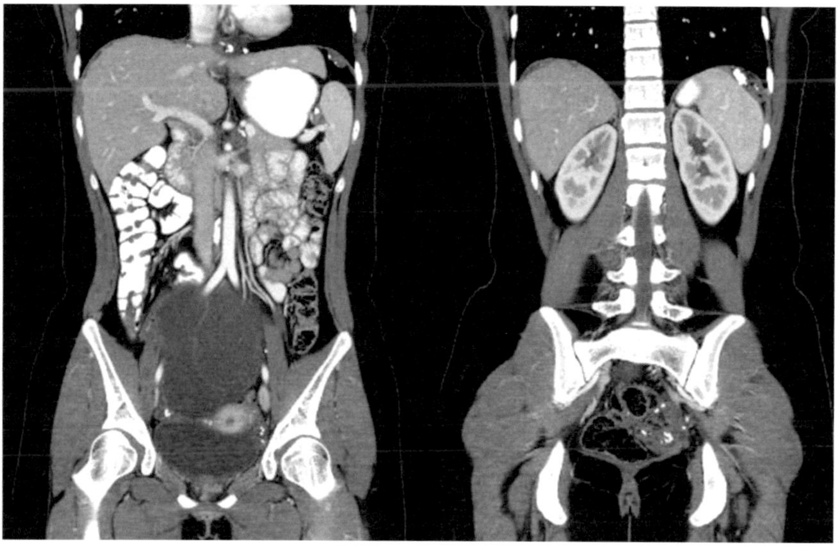

What is the most likely diagnosis:

a) Neuroblastoma
b) Mature Teratoma
c) Immature Teratoma
d) Ovarian torsion

Case 201: Immature teratoma

a) Neuroblastoma: Neuroblastomas present more commonly as solid tumors; predominantly cystic neuroblastomas are rare. The age of the patient and the presence of peritoneal seeds would be also unusual.

b) Mature teratoma: The combined cystic and solid pelvic mass with speckled calcifications could be consistent with a mature teratoma. However, the peritoneal seeds would be unusual.

c) Immature teratoma: Correct! The coronal CT scan shows a cystic and solid mass with speckled calcifications in the pelvis. There are multiple peritoneal seeds along the diaphragm, around the liver, at the origin of the celiac trunk and at the hilum of the spleen.

d) Ovarian torsion. The CT images shown here demonstrate an inhomogeneous cystic and solid pelvic mass.

Case 202: Teenage male with testicular pain
Author: Heike E. Daldrup-Link, M.D.

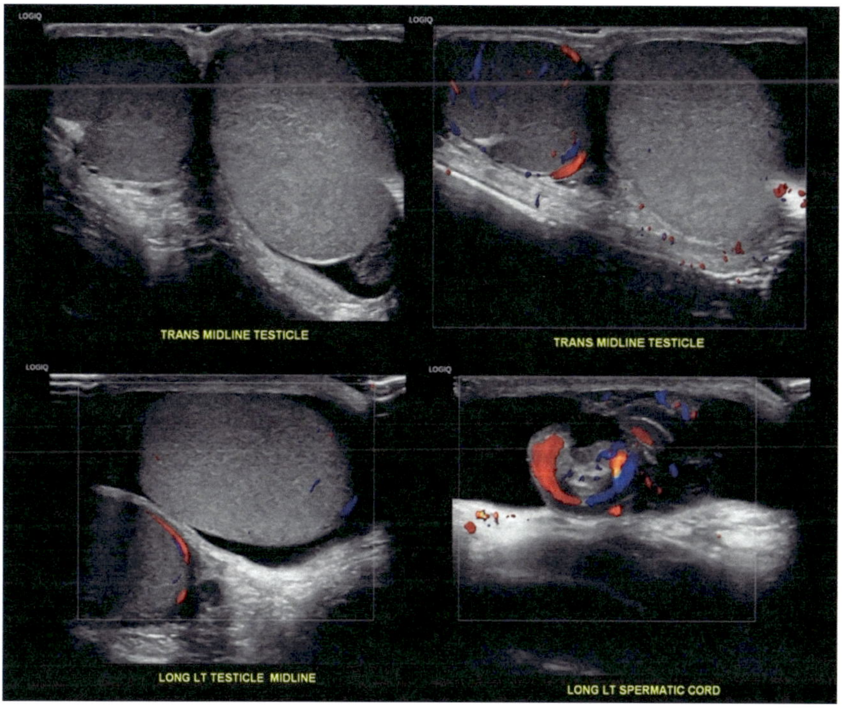

What is the most likely diagnosis:

a) Leukemia
b) Seminoma
c) Testicular Teratoma
d) Testicular Torsion

Case 202: Testicular Torsion

a) Leukemia: Leukemic infiltration of the testicle can you present as unilateral or bilateral enlargement. The blood-testis barrier impairs delivery of chemotherapeutic drugs to the testis, which can serve as a sanctuary for leukemic cells. However, doppler ultrasound typically demonstrates vessels within the testicle.

b) Seminoma presents as an inhomogeneous, vascularized mass of the testicle. Doppler ultrasound typically demonstrates vessels within the testicle.

c) Testicular teratoma presents as an inhomogeneous mass of the testicle with vascularized soft tissue, cystic areas, hypoechogenic and hyperechogenic fat components.

d) Testicular torsion: Correct! The ultrasound images shown here demonstrate marked enlargement and hyperechogenicity of the left testis compared to the normal right testis. The doppler exam shows normal blood flow of the right testis and absent blood flow of the left testis. The spermatic cord displays the whirlpool sign, a spiral twist of the spermatic cord.

Patient 203: Four-month-old male, antenatally noted hydronephrosis

Author: Marcello Chang, Michael F. Fadell, M.D.

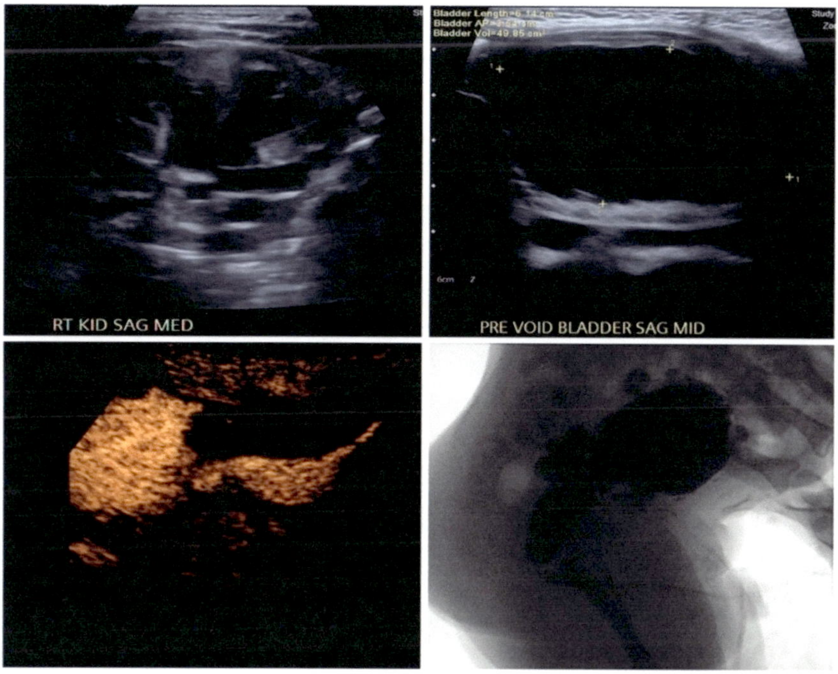

What is the most likely diagnosis:

a) Posterior urethral valve
b) Vesicoureteral reflux
c) Neurogenic bladder
d) Ureterocele

Case 203: Posterior Urethral Valves

a) Posterior urethral valves (PUV): Correct! The ultrasound shows pelvocaliectasis of the right kidney, dilated distal ureters behind the urinary bladder and with a bladder wall that is thickened and trabeculated. Microbubble contrast ultrasound and fluoroscopic images of the urinary bladder and urethra show a dilated posterior urethra during the voiding phase. These findings all suggest PUV. Posterior urethral valve result from failure of regression of the mesonephric duct, that courses from the verumontanum to the most distal portion of the prostatic urethra and formation of a valve-like membrane. Typically, this leads to dilation of upstream structures. The finding of a distended bladder and distended dilated posterior urethra on voiding cystourethrogram (VCUG) is classically known as the keyhole sign.

b) Vesicoureteral reflux would require a dynamic voiding cystourethrogram (VCUG). The images presented do not show findings that suggest reflux of contrast material from the urinary bladder into the ureters or collecting system of the kidneys.

c) A neurogenic bladder would be also associated with trabeculation and thickening of the urinary bladder. However, the proximal urethra would not be dilated.

d) A ureterocele would demonstrate as a cystic protrusion of the ureter into the urinary bladder near the vesicoureteral junction (VUJ). A ureterocele is frequently associated with a duplicated collecting system. While pelvocaliectasis might be present, bladder trabeculation and urethra abnormalities would not be expected.

Case 204: 6-month-old male infant

Author: Heike E. Daldrup-Link, M.D.

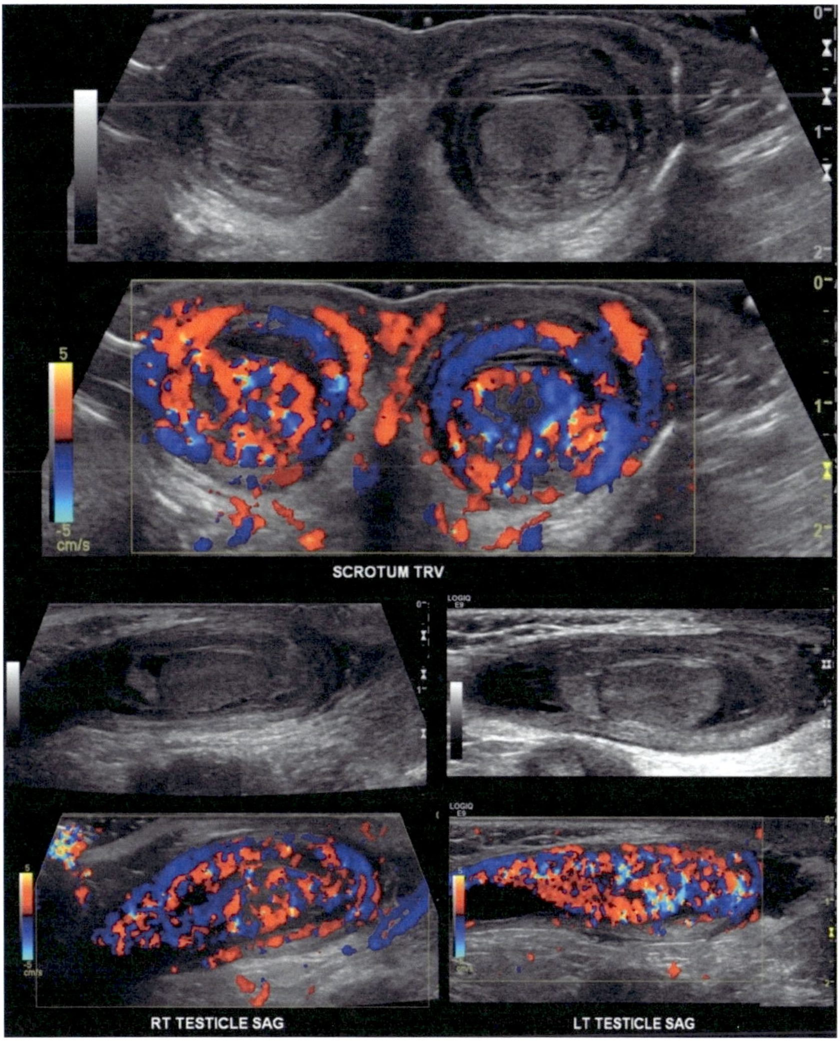

What is the most likely diagnosis:

a) Epididymitis
b) Epididymo-Orchitis
c) Testicular Teratoma
d) Testicular Torsion

Case 204: Epididymo-Orchitis

a) Epididymitis presents with increased blood flow and perfusion of the epididymis, while the testis remains normal. A reactive hydrocele can be present as well. This is not the case here.

b) Epididymo-Orchitis: Correct! The color doppler ultrasound images demonstrate increased blood flow and perfusion of the bilateral testis and epididymis. Grey scale images demonstrate swelling of the subcutaneous soft tissues. The findings are characteristic of combined inflammation of the epididymitis and testis, called epididymo-orchitis. Underlying causes can be bacterial or viral infections.

c) Testicular teratoma presents as an inhomogeneous mass of the testicle with vascularized soft tissue, cystic areas, hypoechogenic and hyperechogenic fat components.

d) Testicular torsion presents with marked asymmetric enlargement and hyperechogenicity of the affected testis compared to the contralateral normal right testis. The doppler exam shows absent blood flow of the affected testis and normal blood flow of the contralateral normal testis. The spermatic cord displays the whirlpool sign, a spiral twist of the spermatic cord.

Case 205: 10-year-old male with testicular pain

Author: Heike E. Daldrup-Link, M.D.

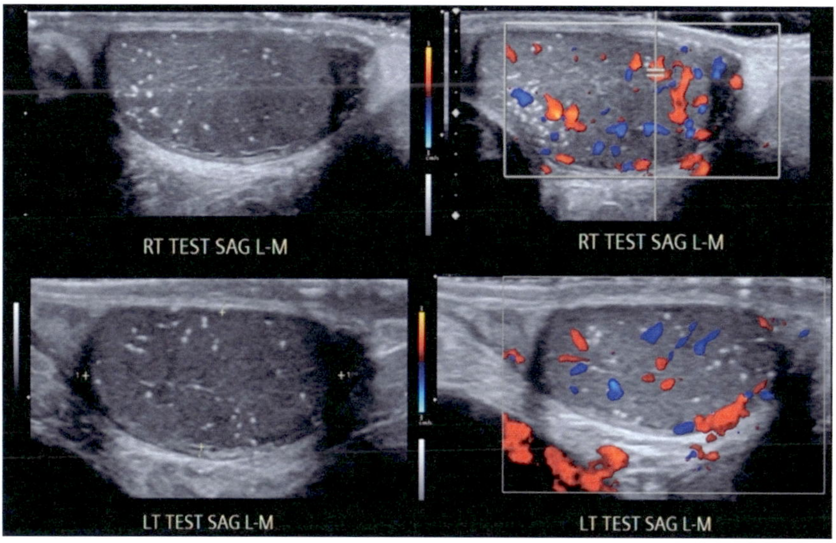

What is the most likely diagnosis:

a) Leukemia
b) Testicular Microlithiasis
c) Testicular Teratoma
d) Varicocele

Case 205: Testicular Microlithiasis

a) Leukemia can be associated with painless unilateral or bilateral testicular enlargement, often with one or more focal lesions. However, microcalcifications are not associated with leukemia.

b) Testicular Microlithiasis: Correct! The ultrasound shows multiple (more than 5) small non-shadowing hyperechoic foci in the bilateral testis with diameters of 1-2 mm, consistent with bilateral microlithiasis. An increased incidence is noted in patients with Klinefelter syndrome, Down syndrome, and cryptorchidism, among a few others. A potential association with the development of testicular germ cell tumors is controversial.

c) Testicular teratoma presents as an inhomogeneous, usually unilateral lesion of the testicle. The lesion is typically inhomogeneous, with vascularized soft tissue, cystic areas, hypoechogenic areas and hyperechogenic fat components.

d) A varicocele presents with dilated, serpiginous veins (> 2-3 mm) beside the testis and in the spermatic cord. An associated swelling or atrophy of the testis might be noted. During a Valsalva maneuver the diameter of the varicocele increases and the venous flow reverses. Primary varicoceles are due to incontinent venous valves in the internal spermatic vein which lead to venous reflux into the pampiniform plexus. 85% affect the left scrotum. The left internal spermatic vein drains into the left renal vein at a 90-degree angle, which leads to high pressure in the internal spermatic vein. On the right side, the internal spermatic vein merges with the inferior cava via a more acute angle. Secondary varicoceles are the result of increased pressure in the testicular vein, e.g., in patients with hydronephrosis, portal hypertension, abdominal tumors and compression of the left renal vein between the superior mesenteric artery and aorta.

Case 206: Teenage male with painless mass in the left testicle

Author: Heike E. Daldrup-Link, M.D.

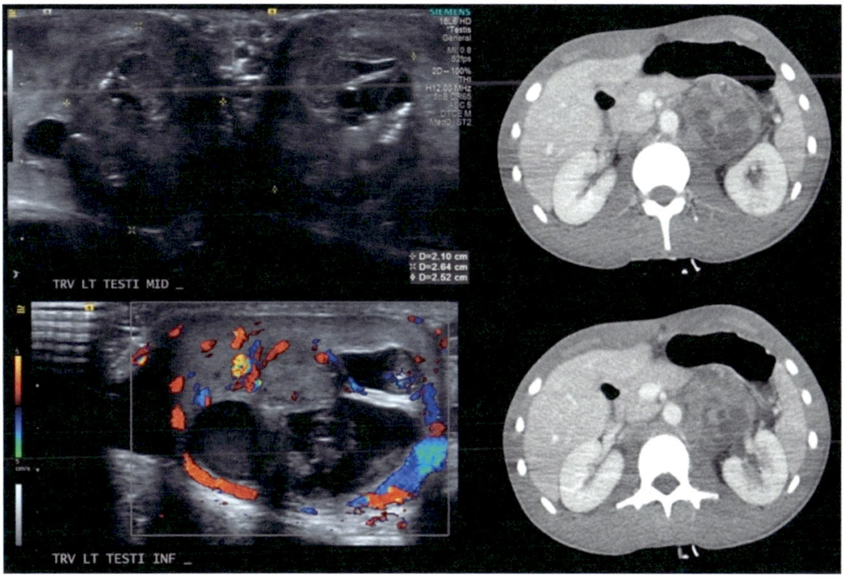

What is the most likely diagnosis:

a) Leukemia
b) Neuroblastoma
c) Germ Cell Tumor
d) Cystic Dysplasia

Case 206: Testicular Non-Seminomatous Germ Cell Tumor

a) Leukemia: Leukemic infiltration of the testicle can present as unilateral or bilateral testicular enlargement, with or without focal lesions. However, the retroperitoneal lymphadenopathy seen on the CT scan suggests a different differential diagnosis.

b) A neuroblastoma could potentially metastasize into the testis. However, this would be very uncommon. In addition, the age of the patient would be uncommon as well for a neuroblastoma diagnosis. Take home point: If you think that you see an atypical something consider that it might be a typical something else.

c) Germ Cell Tumor: Correct! The ultrasound images demonstrate an inhomogeneous mass of the left testis with vascularized soft tissue, hypoechogenic cystic areas and hyperechogenic fat components. The CT scan demonstrates an inhomogeneous mass at the left renal hilum, consistent with lymph node metastases at a typical location, at the insertion site of the left testicular vein into the left renal vein. Note that serum biomarkers can be helpful in the differential diagnosis of patients with testicular masses. In this patient, the alpha fetoprotein (AFP) was moderately elevated, which suggests the diagnosis of a non-seminomatous germ cell tumor. A moderately elevated AFP excluded the differential diagnosis of a seminoma (which are AFP negative) and made a yolk sac tumor much less likely (would have high AFP).

d) Cystic dysplasia of the rete testis presents as a rare, benign, unilateral multicystic lesion. In some cases, the lesion can exert mass effect on the mediastinum testis and cause testicular atrophy due to chronic vascular compression. Cystic dysplasia of the rete testis has been associated with ipsilateral renal anomalies, including renal agenesis, multicystic dysplastic kidney and vesicoureteral reflux.

Case 207: 14-year-old female with increasing abdominal girth
Author: Heike E. Daldrup-Link

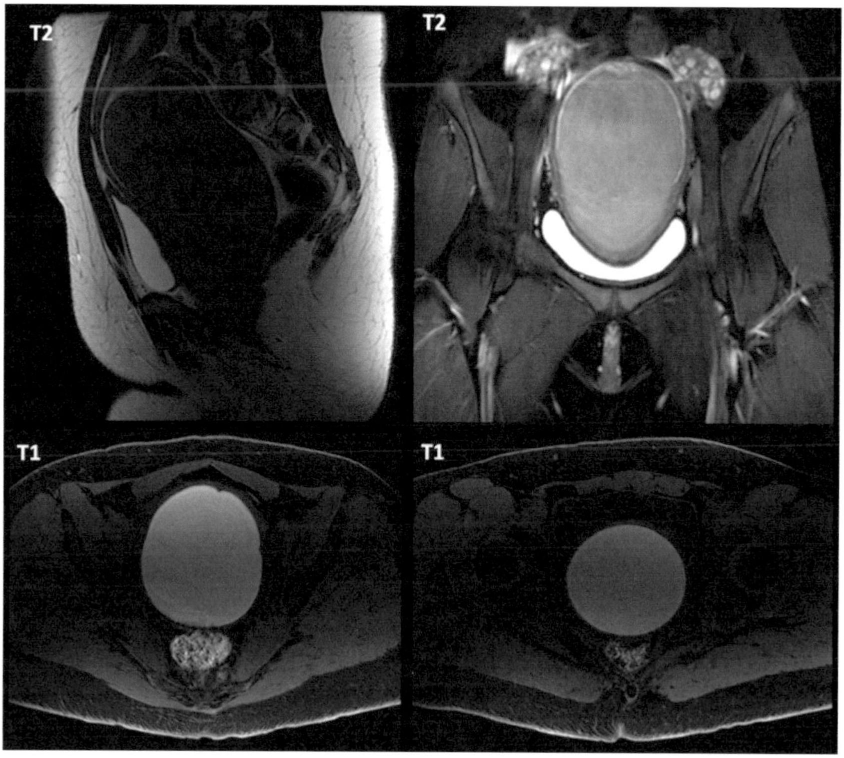

What is the most likely diagnosis:

a) Hematocolpos
b) Ovarian Dermoid Cyst
c) Immature Teratoma
d) Hemorrhagic Ovarian Cyst

Case 207: Hematocolpos

a) Hematocolpos: Correct! The MRI scan demonstrates an elongated, well defined fluid containing lesion between the urinary bladder and the rectum. The lesion contains T2-hypointense and T1-hyperintense fluid, consistent with blood. The first sagittal image shows that the lesion is located below the uterus and connected with the uterus, consistent with a dilated vagina which is filled with menstrual blood (hematocolpos). The underlying cause is most commonly a transverse vaginal septum or an imperforate hymen. If the blood accumulation extends from the vagina into the uterine cavity, it is termed "hematometrocolpos". It is important to look for associated Mullerian duct anomalies, such as a bicornuate uterus or uterus didelphys, which is not noted in this case here.

b) An ovarian dermoid cyst presents as a large cystic mass in the abdomen and pelvis, which can be connected to one of the ovaries. The ovaries in this case here contain multiple follicle cysts and are normal. Mature cystic teratomas can present with identical imaging findings. Histologically, mature cystic teratomas can present as more inhomogeneous lesions, with internal calcifications, bone, teeth, hair, macroscopic fat, etc.

c) An immature teratoma would typically present as an inhomogeneous, cystic, and solid mass with internal areas of fat and calcifications. Immature teratomas can metastasize.

d) Hemorrhagic Ovarian Cyst. The bilateral ovaries are normal. The cystic lesion shown here is not connected to the ovaries. The longitudinal shape of the lesion would also be unusual for an ovarian cyst. The key to the diagnosis here is to note that the lesion is in the anatomical space of the vagina.

Case 208: Two-year old male, painless mass in the right testicle

Author: Heike E. Daldrup-Link

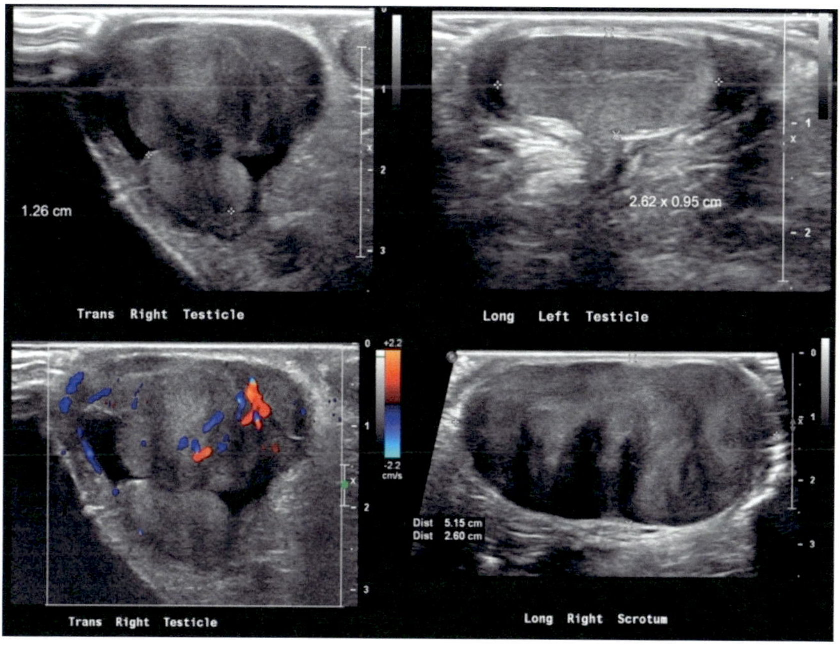

What is the most likely diagnosis:

a) Leukemia
b) Neuroblastoma
c) Germ Cell Tumor
d) Rhabdomyosarcoma

Case 208: Paratesticular Rhabdomyosarcoma

a) Leukemia: Leukemic infiltration of the testicle can present as unilateral or bilateral testicular enlargement, with or without focal lesions. However, the lesion shown here is located beside the testicle.

b) A neuroblastoma could potentially metastasize into the testis. However, this would be very uncommon. The lesion shown here is located in the scrotum but outside of the testicle.

c) A germ cell tumor would present as an inhomogeneous mass of the testis with vascularized soft tissue, hypoechogenic cystic areas and hyperechogenic fat components on ultrasound scans. However, the lesion shown here is located beside the testicle.

d) Rhabdomyosarcoma: Correct! The ultrasound images show an inhomogeneous, vascularized soft tissue mass in the right scrotum. A normal right testicle is seen below the mass on transaxial images. A rhabdomyosarcoma is the most common diagnosis of paratesticular soft tissue masses in young children.

GI, GU, and Interventional

8) Vascular and Interventional

Patient 209: History withheld

Author: Heike E. Daldrup-Link, M.D.

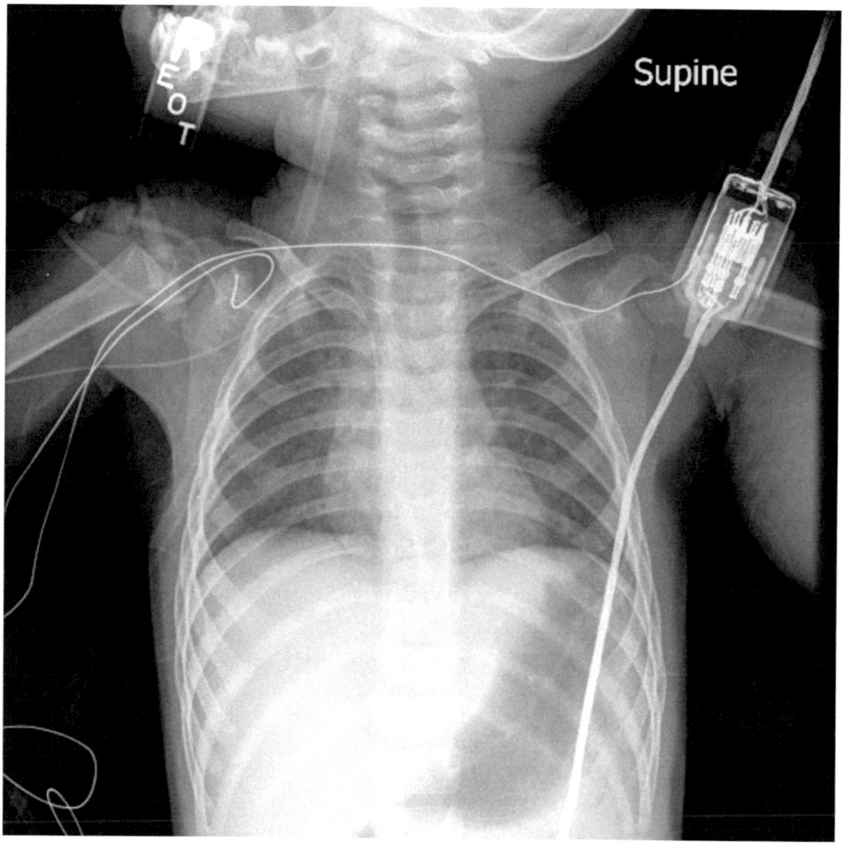

Where is the abnormality:

a) Lungs
b) Mediastinum
c) Musculoskeletal
d) Normal Radiograph

Case 209: Lymphatic Malformation

a) The lungs are normal.

b) The mediastinum is normal.

c) Musculoskeletal: Correct! The radiograph shows marked soft tissue swelling of the left arm. The MRI of this patient (shown below) demonstrates a T2-hyperintense, T1-hypointense lesion with fluid-equivalent signal intensity and septal enhancement after intravenous Gd-chelate injection. Findings are consistent with a lymphatic malformation.

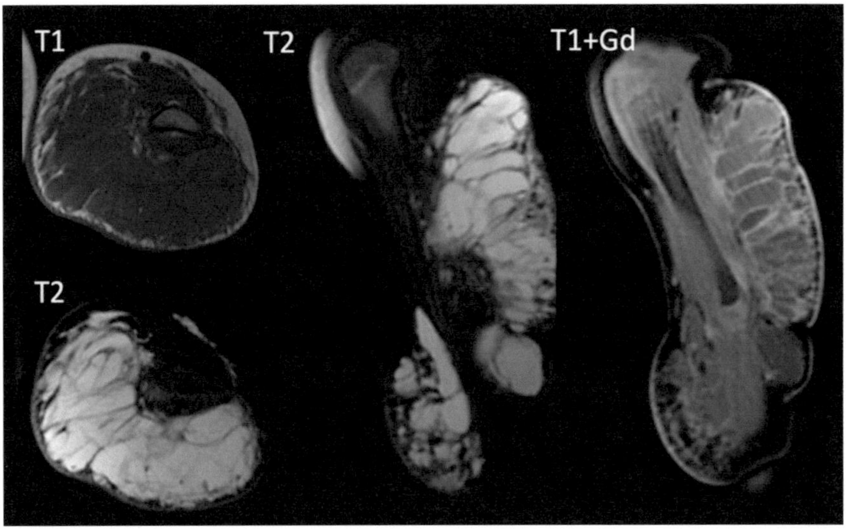

d) This radiograph is not normal, see above.

Patient 210: 16-year-old female, palpable thrill after radial artery catheter

Author: Heike E. Daldrup-Link, M.D.

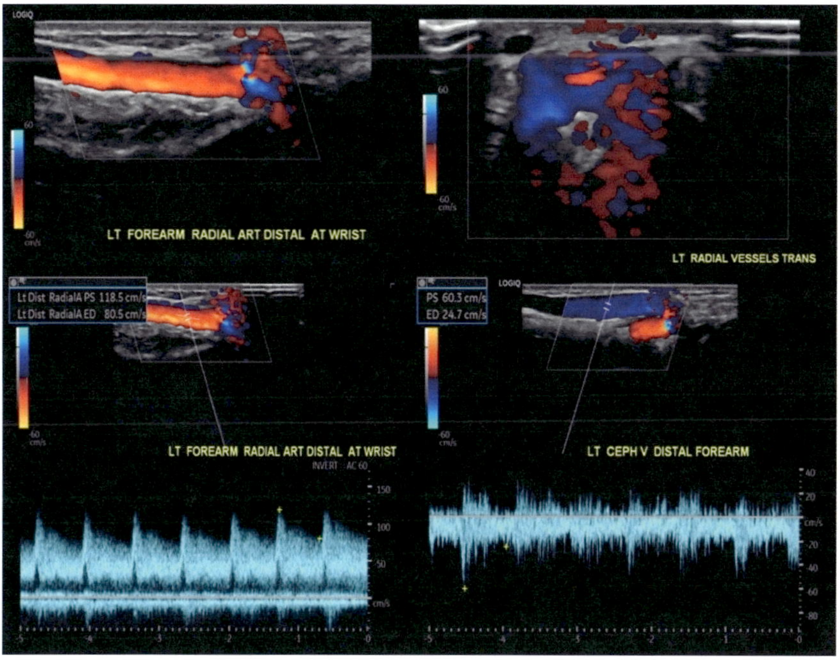

What is the most likely diagnosis:

a) Arteriovenous Malformation
b) Pseudoaneurysm
c) True aneurysm
d) Arteriovenous Fistula

Case 210: Arteriovenous Fistula

a) An arteriovenous malformation represents one or multiple connections between arteries and veins. It represents a developmental anomaly rather than an acquired abnormality.

b) A pseudoaneurysm or false aneurysm can occur after an injury of the vessel wall, either after a trauma or vessel puncture, leading to a blind ending outpouch of the vessel which is only lined by a thin layer of the tunica adventitia. Color doppler ultrasound demonstrates a "to and fro" pattern of turbulent blood flow within the aneurysm.

c) A true aneurysm is defined as a blind ending outpouch of a vessel outlined by all three layers of the vessel wall. Color doppler ultrasound demonstrates a "to and fro" pattern of turbulent blood flow within the aneurysm.

d) Arteriovenous Fistula: Correct! The ultrasound demonstrates an abnormal communication of the distal radial artery and cephalic vein with increased diastolic flow within the the distal radial artery and arterialization of venous blood flow in the distal cephalic vein.

Patient 211: Adolescent male with left hip pain
Author: Heike E. Daldrup-Link, M.D.

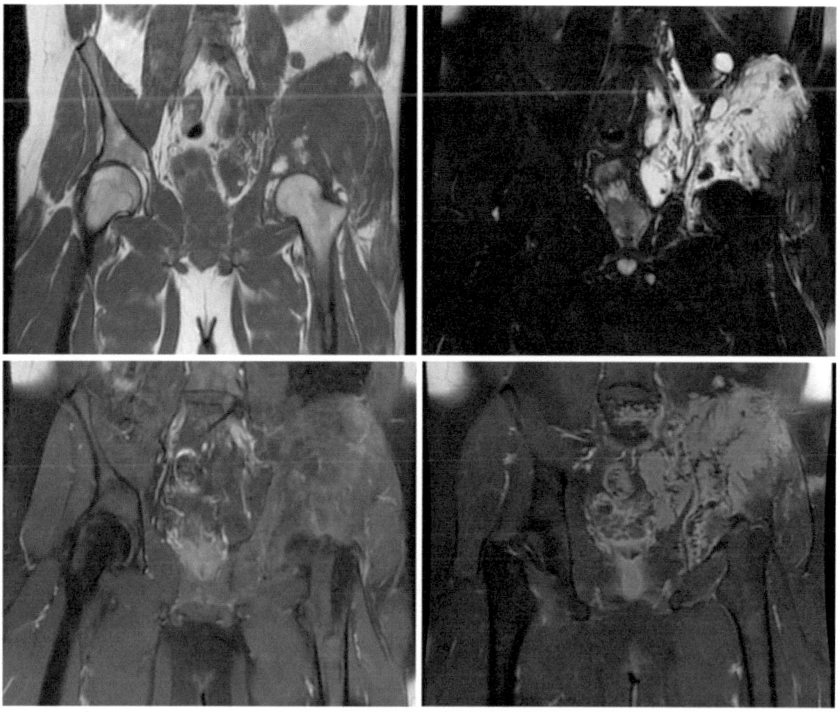

What is the most likely diagnosis:

a) Osteosarcoma
b) Osteomyelitis
c) Gorham Disease
d) Lymphatic Malformation

Case 211: Gorham Disease

a) An osteosarcoma would present as a localized soft tissue mass with an intraosseous and extraosseous component, moderate signal on T2-weighted MR images and imhomogenous contrast enhancement on contrast-enhanced MRI scans. The high T2-signal of the lesion show here suggests an underlying highly vascular lesion. A telangiectatic osteosarcoma can present with multiple T2-hyperintense fluid spaces, but these would typically show fluid-fluid levels and peripheral/septal enhancement.

b) Osteomyelitis would present as an intraosseous pathology. The surrounding soft tissues can demonstrate an edema or adjacent abscesses, but the extraosseous extension of the lesion noted here suggests a different diagnosis.

c) Gorham disease or Gorham-Stout disease: Correct! The coronal MRI scans of the pelvis demonstrates a large lesion in the left ilium, which is hypointense to adjacent muscle on unenhanced T1-weighted MRI scans, demonstrates fluid-equivalent hyperintense signal on T2 weighted MRI images and marked enhancement on contrast-enhanced MRI. The lesion is locally aggressive and infiltrates the gluteus muscles, the left hip joint, the proximal left femur, the iliopsoas muscle, the left paravertebral soft tissues and the 5th lumbar vertebral body. The underlying cause is non-hereditary and likely multifactorial, but otherwise poorly understood. Histologically, an aggressive, expansile, non-neoplastic proliferation of capillary or cavernous blood vessels leads to replacement of normal bone by fibrovascular tissue and activation of osteoclasts such that the underlying bone can completely dissapear, a process referred to as "vanishing bone disease."

d) A lymphatic malformation is primarily composed of fluid-filled spaces which are hyperintense on T2 weighted MRI images, but does not enhance on contrast-enhanced MRI.

Patient 212: Premature newborn baby boy

Author: Heike E. Daldrup-Link, M.D.

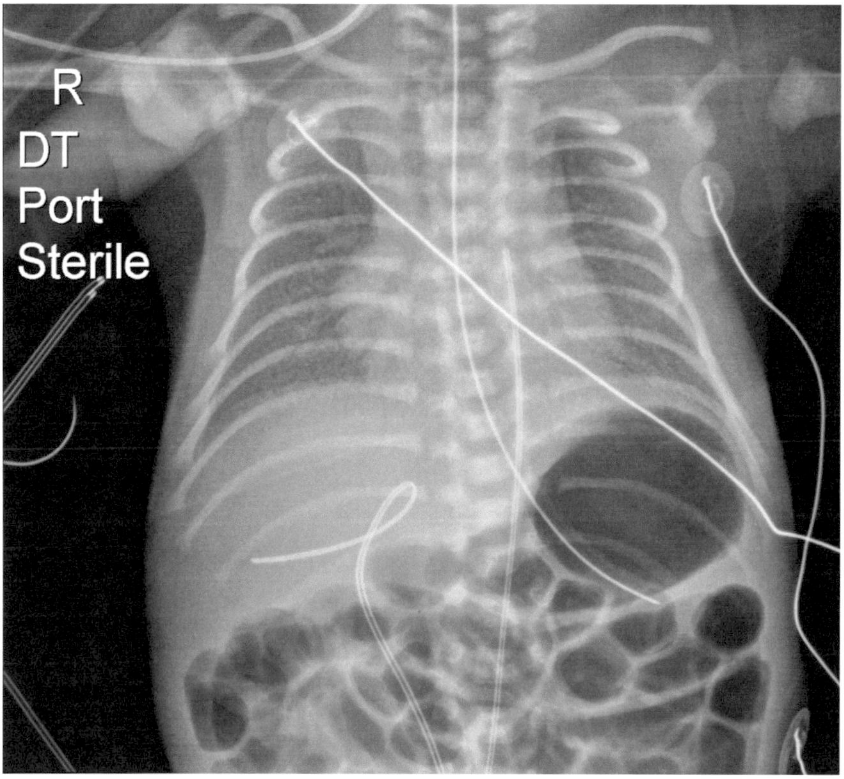

What is the most likely diagnosis:

a) Malpositioned biliary drain
b) Malpositioned peritoneal drain
c) Malpositioned umbilical venous catheter
d) All lines and tubes in appropriate position

Case 212: Malpositioned Umbilical Venous Catheter (UVC)

a) Malpositioned biliary drain: There is no biliary drain shown here. Placement of a biliary drain in a newborn would be very unusual.

b) Malpositioned peritoneal drain: There is no peritoneal drain shown here.

c) Malpositioned umbilical venous catheter (UVC): Correct! The frontal x-ray of the chest and upper abdomen demonstrates a UVC, which can be followed from the left portal vein to the right portal vein. The tip of the catheter ends in the right portal vein. The expected normal course of the catheter would be from the left portal vein superiorly through the venous duct towards the lower cavoatrial junction.

d) Lines and tubes are not in appropriate position. The UVC is misplaced in the right portal vein (see above). In addition, the umbilical artery catheter ends relatively high, at the level of T5. It is usually expected to terminate at the level of T6 (high position) or below the level of L2 (low position below the level of the renal arteries). These positions are favored in order to avoid potential thrombus material along the catheter to enter the branches of the thoracic or abdominal aorta. Note that there are also diffuse hazy airspace opacities of the bilateral lungs, consistent with microatelectasis and respiratory distress syndrome in this preterm newborn.

ACKNOWLEDGMENTS

An accurate and timely medical diagnosis can improve health outcomes and safe lives by referring patients to the appropriate treatment in a timely manner. Medical imaging is particularly important in the evaluation of children, who may not be able to localize or articulate a clinical problem. I am grateful to everyone who invested time and effort in creating this case series so that trainees and practitioners alike can expand their knowledge and provide more accurate diagnoses.

Of course, a book such as this does not happen in a vacuum. I would like to thank the American Board of Radiology for providing the Pediatric Radiology study guide, which served as a general outline for this book. I would like to extend my gratitude to the trainees and Radiology colleagues who contributed cases to this series and provided important feedback. A big thanks also to the technologists, nurses and ultrasonographers who helped creating the images shown in this book. Thank you for serving our community as a healthcare worker!

Our entire team sincerely thanks our patients and families who inspire us every day. An illness of a child can be scary, stressful, demanding and exhausting. We hope that our swift imaging diagnosis will help our young patients to get back on their feet quickly. That's what our work is all about.

I would like to specifically thank my awesome husband, Dr. Thomas Link, who critically reviewed all cases and provided specific input for the musculoskeletal imaging chapter. And a big thanks to Hendrik Daldrup for helping with the creation of the book cover and the book website.

To everyone who contributed to this case collection directly or indirectly: Thank you!

A NOTE FOR THE READER

Thank you for reading an authorized copy of this book. Monasteria Press LLC is a startup company, which is subsidized by its entrepreneurial founders. By purchasing our publications, you are supporting our authors and allowing Monasteria Press to continue to publish new books for future readers.

If you found this case collection helpful for your studies, please consider submitting a review about the book on Amazon, Barnes & Noble, Powells, Goodreads or Twitter. Reviews are very important. They help to spread the word about great books and can make an author's day. A great review is a wonderful reward for the hard work, long weekends, and sleepless nights that the editor and authors invested to share their experience.

If you would like to read additional books from Monasteria Press, you can find our newest publications on our website: monasteria-press.com

Thank you for being part of our amazing community!
We look forward to welcoming you back soon!

The Monasteria Press Team

AUTHOR INDEX

Lisa Adams, M.D., Research Fellow, Pediatric Radiology, Lucile Packard Children's Hospital, Stanford University School of Medicine

Joe B. Baker, M.D., Instructor, Pediatric Radiology, Lurie Children's Hospital, Northwestern University School of Medicine

Marcello Kendrew Chang, Medical Student, Stanford University School of Medicine

Soni C. Chawla, M.D., Health Sciences Clinical Professor, Department of Radiological Sciences, David Geffen School of Medicine at the University of California Los Angeles (UCLA), Attending Pediatric Radiologist, Olive View - UCLA Medical Center

Heike E. Daldrup-Link, M.D., Ph.D., Professor of Radiology, Pediatric Radiology, Lucile Packard Children's Hospital, Stanford University School of Medicine

Desiree R. Eshraghi, Undergraduate Student, University of California Los Angeles (UCLA).

Michael Fadell, M.D., Clinical Associate Professor, Pediatric Radiology, Lucile Packard Children's Hospital, Stanford University School of Medicine

Wipawee Marakote, M.D., Visiting Instructor, Pediatric Radiology, Lucile Packard Children's Hospital, Stanford University School of Medicine and Pediatric Radiologist, Department of Radiology, Faculty of Medicine, Chiang Mai University, Thailand

Praveen Jayapal, M.D., Clinical Instructor, Pediatric Radiology, Lucile Packard Children's Hospital, Stanford University School of Medicine

AUTHOR INDEX

Shelby Payne, M.D., Radiology resident, Department of Radiology, Stanford University School of Medicine

Ali Rashidi, M.D., Research Fellow, Pediatric Radiology, Lucile Packard Children's Hospital, Stanford University School of Medicine

Shakthi Kumaran Ramasamy, M.D., Research Fellow, Pediatric Radiology, Lucile Packard Children's Hospital, Stanford University School of Medicine

Jayne Seekins, M.D., Clinical Assistant Professor, Pediatric Radiology, Lucile Packard Children's Hospital, Stanford University School of Medicine

Pannee Visrutaratna, M.D., Pediatric Radiologist, Department of Radiology, Faculty of Medicine, Chiang Mai University, Thailand

..with our best wishes

for a successful exam!

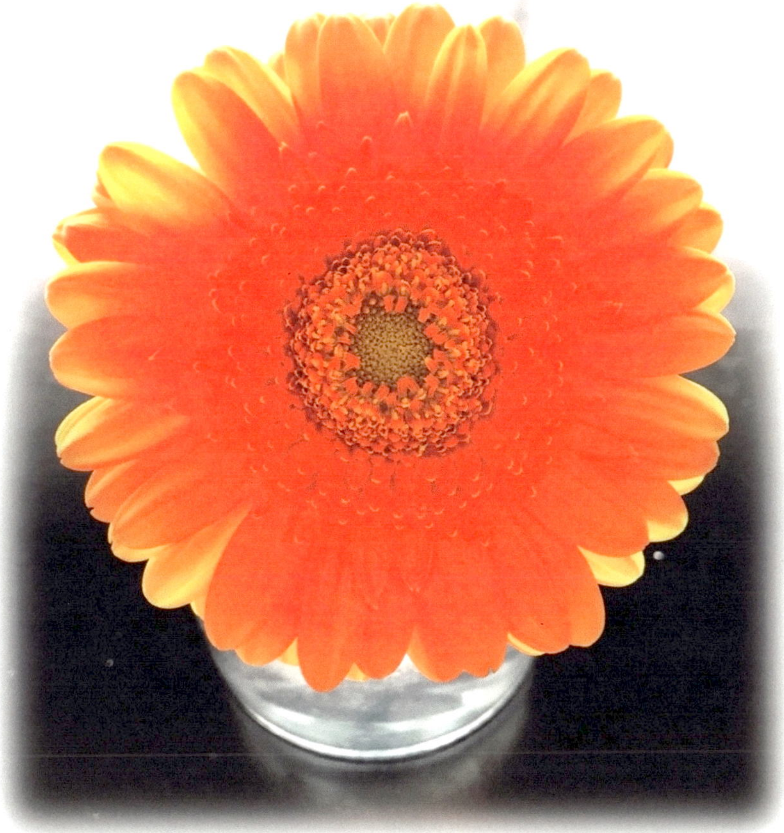

The Monasteria Press Team

Made in the USA
Las Vegas, NV
03 November 2026

57423531R00264